For Stephen,
To your Greatest
Health, Wealth &
Longevity ...

Salud,   Matthew

January,
2013

WHAT PEOPLE ARE SAYING ABOUT...

The Golden Ratio Lifestyle Diet is a masterpiece. By uncovering the universal key to health, healing, and beauty, Dr. Friedman and Matthew Cross have unlocked a "secret" formula that can help us transform each area of our lives so that quality longevity is within the reach of every human being. This book deserves a Nobel Prize in medicine.

Ann Louise Gittleman, Ph.D., C.N.S., NY Times Bestselling Author of
The Fat Flush Plan* and *Your Body Knows Best

For millennia scientists have noted significant mathematical relationships that seem to optimize function. In this landmark book, these relationships have been extended to optimizing our lifestyle. Obviously, we are all genetically unique, so one size does not fit all. However there are limits beyond certain mathematical relationships where performance drops. This book provides an excellent starting point to retake control of your life by finding those limits. I strongly recommend it.

Dr. Barry Sears, Bestselling Author of *The Zone*

If Leonardo Da Vinci and Thomas Edison were alive today, they would no doubt be impressed to see how Dr. Robert Friedman and Matthew Cross have ingeniously utilized the Golden Ratio in the pursuit of health and longevity.

Michael J. Gelb, Bestselling Author of
How to Think Like Leonardo DaVinci* and *Innovate Like Edison

The key to improving and maintaining health is to approach the challenge from all sides. This book is genius because it does exactly that. The Golden Ratio Lifestyle Diet considers all the angles in a unique and proactive manner that will work wonders for those willing to apply its secrets.

Dennis Schumacher, M.D., Body, Mind and Wilderness Medicine Expert

The Golden Ratio Lifestyle Diet is a germinal work which can lead to a renaissance of well-being for the reader. Friedman and Cross clearly show how the Golden Ratio will impact every aspect of your life in powerful ways that seem miraculous. This book is a "must read" for everyone serious about creating an amazing life.

Dr. Phil Nuernberger, President, Strategic Intelligence Skills;
Author of *The Warrior Sage*

THE GOLDEN RATIO LIFESTYLE DIET

I have been in the health and fitness industry for almost 30 years and your Golden Ratio Lifestyle Diet is one of the most comprehensive resources that I have ever seen. It is simple, thought provoking and covers all the basics to live a life of health & happiness! The thing I like most about your book is its balance and hierarchy of needs. It covers the essentials of living a life in balance with optimal health! So much more than your typical "Diet Book." I recommend this book to everyone who wants to lead a life with more energy, better health and VITALITY! Well done—this is an excellent book!

Chris Johnson, Performance Coach and CEO, OnTarget Living;
Author of *On Target Living Nutrition* and *Let's Get Moving*

The Golden Ratio Lifestyle Diet teaches us that by mimicking and adopting Nature's mathematical proportions of perfection, each of us holds the key to our own healthy lifestyle, happiness, and inner peace. This book shows us, for the first time, how "Nature's Secret Nutrient" aligns our bodies and minds to achieve perfect balance, good health and insured longevity. Follow the truths in this book and change your life!

Joan Andrews, Founder & President, Foundation for the American Indian

After reading and considering the theories in this book, I have begun the journey of making changes in my life patterns and have already seen profound improvements in my energy level, skin, hair and creativity. This is a fantastic resource, simply explained and results in positive outcomes within the first 24 hours of adopting the new behaviors. Absolutely amazing.

Shirley Cahill, Quality Process Medical Consultant

This is a book that really lives up to its title. Immensely readable, it takes you through small, doable, yet extremely effective changes you can make in your lifestyle that have an IMMEDIATE effect on your health, state of mind, and well-being. I started implementing the ideas as I read, and could feel the changes right away. Using the Golden Ratio as the common denominator among all the suggestions seems to line everything up with an underlying harmony in the world. I can't recommend this book highly enough.

Victoria Morse, Schoolteacher

WHAT PEOPLE ARE SAYING ABOUT THE DIVINE CODE/GOLDEN RATIO

In The Divine Code of Da Vinci, Fibonacci, Einstein & YOU, Matthew Cross and Dr. Robert Friedman take one of Creation's great secrets [the Golden Ratio] and make it accessible, engaging and fun. This book offers you a cornucopia of delightful insights, enlivening practices and inspiring "A-ha's"!

Michael J. Gelb, Bestselling Author,
How to Think Like Leonardo Da Vinci** and **Da Vinci Decoded

I just re-read the The Divine Code, this time to savor its exquisite intricacies. It is a stunning masterpiece. The code is interwoven into all of life, into everything we are, into everything we do. To understand it is to understand the very fabric of our being. To live its principals is to live in harmony with all that is. Cross and Friedman have created a timeless resource and a grand guide - the ultimate guide - to success in all we endeavor to experience and accomplish in our lives.

Walter R. Hampton, Jr., Attorney and Author,
Journeys On The Edge: Living A Life That Matters

The Divine Code of Da Vinci, Fibonacci, Einstein & YOU is a profound accomplishment and contribution to the future of humanity. It is great that all this information is compiled in one place and provides the foundation and inspiration for us to apply the power of the Golden Ratio.

Debra Reynolds, Founder, The Children's Dignity Project

The Divine Proportion is a scale of proportions which makes the bad difficult [to produce] and the good easy.

Albert Einstein

(The Golden Ratio is) The Secret of the Universe.

Pythagoras

...PHI (1.618) is the Most Beautiful Number in the Universe...

Dan Brown, *The Da Vinci Code*

Nature's Path of Least Resistance and Maximum Performance follows the Golden Mean.
Dr. Ronald Sandler, Golden Ratio Peak Performance Pioneer

The Fibonacci Sequence is a metaphor of the human quest for order and harmony among chaos.
Mario Merz, Modern Italian Golden Ratio Artist

4

In response to the question 'Are you a fan of the Fibonacci Sequence?' Bono replied:
'How can you not be? It's everywhere; it's all around.'

Bono, Lead Singer, U2

...The Fibonacci Series... shows up all over the place in Nature; nobody knows exactly why...

Noam Chomsky, MIT Professor, World-renowned Linguist,
Political Analyst and Author, *Manufacturing Consent*

I learned about the Golden Mean when I was about five years old... it greatly fascinated me.

Dr. Murray Gell-Mann, World-renowned Physicist,
Nobel Prize Winner and Author, *The Quark and the Jaguar*

The single most important biological structure, the DNA molecule, is in PHI
(Golden Ratio) proportion.

Stephen McIntosh, Leading Integral Theorist and Author,
Integral Consciousness and the Future of Evolution

The great Golden Spiral seems to be Nature's way of building quantity, without sacrificing quality.

William Hoffer, Author, *Midnight Express* and *Not Without My Daughter*

[The Golden Mean] is a reminder of the relatedness of the created world to the perfection of its
source and of its potential future evolution.

Robert Lawlor, Sacred Geometer and Author, *Sacred Geometry: Philosophy and Practice*

The [Golden] ratio is always the same: 1 to 1.618 over and over and over again. The patterns,
mathematical in design, are hidden in plain sight. You just have to know where to look.
Things most people see as chaos actually follow subtle laws of behavior. Galaxies, plants,
seashells; these patterns never lie. Only some of us can see how the pieces fit together...

Actor David Mazouz (as Jake) from the 2012 Fox Television Series *Touch*,
Starring Kiefer Sutherland and Danny Glover

The Fibonacci Sequence is a mathematical sequence discovered by a 12th century mathematician
named Fibonacci. [it frames] the patterns found in nature over and over again: the curve of a
wave, the spiral of a shell, the segments of a pineapple. The universe is made up of precise ratios
and patterns all around us. You and I, we don't see them, but if we could, life would be magical
beyond our wildest dreams, a quantum entanglement of cause and effect where everything and
everyone reflects on each other, every action, every breath, every conscious thought connected.
Imagine the unspeakable beauty of [such a] universe...

Actor Danny Glover (as Arthur) from the 2012 Fox Television Series *Touch*,
Starring Kiefer Sutherland, David Mazouz and Danny Glover

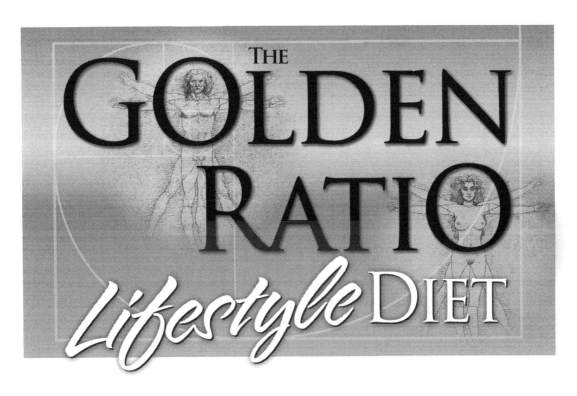

THE GOLDEN RATIO Lifestyle DIET

Upgrade Your Life & Tap Your Genetic Potential for

ULTIMATE HEALTH, BEAUTY & LONGEVITY

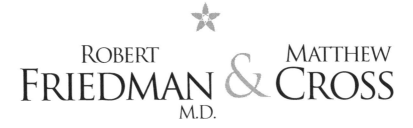

ROBERT
FRIEDMAN
M.D.

&

MATTHEW
CROSS

WWW.GOLDENRATIOLIFESTYLE.COM

DEDICATION

To our superstar parents,

Maxine & Jerry (Robert's)
Jan & Matt (Matthew's)

*For helping us to upgrade our lives, tap our genetic
potential and strive to make a difference.*

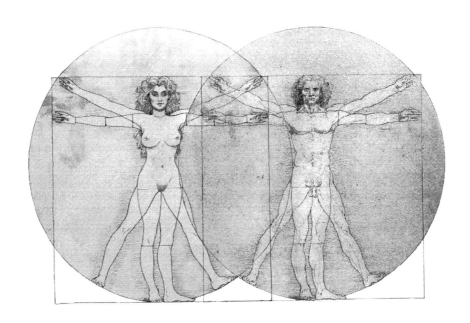

The First Wealth is Health.

Ralph Waldo Emerson, American Poet

True Health is a Lifestyle.

Anatol Vartosu, Romanian Olympic Marathon Qualifier

Health is the First Secret of Success.

Charles Atlas, Health and Bodybuilding Pioneer

*When Health is absent, Wisdom cannot reveal itself,
Art cannot become manifest, Strength cannot be
exerted, Wealth is useless and Reason is powerless.*

Herophilies, 300 B.C., Physician to Alexander the Great

Get Busy Living, or Get Busy Dying.

Andy Dufresne (Tim Robbins), *The Shawshank Redemption*

DISCLAIMER ~ NOTA BENE

The information and/or recommendations in this book are not meant to diagnose, treat or cure any medical condition. None of the statements accompanying any of the products/practices listed in this book have been evaluated by the Food and Drug Administration. None of the products/practices in this book are intended to diagnose, treat or cure any disease. Before beginning or following any of the nutritional recommendations, exercise protocols, training techniques, health improvement or any other health-related suggestions described in this book, please consult your physician or health care professional. The reader assumes 100% complete responsibility for any/all interpretations they may have and/or actions they may take and/or results they may enjoy as a result of reading this book. Neither the Publisher nor the Authors are liable for any loss, injury, damage or misunderstanding, which may occur from any interpretation and/or application of any of the information within this book.

The quotes featured within this book are from numerous sources, and are assumed to be accurate as quoted in their original and/or previously published formats. While every effort has been made to verify the accuracy of the featured quotes, neither the Publisher nor the Authors can guarantee or be responsible for their perfect accuracy. All websites, URLs and telephone numbers within this book were accurate at time of publication. However, websites may be modified or shut down and URLs or telephone numbers may change after publication without any notice. Therefore, the Publisher and Authors are not responsible in any way for the content contained in or missing/modified within any specific web site featured within this book.

The authors' insights and conclusions reached within this book are theirs alone, and—however provocative and mind-expanding they may be—may not be endorsed by any of the people, companies or organizations referenced within this book. The reader should know that this book is intended to be a holographic, gestalt approach to understanding and applying the principles explored within it. Last yet not least, the authors are not responsible for any improvement, however small or great, in one's condition or for any sense of enlightenment or wonder that might result from reading, enjoying and applying the principles explored in this book.

Publishing Data: Published in the United States of America by:
Hoshin Media Company • P.O. Box 16791, Stamford, Connecticut 06905 USA • ISBN: 0-9752802-5-2

Special acknowledgement to artist Chloe Hedden for her masterful rendition of the commissioned *Divine Code Vitruvian Woman*.
Visit: www.ChloeHedden.com

Made on a Mac. This book was written and designed on the incomparable computers made by the talented people of Apple Inc. Thank you Steve & Steve and team for your delightfully timeless genius.

The cover title of this book is set in the Golden Ratio-resonant TRAJAN FONT, directly based on the letters inscribed on the still-standing 98-foot high Trajan's column in Rome, completed 113 A.D. Constructed by the architect Apollodorus of Damascus by order of the Imperial Roman Senate, the column honors Roman Emperor Trajan and his victorious campaigns, e.g., against the Dacians, the pre-Roman inhabitants of present-day Romania. 2000 years later, Trajan's font has become the most popular choice for the world's top movie posters (e.g., the all-time #1 *Titanic*), television show titles and book covers.

CONTENTS

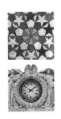

2. WATER & HYDRATION   73

3. SLEEP, REST & RECOVERY 89

4. NUTRITION: FOOD & BEYOND 109

5. POSTURE: GOLDEN RATIO STRUCTURE 157

6. EXERCISE: GOLDEN RATIO MOTION 179

7. DETOXIFICATION 211

Breathing as Detoxification

Water, The Alkahest: Nature's Universal Solvent

Der Goldene "Schnitt": The Golden Bowel Movement

Insoluble/soluble Fiber Ratios

In Search of the "Golden Schnitt"

Radiation Protection and Detoxification 101

8. HAPPINESS & INNER PEACE 229

DNA and the Golden Ratio of Happiness

Our DNA is Modifiable

Our Hardwired 62/38 Golden Ratio Perspective

Sleep Deprivation: A Major Cause of Unhappiness

The 90% Happiness Ratio

Inner Peace and Mona Lisa's Smile

9. NATURAL BEAUTY & ATTRACTION   263

10. VIBRANT HEALTH & LONGEVITY 297

Vibrant Health & Longevity Rx's

1. *Golden Prime Zone Holodeck Meditation/The TimeMap™ Graph: Blueprint for Activating Your Inner Fountain of Youth*
2. *Chocolate: Longevity Food of the Gods*
3. *The Master Golden Ratio Lifestyle Diet Prescription*

11. 21-DAY QUICK-START CHECKLIST SYSTEM　327

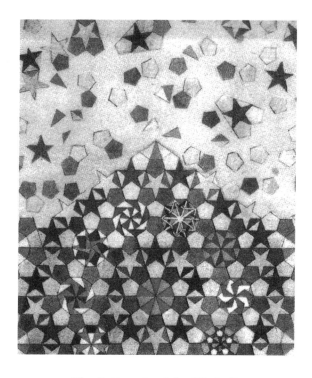

The Pattern, by John Michell.

Look beyond the chaos of existence and you see order.

It is not utopian or fascistical or like any kind of man-made

order, but divine and perfect, and it existed before time.

Socrates called it the 'Heavenly Pattern' which anyone

can discover, and once they have found it

they can establish it in themselves.

John Michell, Golden Ratio genius
and author of *The New View Over Atlantis*.

AUTHORS' NOTES

Within each of us lies a vast treasure: the opportunity to achieve and maintain vibrant health and longevity, live our full potential and make a difference. From personal experience, I know that the easy-to-apply principles you'll discover within these pages can help you bring this treasure to life—your life. I began researching the Golden Ratio at age 12. My knowledge and application of this universal synergy principle is a golden key to true success in my health and life. As the authors of this book we are constantly testing, on ourselves and others, what we write about. For example, I've been a competitive runner for decades. After hundreds of races, I credit my first win to the Golden Ratio Lifestyle Diet principles. These include Golden Ratio breathing, hydration, sleep, nutrition, posture, detoxification and of course, exercise. I've found that the ongoing results of applying this predictive knowledge is a solid increase in health and performance, on all levels of my life. I know that you can enjoy greater health, energy, fulfillment and enhanced longevity through learning and beginning to apply the priceless life knowledge in the pages ahead.

To your greatest health and happiness,
Matthew Cross, New Canaan, Connecticut ☆ September, 2011

This book contains some of the most fundamental tips and tricks for health, longevity and peace of mind that I've distilled from twenty-five years of medical practice. What makes these particular insights most valuable is that they contain the essence of Nature's healing secrets—nothing less than the wisdom of the ages—variably known as Divine Proportion, Golden Mean or Golden Ratio. In spite of the miraculous advances in pharmaceutical and high tech medicine, the simple wisdom in *The Golden Ratio Lifestyle Diet* may be the most valuable health and longevity information you will ever receive. I have found through trial and error in my own life and through treating thousands of patients that these simple principles are the absolute foundation of my health and healing regimen that will guide me to becoming a super-centenarian+.

To 100 and beyond,
Robert D. Friedman, M.D., Santa Fe, New Mexico ☆ September, 2011

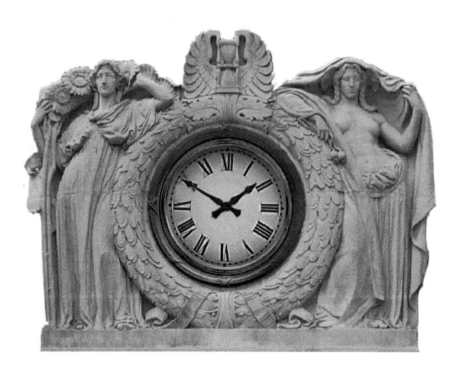

The Golden Ratio Lifestyle Diet encompasses and strengthens *all* key health and longevity drivers in our day and night. Indeed, the word *Diet* literally means *way of living, thinking; a day's journey*. This concept is beautifully captured in Adolph Weinman's *Day and Night* clock maidens, from New York City's magnificent original Penn Station (1910–1963).

Note how Day (left) is looking up with open sunflowers behind her, while the hooded Night (right) and the flower in her hand appear to be sleeping; also, the winged hourglass between them.

INTRODUCTION

The beginning is the most important part.

Plato

Congratulations: you're holding the first book of its kind in history. This book offers a paradigm jump in how you'll view and enhance your diet, health and longevity. It also offers a new and refreshing approach for anyone with virtually any health concern: obesity, high blood pressure, diabetes, cardiovascular disease, cancer, auto-immune issues, stress, cholesterol imbalances, arthritis, osteoporosis, insomnia, chronic pain, digestive troubles, asthma, allergies, hot flashes, depression—the list goes on. Whatever your present condition, you'll learn to access and apply Nature's Master Code for efficiency, harmony, quality and health: the Golden Ratio. You'll be empowered to apply it in your life for increased immunity to disease, while simultaneously manifesting the vibrant health and happiness that is your birthright.

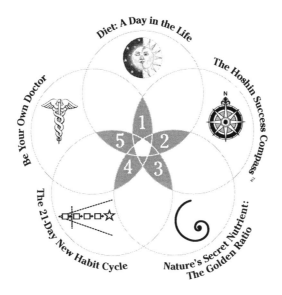

The 5 Organizing Principles of the Diet

The Golden Ratio Lifestyle Diet is a revolutionary yet easy-to-apply health and longevity program. It integrates cutting edge insights into modern physiology, nutrition and human performance with powerful quality achievement principles used by leading companies. We also introduce a never before recognized essential

23

ingredient of optimum health: The Golden Ratio, a.k.a. Nature's Secret Nutrient (NSN). This unique, synergistic system supports vibrant health, increased immunity to disease and enhanced longevity. Here's a quick look at the 5 core principles of the Golden Ratio Lifestyle Diet:

1. DIET: A DAY IN THE LIFE

The powerful hidden meaning in the word *Diet* offers a new, synergistic approach to achieving your birthright of vibrant health and longevity.

2. THE HOSHIN SUCCESS COMPASS™

The master strategic Planning/Action/Results Hoshin process (Japanese, *Inner Compass/Guiding Star*) revealed the sequenced priorities of the health success drivers in this book, and the chapter order in which these drivers are presented. Once activated, the optimal sequence of these health drivers can transform your ability to achieve vibrant health and longevity.

3. THE GOLDEN RATIO: NATURE'S SECRET NUTRIENT (NSN)

Nature's blueprint for virtually all biologic processes, including human anatomy, physiology and nutritional biochemistry. Geniuses like Leonardo Da Vinci and Albert Einstein were inspired by and used this code in their work. In this book, we show how to harness Nature's Secret Nutrient (NSN)—the Golden Ratio—to attain and sustain maximal health and peak performance. This is the first time in history this priceless information has been made available for practical application to health and longevity.

4. THE 21-DAY NEW HABIT CYCLE

A literal *lifestyle upgrade* is necessary in order for you to benefit from this new paradigm of health and longevity. With the 21-Day New Habit Cycle and the Quick Start Rx's at the end of every chapter, you will be able to harness and sustain the Golden Ratio in establishing your new, healthy lifestyle.

5. BE YOUR OWN DOCTOR

A simple and profound truth of health and healing is: *You are always your own doctor,* as it's your body that has the innate intelligence to perform its own health maintenance and healing. You must simply reclaim and exercise your innate wisdom to restore and strengthen your health. Let's explore these 5 key principles of the Diet in a little more detail...

1. DIET: A DAY IN THE LIFE

I read the news today, oh boy...
The Beatles, *A Day in the Life*

For most of us, the word *Diet* does not bring a smile to our face. Thoughts of deprivation, struggle and failure usually abound. Yet like many commonly misunderstood words, the word *Diet* contains a vast treasure. Its true meaning opens a vast window of opportunity, especially when merged with the Golden Ratio Lifestyle Diet. According to the *Dictionary of Word Origins*, the word Diet comes,

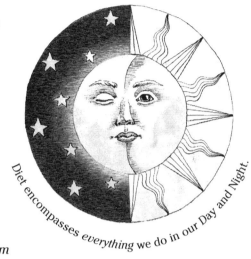

Diet encompasses everything we do in our Day and Night.

Via Old French diete and Latin diaeta, from Greek diaita **'mode [or way] of life.'** *This was used by medical writers, such as Hippocrates, in the specific sense of 'prescribed mode of life.'* Thus, our Diet—our *mode* or *way of life*—encompasses *everything* we do in our daily lives—not just what we eat!

In fact, the other key elements of our daily *Diet*—beyond what we eat—have every bit as much impact on our total health, energy, beauty, sexual vitality and longevity.

> Actress and author Alicia Silverstone underscores the full meaning of Diet in her inspiring book *The Kind Diet*:
>
> *When the word Diet entered the English language in the 1600's, it originally meant A Way of Living, or Thinking, a Day's Journey... ...we are returning the word to its original definitions, for this journey is about changing how you think and live, one day at a time. And by allowing your mind and your choices to change, you will see amazing—even magical—results.*

This includes our breathing, hydration, sleep, exercise, detoxification, emotions, mindset, relationships—and yes, what, how much and when we eat. Herein lies the true power of the concept and word *Diet*, applied holistically to enhancing the total quality of our life. This expanded, accurate definition is the foundation upon which we'll build a powerful and easy-to-follow health enhancement system that will transform your life, one step at a time. Making some small, targeted upgrades to your total *Diet* holds the golden key to upgrading the whole of your life. In the final analysis, *Lifestyle* is really the best single synonym for the all-encompassing spirit and meaning behind the often-misinterpreted word *Diet*.

2. THE HOSHIN SUCCESS COMPASS™

The sequenced priorities of the key health and longevity drivers in this book were determined through the Hoshin Kanri strategic planning process. Hoshin allows one to identify and prioritize key issues around any goal. Due to the complex and multifaceted nature of problems, challenges and opportunities in business (and health) the most efficient means to identify and deal with them is not always clear. Hoshin has a magical ability to clarify the true success "drivers" and their relative influence on a given subject or challenge.

This Japanese strategic Planning/Action/Results system was inspired by the Einstein of Quality, Dr. W. Edwards Deming. Hoshin Kanri translates roughly as: *shiny compass needle + management towards the revealed best direction.* This is the "GPS Quality Navigational System" behind many of the world's leading corporations. It is a key element of co-author Matthew Cross' consulting alliance, detailed in his book *Get Your Priorities Straight with the Hoshin Success Compass,*™ designed for individuals and organizations to achieve breakthrough success. Regarding Hoshin Kanri, Japanese Deming Quality Prize winner Dr. Yoji Akao notes,

> *Hoshin Kanri is a method devised to capture and cement strategic goals as well as flashes of insight about the future and develop the means to bring these into reality.*

The magic of Hoshin is the way it reveals the most efficient way to address any goal or problem, through correctly prioritizing the key issues involved. In this book we utilized this Hoshin master process for successful business leadership and adapted it to decoding the mysteries of health and longevity. We thus identified the vital catalysts that set the stage for more predictable, fulfilling results. Achieving greater predictability in desired outcomes is Hoshin's promise. It was vital that we prioritized the main drivers of health and longevity, for as Dr. Deming said:

It is not enough to just do your best or work hard. You must know what to work on.

The Hoshin process, as applied to our aim for this book,

1. Identified and defined the key priority factors necessary for achieving, maintaining and enjoying optimal health and longevity.
2. Revealed the best action sequence to implement the Golden Ratio Lifestyle Diet.

The 9 key priorities we surfaced as vital drivers of health and longevity were:

**Nutrition • Exercise • Air • Posture • Happiness & Inner Peace
Sleep • Water • Detoxification • Natural Beauty & Attraction**

All of these priorities are clearly important for health and longevity. We wanted to know which of them were the key foundational factors, deserving greater consideration—*and in what prioritized order.* Before we show you how we came to our conclusions, take a moment now and review the above 9 priorities. Which would *you* rank as the top 4 health and longevity influences? List your answers below:

1. _____   3. _____

2. _____   4. _____

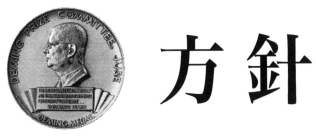

(left): Dr. W. Edwards Deming (1900-1993), the quality Einstein of success. His work is the foundation of the Hoshin Success Compass™ strategic alignment process. (right): The Japanese characters for Hoshin Kanri. Note the delightful similarity to a person with an arrow aimed at a target.

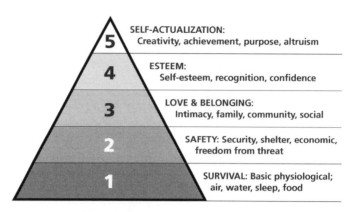

Maslow's Hierarchy of Human Needs Pyramid. Just as humanistic psychologist Abraham Maslow's hierarchy (above) highlights the satisfaction of the lower drivers before the upper ones, so it is with the Golden Ratio Lifestyle Diet health and longevity drivers (see Hoshin Success Compass FAR Pyramid™, following page).

What questions did you consider to determine the top 4 priorities? The criteria we used to determine the priorities and their optimal sequence were drawn from the Hoshin process. Here are the three key questions that gave us insight into prioritizing the most influential elements for health and longevity:

- *Which category is more causal or foundational, in relation to the others?*
- *Which category seemed like a more supportive, stronger starting point in relation to the others?*
- *How long can a human thrive/survive without it?*

Decoding the 9 Golden Ratio Lifestyle Diet Success Drivers

SPOILER ALERT: Don't read any further until you choose your top 4 priorities on the previous page. Done? OK, take a moment and review the Hoshin Success Compass FAR Pyramid™ on the next page. This pyramid succinctly summarizes the optimal sequence of the 9 key health and longevity drivers of The Golden Ratio Lifestyle Diet. Air is clearly the #1 health driver, as death results from mere minutes of deprivation. Yet some people

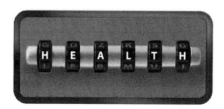

Like a combination lock, all health drivers must be lined up in the proper sequence to open the vault to optimal health and longevity.

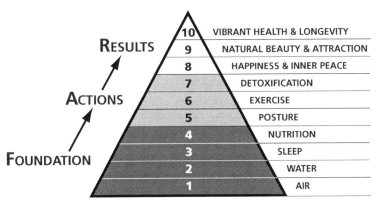

RESULTS	10	VIBRANT HEALTH & LONGEVITY
	9	NATURAL BEAUTY & ATTRACTION
	8	HAPPINESS & INNER PEACE
	7	DETOXIFICATION
ACTIONS	6	EXERCISE
	5	POSTURE
	4	NUTRITION
FOUNDATION	3	SLEEP
	2	WATER
	1	AIR

The Hoshin Success Compass FAR Pyramid™, the Golden Ratio Lifestyle Diet's bottom-up ladder for achieving optimal health and longevity: **F**oundation, **A**ctions, **R**esults (FAR).

can go 4 days+ without water before succumbing to dehydration. Sleeplessness becomes metabolically and cognitively deranging after 10 days. People with adequate fat stores can go without food for a month or more. The remaining categories are all important for human life, yet in respect to the three Hoshin discovery questions are less essential for immediate survival. Please note that the sequence we arrived at is a direct reflection of our combined research. Everyone's total Hoshin sequence is always a unique reflection of their individual perspective. This said, we are confident that the priority sequence of the first six drivers is fundamentally the same for all people. Obviously, none of these health and longevity drivers exists in a vacuum. All are at once singularly important, interrelated and continually cross-reinforcing one another. Air is a vital macro-macronutrient in its own right and at the same time is clearly a vital thread woven through every driver. Adequate hydration is necessary for proper respiratory function and oxygen uptake, while both adequate hydration and good respiratory function are necessary for refreshing, restorative sleep, and so on.

It may be a surprise to see that Nutrition and Exercise were not in our top 3. However, our top 3 drivers were revealed in relation to the specific Hoshin questions we posed. Alternative rankings are always possible if you ask different starting questions. Diet and exercise are the two prime focus points of the majority of health-conscious people, and the cornerstones of the multi-billion dollar weight-loss/fitness movement. Yet when sequenced through the Hoshin process with our focus, the positions of Nutrition and Exercise came in at #4 and #6 respectively. They are nevertheless obvious vital health drivers interconnected with all other drivers. *The secret of this Lifestyle Diet is in their optimal, cross-reinforcing sequence.*

A good Hoshin analogy is a lock combination code: all combination numbers must be entered in the proper sequence, or the lock will not open. Even if you have all the right numbers, if just *one* is out of sequence the lock will not open. With Hoshin, you discover the optimal sequenced priorities to focus on for best results. This opens the lock to a treasure chest of greater probability of success around your chosen focus. This is how we arrived at the sequence of the key health and longevity drivers—and thus the chapters—in this book. Yet to fully unlock their power and potential all categories must be properly supported by the Foundational Drivers that precede them, e.g., ample clean Air and Water and adequate, restorative Sleep. In the race to monetize people's obsession with their weight and appearance, many foods, supplements, diets, exercise equipment and health programs are touted to achieve "magic bullet" cure-alls. Perhaps this explains that to-date there's been far less focus on proper breathing, hydration, sleep and posture relative to good nutrition and exercise. The fact remains: insufficient oxygen, hydration, sleep and posture are under-appreciated yet vital causal factors related to virtually all disease, including cardiovascular disease, diabetes, cancer, immune dysregulation and obesity. Our Hoshin process resulted in three sequenced success driver categories:

Foundation: must be addressed first *and* always kept top-of-mind.

Actions: continuous action factors best implemented with the support of all preceding drivers.

Results: results or outcomes that can be expected when the proper sequence of the preceding drivers is honored.

The FAR sequence holds enormous power when revealed and followed. This is why it guides the chapter sequence in this book and is woven throughout its structure and content: to travel FAR (and fast) towards optimal health and longevity, discover and follow the optimal FAR sequence as revealed though the Hoshin process.

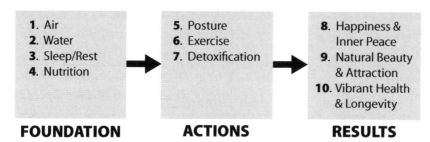

The essential Golden Ratio Lifestyle Diet's Hoshin FAR (Foundation > Actions > Results) sequence for optimal health and longevity.

3. THE GOLDEN RATIO: NATURE'S SECRET NUTRIENT (NSN)

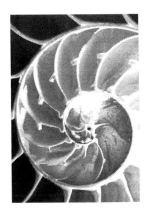

Nutrients are usually thought of as being something you can eat for sustenance, like what you had for dinner last night. They can also fall into the category of supplements, like vitamins, minerals or herbs that strengthen your immune system and give you increased energy. All of these nutrients have substance to them: you can eat, taste and swallow them. Virtually all diet books and nutritional programs revolve around specific nutrients you can eat or take to improve your health. However, Nature's Secret Nutrient is different from anything that has ever been recommended before, even by the most astute nutritionist or physician. Nature's Secret Nutrient has no mass, no calories, is tasteless, has no expiration date and never spoils, the supply is unlimited and perhaps best of all... it's free.

So, what is Nature's Secret Nutrient (NSN)? It is simply the Golden Ratio applied to the drivers of health and longevity. It's a particular way of structuring or combining complementary physiologic elements, such that their relationship mirrors Nature's formula for maximum efficiency and harmony. Once the Golden Ratio is accessed and activated, one's entire physiological efficiency dramatically improves. Throughout history, artists, architects, notable scientists and stockbrokers have utilized the Golden Ratio to bring harmony, beauty and success into their work. Geniuses such as Leonardo Da Vinci, Leonardo Fibonacci and Albert Einstein were all inspired by and used it in their work. Yet no one has integrated the principle into the fields of physiology, nutrition, health and human performance—until now. The Golden Ratio has remained largely hidden in modern times, although it is an Open Secret—evident for all those who have the eyes to recognize it in the workings of the Universe and in the human body. We have taken the next logical step and turned the principle of the Golden Ratio into an easily accessible and usable Nutrient. When the importance of the Golden Ratio is fully appreciated, it is seen as nothing less than one of mankind's most essential Nutrient, as important for life as any other essential nutrient like vitamins A, B, C, D or E. Just as these vitamins are the catalysts for multiple biochemical reactions, the Golden Ratio is the missing element that brings resonance into *all* factors supporting health and longevity. In this book we will show you how to harness Nature's Secret Nutrient in all areas of your life to obtain maximal health benefits and attain peak performance in the shortest amount of time, with minimal effort. So, what exactly is the Golden Ratio, a.k.a. the Divine Code?

The Secret Code of the Universe: The Golden Ratio/Divine Code

The Golden Ratio is a simple universal principle and pattern: the basic geometry of structure, movement and life. As you'll discover, it expresses itself in many wonderful ways, the five primary of which follow. When applied to anything, the Golden Ratio always creates greater efficiency, harmony and success—a greater whole that exceeds the sum of its parts. We refer to the five primary visible facets of the Golden Ratio collectively as the Divine Code:

- The Golden Ratio of 1.618:1
- The Golden Rectangle
- The Golden Spiral
- The Golden Star
- The infinite Fibonacci Sequence: **0, 1, 1, 2, 3, 5, 8, 13, 21...**

These are five integrated facets of the principle which underlies all creation (see the accompanying full-page overview on the Golden Ratio/Divine Code for more insight). This Code can be simply and ingeniously utilized in many ways. It's like rediscovering an Open Sesame to a higher quality of health and life. Consider the historical impact and applications of the Golden Ratio/Divine Code:

- The form and function of the Universe are based on it: the Golden Ratio guides the structure of matter, movement of energy and growth throughout the cosmos.

- It has been a key inspiration for many geniuses throughout history. From Leonardo Fibonacci, to Leonardo Da Vinci, to Albert Einstein, the essence of the Golden Ratio has been kept alive and passed down through the centuries.

- The secrets of success in health, nutrition, exercise, longevity, wealth and peak performance can be unlocked through its simple application.

- Relationships and intimacy can be enhanced through its conscious application.

- Is the golden key to greater self-understanding, creativity and spiritual growth.

> *The single most important biological structure,*
> *the DNA molecule, is in PHI Φ (Golden Ratio) proportion.*
> **Stephen McIntosh, Golden Ratio genius and author of**
> ***Integral Consciousness and the Future of Evolution***

The Divine Code and the Golden Ratio (Phi Φ =1.618:1)

The Divine Code is a synthesis of the 5 key visible aspects of the Golden Ratio. Clearly evident as Nature's unifying principle, the Code guides the structure of matter, movement of energy and growth throughout the Universe. The term *Divine Code* integrates the 5 individual yet interrelated facets of the Golden Ratio, uniting them under one umbrella. The word *Divine* refers to the transcendent qualities that permeate the cosmos and also the ability to foresee or foretell with increased accuracy. By harnessing the Divine Code, we can increase the probability of creating and sustaining greater health, harmony and success in our lives. The Golden Ratio's 5 facets—the Divine Code—its history, inspired geniuses and practical applications are explored in depth in *The Divine Code of Da Vinci, Fibonacci, Einstein & You.*

1. Golden RATIO

Appears when any unit is divided such that the small and large parts are in 1.618:1 ratio to one another, or simply 62:38. Ubiquitous, infinite, the ratio is the Universal Code for harmonious structure, movement and life.

1.618   1.0
62   38
A   B

A + B
A + B is to A as A is to B

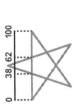
Hand

Heart Placement

The Proportion of Beauty: Golden Ratios in the Face

Proportions of the Body at all scales, from micro to macro
38   62

Humans are naturally drawn to the Golden Sleep Ratio of 9:15— 9 hrs. sleep/rest to 15 hrs. waking (62:38)

62% 38%

Sunflower's Golden Ratio face (linear); seeds are placed in alternating nonlinear Golden Ratio spirals

Planetary distance Golden Ratios

2. Golden RECTANGLE

Any rectangle whose length and width are in 1.618:1 ratio to one another.

1.0
1.618
62
8
3 2
5
38

One complete revolution of DNA fits neatly within a Golden Rectangle

Natural ellipses, e.g., Eggs
1.0
.382 .618
.618
Credit/ ATM Cards

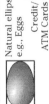
iPod®
Playing Cards

16:9 Screens mirror our natural Golden Rectangle visual field

Flags

The Parthenon

3. Golden SPIRAL

Any spiral whose each complete revolution is 1.618 times larger than the previous one.

1.618
62
1.0
38

Neutrinos dancing in Golden Spirals at the atomic level

Humans begin their journey of life unfolding in a gentle Golden Spiral

Heart Muscle design supports its Golden Spiral corkscrew action, for maximum efficiency

Curl of every Arm, Hand and Finger

Roses
Ocean Waves

Hurricanes
Galaxies

4. Golden STAR

A 5-pointed star where each of the star's lines cross each other at their precise Golden Ratio cut points: the .38 and .62 marks.

0   38 62   100

DNA cross section is a dodecahedron: 2 overlapping 5-pointed Stars

Back of Rose
Pentagonal Leaf growth

Apple Blossoms and Apple Cores (X-section)

Starfish, Sand Dollars and many Flowers

Our Body: a natural star
Wash. D.C. Street Plan

Venus' orbit dances around the Earth in pentagonal symmetry

5. FIBONACCI SEQUENCE

An infinite sequence starting at 0, where each successive term is the sum of the previous two: **0,1,1,2,3,5,8,13,21,34,55,89...** As the numbers grow, the *ratio between them* approaches yet never actually reaches the infinite Golden Ratio 1.618... e.g., 21/13=1.615; 34/21=1.619; 55/34=1.617; 89/55= **1.618...** 13th century discovery by Leonardo Fibonacci, Genius of Pisa.

Leonardo Fibonacci, c. 1170–1250, A.D.; also introduced 1-2-3 Arabic numbers, the decimal and zero (0) to the West

DNA height:width = 34:21 angstroms

Daisy petal counts follow the *sequence*; Einstein was fascinated by this phenomenon as a boy

Plant growth and leaf placement is guided by the *sequence* for maximum efficiency and sun and rain exposure

Pinecone's Golden Fibonacci Growth Ratios: 8 spirals in one direction, 13 in the other

Elliott Wave, basis of Prechter's *Socionomics* and Sandler's *Workout Wave*: Fibonacci Ratios in motion

5 Waves Up   3 Waves Down
8 Waves Total

If there were such a thing as a Master Code that blueprints the Universe at every level, the Golden Ratio would have to be it. Within the realm of man, this pervasive principle underscores all creative endeavors. It underlies successful and fulfilling art, architecture, music, science, medicine, relationships, business, athletic achievement and spirituality. The reason anyone is successful at anything—even though they may not know why or may attribute it to other causes—is that they have accessed and applied Golden Ratio principles in some way to whatever they think, make or do. The evidence increasingly points to the reason that we consider anything to be good, true or beautiful is that it awakens and delights our inherent Golden Ratio nature.

The Fibonacci Sequence and the Golden Ratio

The following simple yet magical Sequence of numbers was introduced in Leonardo Fibonacci's classic book, *Liber Abaci* (1202) and later named in his honor. This infinite Sequence is formed by adding one number to the next, beginning with zero:

> **0, 1, 1, 2, 3, 5, 8, 13, 21, 34, 55, 89, 144, 233, 377...**

The Golden Ratio or Phi Φ is a special, infinite value, closely related to the Fibonacci Sequence and is very close to the ratio of its successive terms. If you graph the ratios of adjacent numbers in the Sequence, you'll see that they converge on the Golden Ratio: 1.618... The ratios actually "dance" around the Golden Ratio, with the first ratio lower than 1.618 and the next ratio higher than 1.618, ad infinitum.

> **1/1=1, 2/1=2, 3/2=1.5, 5/3=1.66, 8/5=1.6, 13/8=1.625,**
> **21/13=1.615, 34/21=1.619, 55/34=1.617, 89/55=1.618...**

This is Nature's way of honing in on the elusive Golden Ratio, which doesn't actually exist in this dimension, as it's an infinite or irrational number. Either way, we arrive at two very special numbers: 1.618, or 0.618 if you invert the ratio. We could say that the Golden Ratio is an ideal, like perfection; we are always striving for it, even if we may never reach it. In this sense, the Golden Ratio is like a guiding star.

Nature's Heartbeat: The Golden Ratio Pulse

The Golden Ratio pulse graph uses progressive Fibonacci Ratios to illustrate how Nature continually strives for dynamic balance. Virtually all living systems, from atoms to galaxies, from the human heartbeat to DNA, tend to cluster around the

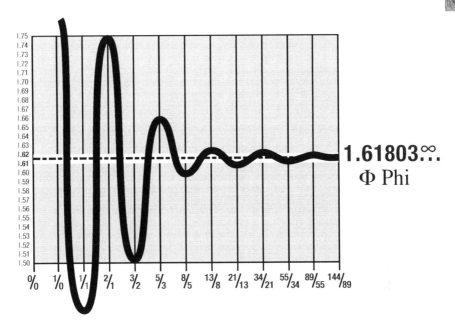

Golden Ratio pulse graph,. Note how the Fibonacci ratios move infinitely closer to the Golden Ratio between each adjacent number in the Fibonacci Sequence.

ubiquitous Golden Ratio. The points on the graph pulse above and below the ethereal Golden Ratio, like a Divine Heartbeat. Life circumstances are constantly introducing chaos into living systems, only to have the systems strive to right themselves, much like finely tuned gyroscopes that automatically return to Golden Ratio balance. Over time this Golden Ratio pulse tends to refine itself, gravitating ever closer to the idealized Golden Ratio, yet never actually reaching it. We can think of the Golden Ratio as Nature's Universal *Set-Point*—that optimal point of homeostatic balance where structure and function are unified in maximum efficiency and harmony. This universal pattern of efficiency is easily applicable to all of the facets of the Golden Ratio Lifestyle Diet. In order to achieve and maintain maximum health with minimum effort, we need to closely *Match* our daily lifestyle choices and habits with easily identified Golden Ratio *Set-Points* in the key health drivers. This process of upgrading our lifestyle habits is remarkably simple, and can deliver profound results in all areas of our life. The double entendre from the game of tennis of "*Set-Point, Match*" is an easy reminder for adjusting/upgrading our lifestyle choices towards Golden Ratio balance. When we consciously realign ourselves with the Golden Ratio we can more effortlessly move away from limiting behavioral patterns and create new healthy habits, habits invariably more attuned to our natural Golden Ratio blueprint.

4. THE 21-DAY NEW HABIT CYCLE

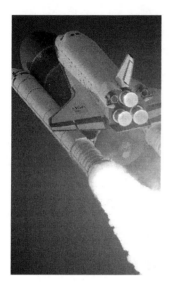

The principles behind the Golden Ratio Lifestyle Diet may seem like simple concepts to grasp. Actually incorporating them into your lifestyle requires behavioral change or "upgrade." We need to move from merely understanding intellectual concepts into the realm of consistent action and sustained momentum. Yet real change for many can often be a difficult task. What may prevent us from making the leap of change are years, even decades, of procrastination, resistance or self-destructive patterning. Futurist Nancy Lieder underscores this challenge:

The common man is more likely to continue to walk in the rut that is their lives, as they have no [visible] alternatives.

Escape Velocity of Day 13.

Luckily, we do have alternatives when it comes to upgrading ingrained behavior patterns and replacing them with healthy ones. Built into the Golden Ratio Lifestyle Diet are both the insights into what the main drivers of health and longevity are along with the means for activating them. Psychologists specializing in habit transformation agree that it takes about 3 weeks or 21 days—both Fibonacci numbers—to set a new habit pattern. Not surprisingly, the code behind our neurophysiology operates according to Fibonacci and Golden Ratio dynamics. Yet it's important to note that a new habit pattern doesn't necessarily erase an old, unwanted one. Habits, new and old, are stored permanently in various places in our holographic brain. As a new habit is learned, the older habit is simply deactivated or overshadowed, much like a dirt road becomes overgrown when unused for a long time. As Dutch renaissance theologian Desiderius Erasmus said,

Habit is Overcome by Habit.

Whether you want to develop a new habit with or without the professional help of a coach or therapist, you can use the Golden Ratio Lifestyle Diet to support your desired new behavior(s). As your brain develops a new neural habit pattern, you acknowledge and affirm your new direction on each of the Fibonacci days in the 21-day new habit cycle: 1, 2, 3, 5, 8, 13, 21. This process is reinforced in the 21-Day Quick-Start Checklist system in chapter 11. Affirming these special days of new neuronal growth and repatterning consciously reinforces your desired new habit patterns. This occurs through positive self-acknowledgment amplified through the Golden Ratio. Dietary research reveals that many people go off their nutritional diets on or about day 13—again, a Fibonacci number. Yet if they can pass this critical day and make it through to their 21st day, they usually will succeed in losing weight and establishing the new habit pattern that allowed them to lose the weight. Day 13 seems to be a crucial threshold. Around that day, it's as if the old habit reasserts itself and tries to sabotage the new. Armed with this knowledge, you can strengthen and intensify your new practice. You can escape the clutches of day 13 and breeze through those final 8 days until the new pattern is securely in place. Finding a way to propel yourself through day 13 is similar to building up what astronauts call "escape velocity"— the tiny percent of additional thrust needed to break the pull of the Earth's gravity and soar into outer space.

The First 15% Principle

We want to make sure that you get to day 13 to have a winning chance to reach escape velocity. So, in order to reinforce your chances of making the jump into living a successful Golden Ratio Lifestyle Diet, we call again on the wisdom of Dr. W. Edwards Deming, quality genius, for an added booster rocket. Deming developed a simple way of turning baby steps into giant steps. His concept of "The First 15%" is an easy, practical way to begin establishing your 21-Day New Habit Cycle. It says that,

85% of the results in any given endeavor are in the First 15%—the front end— of the process or journey.

This means that days 1, 2 and 3 are the most important days in getting off to a good start in hitting the next milestones—days 5, 8, 13 and then day 21. The First 15% of 21 days is about the first 3 days. The First 15% rule is used to point you in

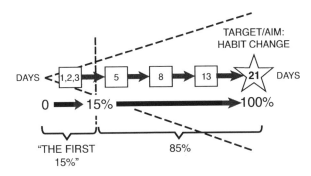

The crucial First 15% sets the stage for successful habit change and long term success.

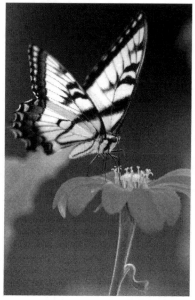

The First 15% principle is reminiscent of the butterfly effect from chaos theory: If the initial conditions are right, tiny imperceptible factors in the beginning of any process—like the flapping of a butterfly's wings in Africa—can have massive effects on the downstream outcome—resulting in a hurricane in Florida. Likewise, small changes in lifestyle can result in huge benefits in health and longevity.

the right direction and Quick-Start your efforts at implementing the Golden Ratio Lifestyle Diet. In the diagram on the previous page, the First 15% is represented from 0–>15%, with the desired result being the Target at 100%. If we properly align and plan best actions in the First 15% on the path to our aim, the odds highly favor our chances of hitting our target of long-term success.

The Fibonacci Number day milestones in the 21-Day Habit Cycle are graphed in the boxes/star in the diagram. Day 22–forward will have maximum probability for success with First 15% days 1-21 properly loaded, locked and aimed. This principle is intuitive common sense for most, yet not a common practice of many. Most operate by the "Just-Do-It" philosophy, also known as "Ready-Fire-Aim." Such an approach might get things going quickly, yet often misfires and delivers less than optimal results, especially long term. The First 15% approach can be understood as *Ready-Ready-Ready... Aim-Fire-Direct Hit*. This is a key lesson Dr. Deming taught the Japanese. The First 15% offers a different approach, which leads to different actions and profoundly different results. It mirrors the unfolding of a Golden Spiral, from a tiny beginning point to infinity. To correctly align an upward success spiral around any worthwhile aim, the initial First 15% is crucial. Hard work on the wrong things out of sequence usually does more harm than good, especially in the beginning stages. Working on the right things in the right order at the right time is a natural result of wise application of the First 15% principle. As Teruaki Aoki, a Sony Vice President, observed:

If you do right in the upstream, the downstream will be much easier.

Simply put, the *quality* of your actions is just as important (if not more) as the *quantity* of your actions. The First 15% helps you identify and act more intelligently towards your aim, revealing the critical "first things first" required for short *and* long-term success. We've applied the First 15% principle throughout this book in a simple

> *Every human being is the author of his own health or disease.*
> **Buddha**

way in order to help you on your way to establishing new and healthy habits in 21 days. Each chapter ends with a few easy First 15% starting point prescriptions, or "Rx's." These simple baby steps set the stage for you to quickly align and focus on the vital First 15% factors for each health driver. In this way you can turn baby steps—small steps taken at the right time—into giant steps: results that multiply and cross-reinforce each other over time. You can chart your progress in establishing your positive new habits over a 21-day period in the Quick Start journal/diary section, to visually reinforce your progress.

5. BE YOUR OWN DOCTOR

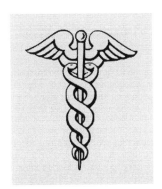

The doctor of the future will give no medicine, but will interest his patients in the care of the human frame, in diet, and in the cause and prevention of disease.

Thomas A. Edison

The best things in life are free, delightful and effective, as are the recommendations for health and longevity in the Golden Ratio Lifestyle Diet.

The "prescriptions" ahead cost little to implement; many can even be done as you read this book. There are no expensive health plans, drugs, weird diets, or years of painstaking study or specialists to consult—with the exception of consulting yourself. After reading and absorbing the information and concepts presented here, you will naturally step into that other, often forgotten role of doctor—that of *Teacher*—the Latin root for *Doctor*. You will learn to harness and teach, yourself first, the core elements of the Diet and extract their essences for vibrant health and longevity.

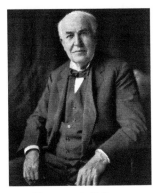

Thomas A. Edison.

Thomas Edison's sage "Doctor of the Future" words from over a century ago are becoming a reality. His astute prediction is being echoed in our time by many enlightened doctors, including Dr. Mehmet Oz, the popular health and wellness advocate (and Golden Ratio aficionado). Dr. Oz's patient empowerment perspective is elegantly elucidated here by his wife, producer and bestselling author Lisa Oz,

...too often the patient sees themselves as the football being tossed around from one caregiver to another. This is not a good situation to be in because the patient needs to be the quarterback... ...more often than not the patient is the passive observer in their care and they totally abdicate all decisions and responsibilities to their physicians. We want to provide them with the education and the motivation to be a key player in their own wellness.

Enlightened doctors/teachers can play a vital role in your health, *if* they honor your pivotal role as being your own doctor *first*. As with that other misinterpreted word Diet, you will now be equipped with a broader perspective on the true role of Doctor, which can empower you to take greater command of your health and longevity.

Enjoy the journey!

There were never so many able, active minds at work on the problems of diseases as now, and all their discoveries are tending to the simple truth—that you can't improve on Nature.
Thomas A. Edison

GOLDEN RATIO LIFESTYLE DIET SELF-TEST

The following is a quick and fun way to see where you stand today regarding key elements of the Golden Ratio Lifestyle Diet. This self-test also provides valuable insights on the next steps to take to upgrade your health, happiness and longevity. Keep in mind that the following questions are only fractal representatives of the many optimal health and longevity practices from the complete Golden Ratio Lifestyle Diet.

Here's how the self-test works:

1. Rate yourself on the 0–4 scale on your practice frequency *today* on the list of key health and longevity factors.

2. Be honest and non-judgmental with yourself when ranking each question. Remember—you're only collecting data to clarify your *starting* position. You're not expected to be perfect yet—this comes later :)

3. When you're finished, tally your final score. Note your lowest scored items with an " * " or by <u>underlining</u> them. The lower your total self-test score at the start, the more you can improve in the coming weeks, as you learn and put into practice key elements of the Diet.

We recommend that you repeat the self-test, *after* your 21-Day Quick-Start launch cycle. You will undoubtedly see positive movement between your *before* and *after* scores. Celebrate your wins first. Then, note any low score items and commit to raising a selected few—even 1 point higher in the coming weeks.

Challenge yourself—this is a game where you're guaranteed to come out a winner—healthier, stronger, more confident and more assured of robust longevity.

Self-Test Scoring:	Never 0	Rarely 1	Occasionally 2	Frequently 3	Always 4

1. _____ I breathe with awareness, deeply and fully: buddha belly + chest-up balloon on inhale; navel-into-spine on exhale (Air—chapter 1).

2. _____ I consciously check my posture throughout the day and keep my shoulders, back and neck tall and open, to support full lung capacity/breaths (Air/Posture).

3. _____ I drink a tall glass of water upon awaking every day (Water).

4. _____ My urine color is consistently in the pale yellow to clear range (Water, proper hydration indicator).

5. _____ I get between 7-9 hours of quality sleep/rest every 24 hrs. (Rest/Recovery).

6. _____ I take a short nap or breaks where I close my eyes and deepen my breath at least once a day (Rest/Recovery).

7. _____ I have a healthy breakfast daily within 90 minutes of arising (Nutrition).

8. _____ I eat to only about 65% of fullness at meals (Nutrition).

9. _____ I include Super Foods in my daily meals such as: greens, high ORAC foods—high antioxidant potential, e.g., kale, blueberries; flax; kombucha tea, etc. (Nutrition).

10. _____ I maintain a slim/flat belly (Nutrition; key health and longevity indicator)

11. _____ I engage in fun, break-a-sweat movement 3–4+ times a week (Exercise).

12. _____ I play with Fibonacci Sequence numbers (1,1,2,3,5,8,13,21,34,55,89…) to demarcate exercise times, reps and rest/recovery periods (Exercise).

13. _____ I have one healthy, easy bowel movement at least once a day or more (Detoxification).

14. _____ I engage in an intestinal cleansing/detoxification program at least twice a year (Detoxification).

15. _____ I hydrate my face at least once a day (Natural Beauty).

16. _____ I am happy with the quality of my intimate life (Attraction).

17. _____ I'm aware of the ratio of my listening/talking time, and strive to really listen 60% and talk 40% of the time (Attraction).

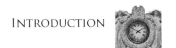

Self-Test	**Never**	**Rarely**	**Occasionally**	**Frequently**	**Always**
Scoring:	**0**	**1**	**2**	**3**	**4**

18. _____ I express gratitude for all the gifts, people and good things in my life at least once a day (Happiness).

19. _____ I choose predominantly positive words to describe both how I feel inside and the world at large (Happiness).

20. _____ I have regular connections with positive, supportive people who genuinely care about me (Happiness).

21. _____ I am happy and fulfilled in my work (Happiness).

22. _____ I am happy with the ratio of work/non-work time in my life (Happiness).

23. _____ I regularly experience feelings of inner peace, contentment and connection to the Divine (Inner Peace).

24. _____ I have a clear, inspiring purpose in my life (Inner Peace).

25. _____ I practice some form of daily meditation, prayer, centering, etc., (Inner Peace).

_____   _____

Initial   **After 21-Day Quick-Start**
Total   **Checklist Total**

Golden Ratio Lifestyle Diet Self-test Scoring Range:

80 to 100 = Great: You're doing *really* well. Strive for the prize by closing any revealed gaps to greater health, happiness and longevity.

62 to 79 = Very Good: You're on track, yet why not kick it up a notch or two? Are you ready to feel your best *and* live long and strong?

46 to 61 = Good: You're hanging in there… but why just hang? Step up to the plate and select the vital 1-3 biggest gaps to close and *go for it!*

31 to 45 = Fair: "Fair"? You can do *much* better than this.

0 to 30 = Help! You do want to *keep* enjoying the miracle of this life, don't you? If so, it's time to get serious—*now.*

Apply the appropriate strategies/Rx(s) inside this book to your low score categories, and be sure to also include them in your 21-Day Quick-Start Checklist at the end of the book.

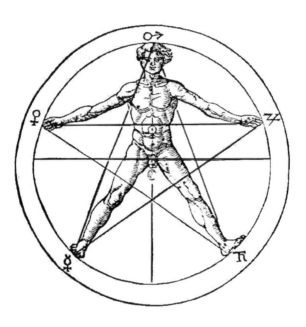

The Golden Ratio is Nature's Universal Thread,

with which optimal health is woven.

Robert Friedman, M.D. and Matthew Cross

Man Star image from *De Occulta Philosophia,*

by Heinrich Cornelius Agrippa.

PREFACE

With the explosion of interest in quantum physics over the last few decades came an understanding of the fractal principle. In 1975, French mathematician Benoît Mandelbrot coined the term fractal, which denotes a geometric shape that retains self-similar properties when broken into ever-smaller fragments. The basic fractal principle can be seen in any head of broccoli, where any smaller piece of broccoli has the same basic shape or pattern as the whole head from which it came. Likewise, the similar cruciferous vegetable Romanesco is fractal to the core, with its beautiful Fibonacci cones spiraling together at many different scales. In the human body, fractal Golden Ratio proportions are found at all levels, from the macro level of our skeleton down to our micro DNA, from the [Golden] Spiral muscle design and pumping action of our heart to the spiral of our arm, hand and fingers as they uncoil.

Fractal relationships are also found throughout our physiology and biochemistry—even in the science of human nutrition. We initially showed how the universal fractal principle of the Golden Ratio could illuminate new principles in health and nutritional science in our 660-page book, *The Divine Code of Da Vinci, Fibonacci, Einstein and YOU.* This book you are reading was born as a fractal seed from that original book—similar, yet different—taking those initial health and nutritional fractal gems to a new and expanded level.

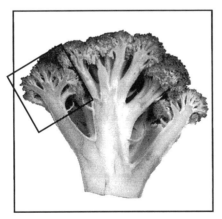

Broccoli's fractal, self-similiar nature, where even the smallest parts always reflect the whole.

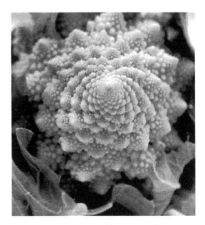

Romanesco cauliflower embodies self-similar Fibonacci Spirals.

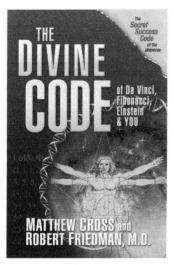

Original seed fractal book for
The Golden Ratio Lifestyle Diet.

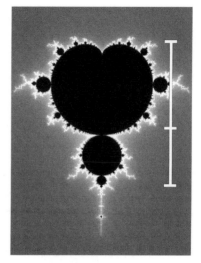

Mandlebrot fractal with
Golden Ratio geometry.

Micro, Macro and Macro-macro Nutrients

The science of nutrition has typically categorized nutrients as being either of a macro or micro class. Simply put, *macro*nutrients are subdivided into either proteins, fats and carbohydrates, whereas *micro*nutrients are vitamins and minerals which are required in far smaller quantities by weight. We have identified another fractal class of essential nutrients—similar, yet different—that we call ***macro-macro*nutrients**. These are needed in much larger amounts than the smaller requirements of the classical macro and micronutrients. Macro-macro nutrients are similar in necessity, yet different than macro and micronutrients in the sheer quantity of their requirements. For instance, we need to breathe around 10,000 liters of air per day and drink around 2 liters (minimum) of water per day. These are really large amounts, compared to the amount of protein, fat and carbohydrates and the lesser amounts of vitamins and minerals that we require for survival. As you will see, the Golden Ratio Lifestyle Diet has identified several other macro-macronutrients that we require in large amounts in order to manifest optimal health and longevity. These other macro-macronutrients are Sleep, Posture and Exercise—all of which you may have never before considered as dietary nutrients. The fact is that if we don't satisfy our Recommended Golden Ratio Allowances (RGRAs) for these macro-macronutrients, our health can suffer on many levels and we will never be able to live a fully vibrant life nor reach our longevity potential.

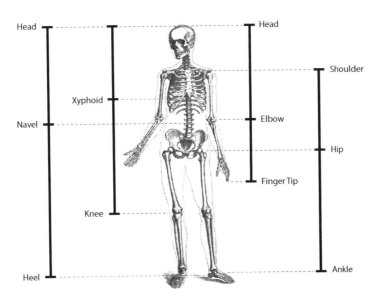

A few of the many Golden Ratio fractals in the human skeleton.

In order to make it easy to re-conceptualize this expanded view of Diet and begin to incorporate the RGRAs into your life, we've embedded cutting edge strategies used by leading international companies for increasing quality and efficiency and achieving sustainable success. You'll be able to become your own doctor, nutritionist, personal trainer and life-coach, lighting a new path of optimal health and maximum longevity. You'll also be able to put these principles to work the first time you pick up this book, by using our 21-Day Quick-Start Checklist system.

The Golden Ratio Lifestyle Diet: Beyond Traditional Diet & Exercise

Obesity is among the greatest health challenges of our time. Most traditional weight loss and diet programs are generally disappointing and have consistently restricted themselves to only addressing nutrition and exercise. Their highly-touted magic bullets for weight loss usually result in temporary improvements at best, with discouraging results in the long run. Could it be that their approach to weight loss and body composition has been too narrowly focused and short-sighted? Perhaps a broader, more synergistic approach—inclusive of other less obvious lifestyle factors—may be where the real magic lies. The Golden Ratio Lifestyle Diet is just such an all-encompassing total lifestyle approach. In addition to the obvious vital factors of diet and exercise, it recognizes and uniquely supports our vital *macro-macro nutrients* such as Air, Water, Sleep, Posture, Happiness, Inner Peace, Beauty and Attraction—even our 5 senses. These macro-macro nutrients are needed in extremely large amounts compared to the typical micronutrients of vitamins, minerals, proteins, fats and carbohydrates needed for our sustenance. The real secret to tapping the power of such a wide variety of macro-macro nutrients is the *sequence* with which they're applied. The upstream drivers supporting nutrition and exercise are often overlooked and don't get the underlying support they need. For example, when oxygen intake is insufficient due to poor breathing habits or sleep is inadequate, digestion suffers and hormones are thrown off, both of which wreak havoc with your ability to exercise effectively and eat and digest properly. Proper oxygenation, hydration, rest and recovery, posture and detoxification all play crucial roles in the causal chain that fosters ideal weight and body composition, not to mention robust health and enhanced longevity.

The final key to the Golden Ratio Lifestyle Diet is learning to access Nature's Secret Nutrient (NSN)—the synergistic ingredient released when all of the aforementioned health drivers are utilized in Golden Ratio. When a large part is to a small part as the whole is to the large part (the essential Golden Ratio formula), a magical synergy is activated and amplified. Synergy—a word often used by Golden Ratio genius Buckminster Fuller—describes,

> *the interaction of two or more substances or agents, which produce a combined effect greater than the sum of their separate effects.*

Maximal synergy can be obtained through the comprehensive approach of the Golden Ratio Lifestyle Diet. Upgrading your total lifestyle invariably leads to better, sustainable results, including optimal weight, ideal body composition and vibrant health, beauty and longevity. These are the promises of the Golden Ratio Lifestyle Diet.

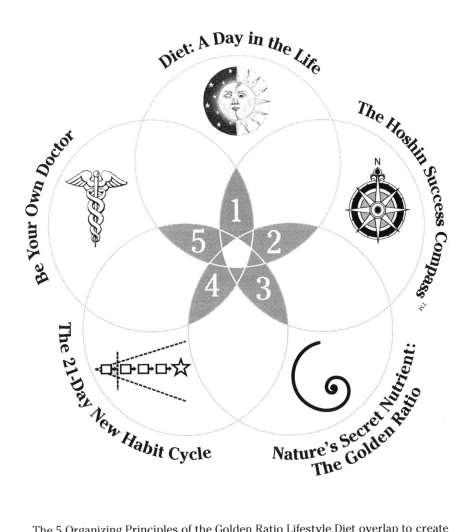

Diet: A Day in the Life

The Hoshin Success Compass™

Nature's Secret Nutrient: The Golden Ratio

The 21-Day New Habit Cycle

Be Your Own Doctor

The 5 Organizing Principles of the Golden Ratio Lifestyle Diet overlap to create
a pentagonal Venn diagram design. The synergistic result is a greater whole which
exceeds the sum of its parts, with the promise of optimal health and longevity.
Note that we've included this design in the upper left corner of every page
as a gentle reminder of the importance of the Diet's 5 foundational principles.

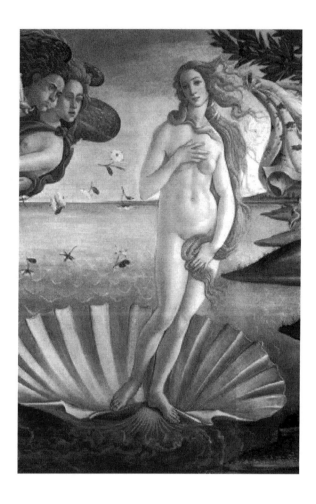

The Birth of Venus, by Sandro Botticelli.

The west wind God and messenger of spring

(Zephyrus and companion) blow the spark

of life-giving air onto Venus.

1.

AIR & BREATH

Oxygen is the giver of life.

Otto H. Warburg, M.D.,
Biochemist & Nobel Prize Winner

Breathing. It's our first action upon entering the world and our last upon leaving. The ancients say that the life-giving oxygen we breathe is also imbued with *prana*, or life force. Perhaps best of all, it's free! Yet insufficient, shallow breathing over time leads to premature aging and early death, with many chronic diseases along the way. In this chapter, we'll explore the profound power of increasing the quality and quantity of oxygen intake in our daily lives, with the Golden Ratio as our super-charging guide.

The ABC's of Healthy Breath & Circulation

Most everyone is familiar with the ABC's of CPR (Cardio-Pulmonary-Resuscitation): Airway, Breathing, Circulation. These are the life-saving techniques used in cases of cardiac arrest or other life-threatening emergencies. Since these three critical aspects of maintaining life are of the utmost importance in an acute situation, it stands to reason that they might also be important, although overlooked, factors in supporting life in every moment of our existence. These automatic and usually unnoticed, unconscious functions of breathing and blood circulation are critical factors in

1

either manifesting robust health or struggling along with less than optimal wellbeing. Our health and longevity are dependent on a cardiopulmonary system (heart and lungs) that can handle constant activity and stress from birth to death. The Golden Ratio Lifestyle Diet will expand the range and efficiency in which your heart, lungs and circulatory system function. Breathing and circulation are intimately connected— bound together in Golden Ratio—and in good health they work together in perfect harmony. Without good respiratory function, a good cardiovascular system isn't of much value, and vice versa.

Since Air & Breath is the number one driver in the Golden Ratio Lifestyle Diet hierarchy, it's imperative to take advantage of this most important energizer and life giver. If there's one thing that you take away from this book, it should be the knowledge of how to access and amplify the Golden Ratio through your breath. Our bodies have set up an ingenious anatomical and physiological leverage system by harnessing the Golden Ratio. Let's start by looking at the operational capacity categories of the lungs. A few definitions are in order and will be made as simple as possible. Please look at the full-page Golden Ratio Lung Volume Graph on page 55 and review the different operational categories. Remember that these categories are functional as opposed to structural, in that they are defined by the amount of air that moves through the lungs during a breath.

Your Vital Capacity (VC): #1 Predictor of Longevity

Through the Hoshin process, Air & Breath was determined to be the #1 driver and thus the vital foundation for optimal health and longevity. Not surprisingly, there is key corroborating data from the science of longevity that supports this theory. As you will learn shortly, your Vital Capacity (VC) is a measurement of how much air you can breathe out, *after* a maximal inhalation. As it turns out, your VC is also your #1 predictor of longevity. By looking at the relationship between Vital Capacity and age, we are immediately drawn to one of the most important studies ever performed in the field of longevity. The Golden Ratio Lung Capacity Graph is adapted from the well-known Framingham study and shows that Vital Capacity decreases in direct relationship with age in both men and women. By continuously investing in increasing your Vital Capacity, you can effectively increase your longevity quality *and* quantity. With this singular direct measure, we are able to make an accurate prediction about a given individual's remaining lifespan. Longevity researcher Roy Walford, M.D. noted the importance of this relationship and the inference that can be drawn from it:

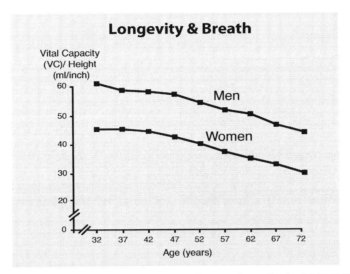

Lung Vital Capacity vs. age, from the Framingham Study, 1948-1968
(after Walford: *Beyond the 120 Year Diet*; originally from Kannel and Hubert, 1982.)

People with low VC for their age did not live as long on the average as those with high VC, and as we have learned, predictability is the most important indicator that a biomarker is measuring true 'functional' age.

"Functional" age is your true physiologic age, as opposed to your chronological age. If you were a 50 year old with a relatively low Vital Capacity, we could extrapolate from the data above and predict that your true functional or physiologic age would be much older. Then we'd want to intervene with some of the recommendations in the Golden Ratio Lifestyle Diet to see if we could lower your "functional" age. Not surprisingly, many studies have documented that Vital Capacity can be increased and presumptive functional age lowered through yoga and breathing exercises. The mechanism for increasing Vital Capacity is through improving chest expansion and strengthening the muscles of respiration.

Golden Ratio Anatomy of Our Lungs

The anatomic structure of our lungs also follows the Golden Ratio. Indeed, our breath moves in spiraling wave motions in our body as it travels through our Golden Ratio-designed airways, mirroring the wind and water currents found throughout Nature. The asymmetrical nature of our anatomy, including our lungs, follows the Fibonacci Ratios embedded in our anatomic structure. We need to reconceptualize

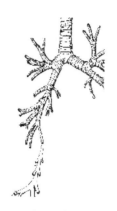

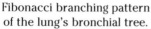

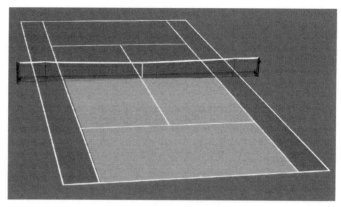

Fibonacci branching pattern of the lung's bronchial tree.

Our lungs have a huge surface area for air exchange, slightly less than half the surface area of a singles tennis court.

ourselves as not being 50/50 creatures. Left and right asymmetry gives rise to the spiraling, dynamic energy that animates us. Indeed, we have left and right lungs that are divided into segments that reflect the Fibonacci Sequence: our left lung has 2 lobes and our right lung has 3 lobes. Remember that 2 and 3 are numbers early in the Fibonacci Sequence: 0,1,1,**2,3**,5,8,13... Not only do the lobes of the lungs reflect the Fibonacci Sequence, but the bronchial tubes do as well. As Robert Prechter, Jr. describes in *Pioneering Studies in Socionomics (2003)*,

> *In the early 1960s, Drs. E.R. Weibel and D.M. Gomez meticulously measured the architecture of the lung and reported that the mean ratio of short to long tube lengths for the fifth through seventh generations of the bronchial tree is 0.62, the Fibonacci ratio. Bruce West and Ary Goldberger have found that the diameters of the first seven generations of the bronchial tubes in the lung decrease in Fibonacci proportion.*

This Fibonacci branching pattern allows for a huge amount of surface area for the exchange of O_2 and CO_2. The surface area of the alveoli (the tiny air sacs at the end of each bronchiole) would be the equivalent of slightly less than half the surface area of a singles tennis court. Even more amazing is the fact that there are close to 620 miles of capillaries surrounding the alveoli to facilitate efficient air exchange (remember that the number 620 is a multiple of the rounded Golden Ratio—0.618 or 0.62).

Each of the top categories in the Golden Ratio Lifestyle Diet has built within it a detoxification phase in order to maintain Golden Ratio balance of intake and output. In the case of the number-one driver, Air, breathing brings in fresh oxygen, while at the same time releasing carbon dioxide—CO_2. The exhalation phase of breathing not

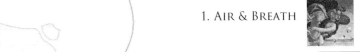

The Ins and Outs of Your Breath and Their Golden Ratio Relationships

As you might expect, there are natural, multiple Golden Ratio divisions between the functional divisions of your breath. The breath has evolved to follow Nature's Path of Least Resistance and Maximum Performance; this is the reason the functional relationships of breathing conform to the Golden Ratio. Of course, our lung capacity graph featured here is a generalized description of the components of an average human breath. Individual variations depend on health, sex, size, body-type, altitude at which a person lives, etc.

Golden Ratio Lung Volume Graph

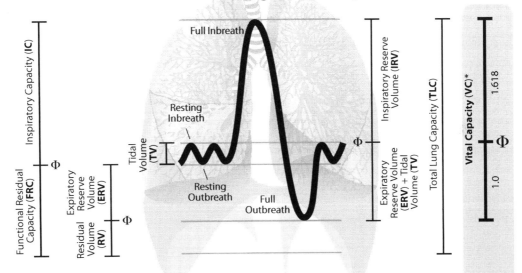

Spirometric lung volume graph, with demarcating Golden Ratio (Φ) divisions of the different functional segments of the breath. The thick undulating line represents inbreaths and outbreaths of different volumes, small and large.

- Inspiratory Capacity (**IC**) / Functional Residual Capacity (**FRC**) = 1.618
- Expiratory Reserve Volume (**ERV**) / Residual Volume (**RV**) = 1.618
- Inspiratory Reserve Volume (**IRV**) / Expiratory Reserve Volume (**ERV**) + Tidal Volume (**TV**) = 1.618

Golden Ratio Lung Volume Graph Key

1. ***Vital Capacity (VC): Total amount of air that can be breathed out, after a maximal inbreath. This one lung function is the #1 predictor of longevity; that is, the higher your Vital Capacity, the greater your longevity.**

2. Total Lung Capacity (**TLC**): Total amount of air that your lungs can hold at maximal inbreath.
3. Inspiratory Capacity (**IC**): Total actual amount of air you can take in on a full breath, starting from a relaxed resting position.
4. Functional Residual Capacity (**FRC**): Air remaining in your lungs after a normal outbreath.
5. Expiratory Reserve Volume (**ERV**): Additional amount of air you can forcefully expel at the end of a normal outbreath.
6. Residual Volume (**RV**): Remaining air in your lungs after you forcefully expel your full breath.
7. Inspiratory Reserve Volume (**IRV**): Extra air that you can inhale on top of a normal inbreath.
8. Tidal Volume (**TV**): Amount of air you breathe in or out during a normal breath.

1

only gets rid of carbon dioxide, it also helps to regulate our vital acid/alkaline balance. Without adequate respiration, not only will our cells be starved of oxygen, but there will be a backup of metabolic acids, causing adverse health effects.

The rate of breathing is of course dependent on whatever our activity demands are at any given time. We continuously sense both oxygen and CO_2 levels. When we're exercising, we breathe faster and when we're at rest we naturally breathe slower. Our body's Divine intelligence has the ability to dynamically change in response to the demands of the moment. With each heartbeat, blood delivers oxygen (O_2) and absorbs carbon dioxide (CO_2) at the cellular level and reverses the process in our lungs. A dynamic interaction between lung and heart activity (breathing and circulation) is required for efficient cellular respiration to occur. At rest, a general rule of thumb is that the ratio of respirations (breaths) to heartbeats x 10 approximates the Golden Ratio of 1.618:

$$\textbf{(Respirations} \div \textbf{Heartbeats) x 10 = 1.6}$$

For example, a person with a respiratory rate of 12 breaths per minute and a resting heart rate of 75 beats per minute will have this ratio:

$$\textbf{12} \div \textbf{75 x 10 = 1.6}$$

This Golden Ratio of respiration to heart rate may not hold during intense exercise or if one crosses the anaerobic threshold, yet the natural Golden Ratio pulse will reestablish itself during the recovery phase. Where most people get into trouble is when they're at rest and tend to *hypo*ventilate or under-breathe. Over-breathing or *hyper*ventilation is a less common, temporary occurrence and is typically caused by anxiety. Under-breathing or hypoventilation is usually exacerbated by poor posture, where rounded shoulders and a caved-in chest inhibit deep and adequate respirations. When one isn't breathing deeply enough, acidity develops in the blood which then forces the kidneys to get rid of the excess acids. Over time, this stress moves even deeper into one's physiology, putting stress on endocrine glands and even dips into mineral buffers in your bones to keep the acid/base balance in your blood normal. The wisdom of your body is programmed with many different physiological Golden Ratio set points (homeostasis/rheostasis). Your body is constantly striving to keep all of your physiologic set points in Golden Ratio balance, including O_2/CO_2, acid/base, blood sugar levels, hormones, blood pressure, temperature, hydration, etc.

> *If you follow your breath, you lose all limitation.*
> **Kathryn Sanford, yoga teacher**

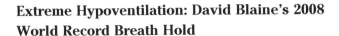

Extreme Hypoventilation: David Blaine's 2008 World Record Breath Hold

Natural Golden Ratio respiratory set points can be artificially changed through training, as is the case in certain athletic endeavors. *The Oprah Winfrey Show* was the stage for the 4/30/08 world record breath-hold by Houdini-inspired magician David Blaine. Blaine demonstrated his skill for oxygen assisted static apnea: the length of time a person can hold their breath after breathing pure oxygen. Blaine's record-setting time was an amazing 17 minutes and 4 seconds, which shattered the previous record of 16 minutes and 32 seconds set by Peter Colat. Blaine was able to suppress his deep-seated respiratory impulse long enough to set a new world record.

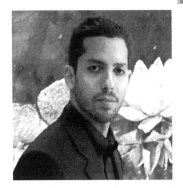

David Blaine, world-renowned magician, illusionist and record-setting breath holder.

David Blaine utilized a technique called air gulping, where he was able to increase the amount of oxygen he could take in to his lungs and thereby hold his breath longer. We don't need to go to that extreme to increase our respiratory capacity. What we're after is simply making sure that we don't hypoventilate and that our lungs are well ventilated with oxygen and that the CO_2 doesn't build up in our system. The most efficient way to do that is by taking full, deep breaths, both inhalation and exhalation. There is a lot of leftover air in our lungs at the end of each breath that we can expel by squeezing our abdominal muscles. Getting rid of that stale air is the only way to make room for the next breath of fresh air. Practicing Lung Yoga, Rx #2 at the end of this chapter, is a simple and effective way to get rid of stale air and build your lung's Vital Capacity.

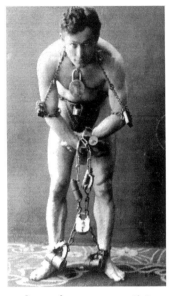

Legendary escape artist and magician Harry Houdini, shown here in 1899. Houdini was the *inspiration* for many of David Blaine's death-defying feats, including his 2008 record-setting breath hold.

There is only one difference between David Blaine's willed apnea and the average person's shallow breathing or hypoventilation: Blaine's respiratory suppression was intentionally trained, while the average person's lack of respiratory drive is largely unconscious and exacerbated by factors like poor posture, polluted air and inactivity. Even though Blaine suffered no apparent ill effects from his stunt, the average person over time will suffer many low-grade symptoms like fatigue, malaise and poor mental and physical performance. Hypoventilation and decreased oxygen levels can also set the stage for many chronic, degenerative conditions. These facts ought to inspire us all to become conscious, mindful breathers as opposed to breathing on autopilot

The Golden Oxygen Ratio

Oxygen is the predominant element found in the human body, at a near-Golden Ratio level of 65% (the remaining 35% is largely composed of a combination of carbon, hydrogen, calcium, phosphorous and potassium). Interestingly, Oxygen is also the predominant element in the Earth's crust. Oxygen is the main area of interest for Ed McCabe, pioneering oxygen researcher and author of *Flood Your Body With Oxygen*. He convincingly argues that the root of all diseases and degenerative conditions, including cancer and AIDS, is oxygen deprivation. Most, if not all, of these diseases thrive in an anaerobic—low or no-oxygen—internal environment. McCabe points out:

The air we breathe today is reported to have only about 21% oxygen. The other 79% is mostly nitrogen... We have shortness of breath when the oxygen level drops into the teens, and below 7% oxygen we cease to live.. Allowing for pollution in the cities, our society as a whole has allowed so much pollution to accumulate, and so much of the environment to be destroyed, that our available oxygen commonly drops below 21% in the air, depending upon the location sampled. This physical machine we walk around in was designed to exist here on the planet within an atmospheric sea full of high-level fresh oxygen...

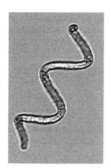 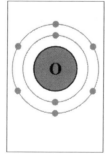 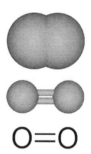

oxygen
8
O
15.999

O=O

(*Left to Right*) 1. The majority of the Earth's oxygen comes from phytoplankton; common types include Diatoms and Spirulina (pictured here) which exhibit Golden Ratio symmetry. 2. Oxygen as featured on the Periodic Table. 3. Oxygen molecule diagram, showing its 8 orbiting electrons. 4. Oxygen molecule or O_2.

> *Peak oxygen is the problem, not peak oil. Oxygen levels in many cities are as low as 10%, creating functional frontal lobotomies in the population.*
>
> **William Deagle, M.D.**

For optimum health and mental functioning, our physical bodies need that Fibonacci number of 21% oxygen, or even more. Oxygen deprivation over a long period of time has been documented to have many deleterious effects. Thomas H. Maugh II, *Los Angeles Times* staff writer describes in Biospherian Roy Walford's obituary the effects of the oxygen deprivation Walford experienced during his time as a Biospherian:

Before ALS caught up with him, he stood 5 feet, 8 inches and weighed 134 pounds. He had a bodybuilder's physique, the product of workouts at a local gym. He got an inadvertent chance to test his theories in humans when he became a member of the Biosphere 2 team. Biosphere 2 (Biosphere 1 being the Earth itself) was a $150 million, 3 acre, glass-enclosed structure built to determine whether humans could live in a self-sustaining environment on another planet, such as Mars. Walford, then 67, was by far the oldest member of the team. The next-oldest was 40, and the rest were about 30. Soon after they were sealed inside in 1991, the group realized that they couldn't grow enough food to provide a normal diet. Walford convinced them to adopt a near-starvation regimen: vegetables and a half-glass of goat's milk every day, meat or fish once a week. They didn't exactly flourish, but they did get healthier. Men lost nearly 20 percent of their body weight and women about 10 percent. Their blood pressure, blood sugar, cholesterol and triglyceride levels all fell by at least 20 percent to extremely healthy levels.

The team members also exhibited an increased capacity to fight off illnesses, such as colds and flu. But levels of nitrous oxide—produced by microorganisms in the soil and normally broken down by sun-light—rose to dangerously high levels, and the crew suffered periods when the oxygen level in the structure was unusually low. Walford later speculated that both problems caused the death of brain cells. 'I remember, when I would talk to him while he was in there, his voice would be slurred, and he would say he would bump into things while he was walking because he was light-headed,' said his Daughter, Lisa Walford. 'The disease started in the Biosphere, even though I wasn't aware of it at the time,' Roy Walford told The Times. 'You can see it on the videos. I was getting a little bit wobbly.'

1

Dr. Roy Walford, Caloric Restriction & Oxygen Malnutrition

Dr. Roy Walford, M.D. (1924-2004) lived to the unripe old age of 79, just slightly above the average life expectancy for U.S. males. He was one of the world's most brilliant life extension scientists, with over 340 published articles. His research showed that simply cutting the caloric intake of laboratory mice in half doubled their expected life span. The Biosphere 2 experiment gave him the opportunity to put caloric restriction to the test on himself and his crew when food stores ran unexpectedly low. When the Biosphere crew severely restricted their calories, they had amazing improvements in their blood pressure, blood sugar and cholesterol levels. The question that arises is: *If caloric restriction is so great, why didn't Walford live to 90, 100 or beyond?*

The answer presents itself when Walford's entire protocol is viewed through the perspective of the Golden Ratio Lifestyle Diet. The prioritization sequence of lifestyle drivers is of the utmost importance. While Walford's main focus was on health and longevity driver #4/Nutrition, he severely compromised the quality and quantity of the Air (driver #1) that he breathed. Since the prioritization of his lifestyle diet drivers was not optimized, Dr. Walford suffered the consequences and ended up dying of a neuro-immune disease—ALS or Lou Gherig's disease. The irony of Walford's untimely death is that not only did he practice caloric restriction, but due to the unforeseen circumstances that developed in the Biosphere, Walford was also forced to practice oxygen restriction as well. Oxygen levels in the Biosphere dropped from around 21% oxygen to 14.5%. While such a spartanesque approach can in fact be beneficial from a nutritional standpoint, it can be deadly when applied to driver #1, Air and Breath. Even being the brilliant scientist that he was, Dr. Walford still had a critical blind spot—not fully recognizing the importance of driver #1, Air and Breath. If *any* of the main health and longevity drivers are out of sequence, this can not only produce inefficiency in your physiology and metabolism—the results can be fatal. The synergistic increase in life force and immune system strength, which arises with the correct prioritization and sequencing of health and lifestyle drivers in conjunction with Golden Ratio balance, is the true life extension therapy.

Oxygen concentration has varied throughout Earth's geologic cycles. It seems logical, as can be inferred from Ed McCabe's oxygen research and Roy Walford's story, that for optimum health and mental functioning our physical bodies need a higher level of oxygen than is presently found in much of the air we breathe. Chronic shallow breathing can result in lowered cellular O_2 levels, suboptimal nutrient assimilation and incomplete cellular detoxification, not to mention lowered mental and emotional function.

The air we breathe is also charged with vital life energy or *prana*, as the ancients called it. One of the scientific correlates of prana is the measurable charge of negative ions. Higher levels of negative ions and prana are always found in natural environments such as mountains, oceans, rivers and are particularly strong near waterfalls. Man-made waterfalls or fountains simulate Nature's pranic and negative ion charge and are a good place to recharge our vital energy when we can't get out in Nature. It is clearly vital on both scientific and energetic levels that we consciously upgrade both the quantity (Vital Capacity) and quality (pranic/negative ion charge) of the air we breathe.

The Biosphere 2

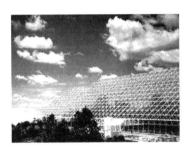

The Biosphere 2 (Biosphere 1 being Earth) is a closed ecological system built in Oracle, Arizona that looks like a giant greenhouse. Its first mission ran from September, 1991 through September, 1993 and was composed of eight people including team leader Roy Walford, M.D. The plants inside the Biosphere 2 didn't produce enough oxygen to keep up with the respiratory demands of the crew and as a result of the constant deficit, oxygen levels fell from 20.9% to 14.5% after the first 16 months. Dr. Walford eventually developed ALS—Lou Gherig's disease—as a result of the prolonged oxygen deprivation.

Oxygen: The Double-Edged Sword

Let's drop down from the anatomic and functional levels to the biochemical level of breath. In order to extract energy from our food, we need a sufficient supply of O_2 or oxygen. The two major pathways of energy production are known as *aerobic* (requiring oxygen), and *anaerobic* (without oxygen). Aerobic respiration is much more efficient than anaerobic. This efficiency is reflected as comfort when you are exercising at a comfortable rate. We all know the lactic acid burn when we cross from aerobic metabolism into anaerobic. Once the "red-line" is crossed, the inefficient anaerobic metabolism can't be sustained for very long.

> *Cancer, above all other diseases, has countless secondary causes. But, even for cancer, there is only one prime cause. Summarized in a few words, the prime cause of cancer is the replacement of the respiration of oxygen in normal body cells by a fermentation of sugar.*
>
> **Otto H. Warburg, M.D.,**
> **Biochemist & Nobel Prize Winner**

The actual chemical that stores energy at the cellular level is called ATP (Adenosine-TriPhosphate). ATP is known as the "universal energy currency" because all cells use it to fire their metabolic processes. The more ATP that we have, the more energized we feel. ATP is made most efficiently by aerobic respiration (oxidative phosphorylation) with a major efficiency ratio over anaerobic fermentation. In this first chapter we've explored the universality and vital importance of oxygen in our health and longevity. It's interesting that another of the top success drivers in the Golden Ratio Lifestyle Diet has been touted as being "universal" as well. Specifically, the second most important substance in the Golden Ratio Lifestyle Diet, Water, is known as the "universal solvent," as we'll explore in the next chapter.

> *Your brain is, on average, less than 3% of your body's weight, yet it uses more than 30% of your body's oxygen. As you become aerobically fit, you double your capacity to process oxygen.*
>
> **Michael J. Gelb, author of**
> ***How to Think Like Leonardo da Vinci***

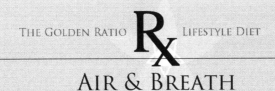

AIR & BREATH

Pick one or more of the following Rx's to add to your daily health regimen.

Interesting note: Leonardo Fibonacci actually originated the R$_X$ symbol, which he used for square roots and which later became used the world over as the universal symbol in prescription writing.

1. Golden Breath Retraining

Since we know that deeper, more efficient breathing is the #1 factor that can improve your health and increase your longevity, it's imperative that the biomechanics of your breathing be correct. The major Golden Ratio division point on the body is at the level of the navel; internally, this is also at the same level as the diaphragm, where the 1st 15% of your breath should always begin. The diaphragm is your main breathing muscle and its ligaments find their origin at the same level as the navel where they attach to the spine. So your every breath actually originates from the main Golden Ratio division point in your body; thus, each breath is actually a subconscious acknowledgement and subtle reminder of the Golden Ratio.

A Full Golden Breath

There are as many ways of breathing as there are people; each breath is truly unique. Since most people breathe with less than optimum awareness and have fallen out of healthy breathing habits, the following example breath is offered as a simple way to begin to restore full, healthy breathing. Try practicing this breath throughout your day. Experiment with variations of timing, focus, mindfulness, mindlessness or any modifications you choose. In actuality your breath is a never-ending, continuous, flowing movement—a recharging of energy and life-enhancing exchange of molecules. For demonstrative purposes, our example of a full, healthy breath is broken down into four basic parts: a two-stage inhalation, followed by a two-stage exhalation, with pauses inserted as desired. This breath begins with:

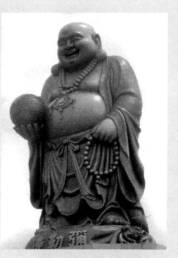

1. A relaxed, full Buddha-belly inhalation, flowing into...

2. A full chest inhalation, while gently pulling in your belly. This supports the rising of your chest, shoulders and head. When you have inhaled just the right amount of air, you will feel a sense of satisfaction and relaxation moving through your entire body. You might choose to linger and enjoy this for a few moments before cresting the breath wave and...

Buddha, demonstrating how his belly moves out during the first phase of inhalation.

3. Letting your breath go completely, allowing your lung's natural elasticity to effortlessly contract and exhale; leading into...

4. Pulling your navel into your spine to complete the full exhalation. When your lungs feel "empty," your belly may naturally relax and return to a neutral position, pausing as desired. This naturally flows into...

5. Your next breath (start over at No. 1)...

Many people have a contrary or paradoxical respiratory motion, where the movement of the diaphragm is reversed. By placing your hand over your navel and assuring its outward, expansive movement as you breathe in and its inward "tacking your belly button to your spine" movement as you breathe out, you will know that your respiratory efficiency is being optimized. To regularly recharge your system, it's a good idea to take a series of deep, Golden Breaths at least hourly. A Golden Ratio Breath is achieved when the time ratio of inhalation-to-exhalation approximates the 38:62 Golden Ratio— about 40% time for the complete inhalation and 60% time for the complete exhalation. This allows for optimal lung oxygen "dwell time"/uptake and carbon dioxide elimination. To easily access this Golden Breath Ratio, breathe IN to the count of any Fibonacci number (e.g., 5), and then breathe OUT to the count of the next higher Fibonacci number, in this example 8. When you have balanced inhalation and exhalation around this simple 3:5 or 5:8 ratio, a unification phenomenon characteristic of the Golden Ratio occurs. At this point of Golden Ratio balance, all of your body's systems are more harmoniously integrated for healthier physiologic functioning.

2. Increase Your Vital Capacity (VC) and Longevity with Golden Ratio Lung Yoga

We can actually do Golden Ratio Lung Yoga: by stretching and strengthening our breathing capacity with deeper inhalations and exhalations. On the lung volume graph below, you can see the dotted lines that have been extended over the top and bottom of the normal Vital Capacity curve. We can expand our Vital Capacity, thereby increasing our health and longevity, by simply including the following easy exercise into our normal breathing several times a day:

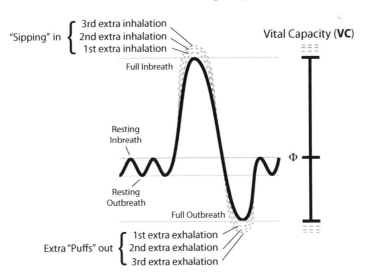

Golden Ratio Lung Yoga Graph

R_X for increasing Vital Capacity (VC), which stretches the lungs and strengthens the diaphragm, chest and abdominal muscles.

- Take three small extra sips of air at the end of a full inbreath. This extra small volume of air gently stretches the lungs and chest cavity and expands lung capacity over time.

- Exhale three extra puffs at the end of a full exhalation. These extra expiratory efforts strengthen chest and diaphragmatic muscles, enabling them to get rid of stale air at the end of each breath.

By doing this 5-8+ times every day, respiratory efficiency is increased. We can stretch and strengthen our respiratory muscles and tissues, regain some of our lost Vital Capacity and increase our vitality, functionality and longevity. Increased Vital Capacity will shift you to the left on the Longevity and Breath/ Vital Capacity graph. By regaining as little as 250-500 ml. of lung volume (roughly between 1 to 2 cups), an age reduction of as much as 5-10 years+ is possible.

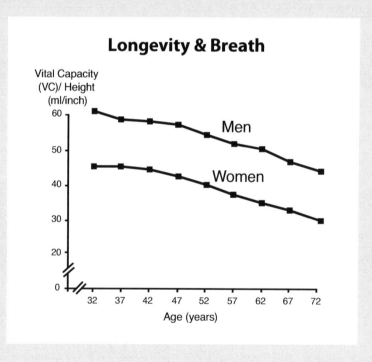

1

3. Golden Ratio Breathing Wake-Up

Upon awakening, find a warm and comfortable place where you can sit comfortably with a straight spine. Inhale fully through your nose and into your abdomen to the count of 3; then exhale to the count of 5. Repeat this breathing pattern for at least 8 cycles. Keep breathing slowly and deeply. As your breathing capacity improves, try inhaling to the count of 5 and exhaling to the count of 8. You might eventually even try inhaling to the count of 8 and exhaling to the count of 13. Go only as far as is comfortable for you. Now your blood is super-oxygenated and you're ready for your day. Feel free to add pauses between inhalations and exhalations, as needed.

4. Fibonacci's Exercise Breath

We have seen that the entire respiratory system is designed around the Golden Ratio, so it makes perfect sense that we would want to adapt our exercise to that code for optimal benefits. While walking or running, you might try inhaling to the count of 3 and exhaling to the count of 5. If you need more air, try a 2:3 ratio of inhalations to exhalations. Find the proportion that feels right for you. This way of breathing offers a valuable alternative to the standard 1:1 inhalation to exhalation ratio. You may keep up the breathing ratio through 3, 5 or 8 breathing cycles, and then let the practice go and breathe in and out without consciously thinking about the ratio for a while. Then try it again, perhaps with a different set of Fibonacci numbers and ratios. See which ratio feels best.

If you are strenuously exercising, you may not be able to keep up with Golden Ratio breathing because your system may try to revert to your habitual 1:1, 2:2 or 3:3 ratio to keep up with maximal oxygen and CO_2 demands. However, if you slow down or stop, you can then resume Golden Ratio breathing. When Golden Ratio breathing is continued for more than 3 minutes it will relax you, lower your blood pressure and calm you down. These breathing exercises can be done anytime, anywhere: driving, lying in bed, at work or exercising. What makes these breathing exercises so effective? Golden Ratio breathing is powerful because it rebalances and repatterns your autonomic nervous system in accordance with the Golden Ratio. This has profound potential for improving your health and restoring overall wellbeing.

5. Pandiculation: The Golden Ratio Reset

Don't like yoga? Well, you may never have thought of it this way, but the yawn and stretch that you do when you're waking up in the morning or perhaps during the day when you're tired is the most natural form of yoga and pranayama. The yawn is a built-in reflex that automatically resets your oxygen and CO_2 levels and equalizes ear pressure. At the same time, a natural stretch occurs that lengthens muscles, relieves stiffness and increases blood and lymphatic circulation. There's even a word for this built-in yawn and stretch reflex: *pandiculation*. Pandiculation is a Golden Ratio reset. Your system is programmed to always try and re-establish internal balance or homeostasis whenever it needs to. You can think of pandiculation or the yawn and stretch as a type of primal yoga. All of the other yoga poses and breathing techniques that have been developed over time are just more complex variations on the basic yawn and stretch. Yawning seems to be contagious, if you've ever noticed how the reflex can spread from one person to another. Pandiculation not only helps you wake-up in the morning, it also has the ability to

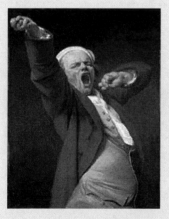 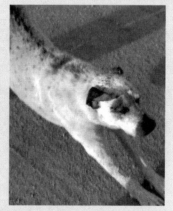

Pandiculation: the essential yawn and stretch. Animals are masters of the yawn and stretch technique.

increase your level of alertness in a boring business meeting. So don't ever be embarrassed when the urge comes, just enjoy it and explain that your body is just doing a Golden Ratio reset, should anyone ask.

6. How to Become a "Thoughtless" Person: Finding the Golden Ratio Space Between Your Breaths

Having discovered where the extremes of breath are in maximal inhalation and exhalation (Rx 2), we can now find the Golden Ratio balance points at the top and bottom of normal inhalation and exhalation. These are the magical pauses at the limits of normal breathing (TV/Tidal Volume), where thought naturally comes to a momentary rest. It makes sense that Golden Ratio breath points would demarcate this long-sought-after state of mental quietude and inner peace.

- The top of a normal, relaxed inhalation—top of Tidal Volume (TV)— marks the Golden Ratio Φ demarcation point of Vital Capacity (VC).

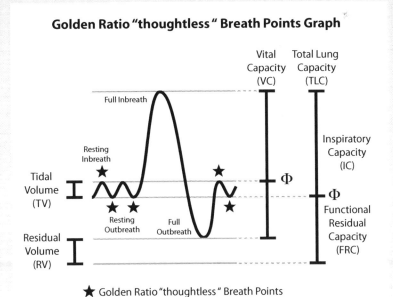

Golden Ratio "thoughtless" Breath Points Graph

★ Golden Ratio "thoughtless" Breath Points

- The bottom of a normal, relaxed exhalation—bottom of Tidal Volume (TV)—marks the Golden Ratio Φ demarcation point of Total Lung Capacity (TLC).

- By spending meditative time at our Golden Ratio breath points, we can temporarily become "thoughtless" people: de-stressed, rejuvenated and regenerated. At the end of a normal inhalation, stop for 3-5 seconds and enjoy the thoughtless state of Golden Ratio balance. Then, repeat after a normal exhalation. You can do this simple exercise throughout the day whenever you need a Golden Ratio tune-up.

7. Golden Ratio Breathwalk

As you walk, try synchronizing your steps and breaths with numbers from the Fibonacci Sequence: 1,2,3,5,8... For example: two steps forward would equal one full inbreath—the next three steps, one full outbreath, for a 2:3 ratio. When Golden Ratio breathing is done at rest, either seated or lying down, you may want to experiment with the larger ratios—3:5 or 5:8—as your lung capacity for longer inhalations and exhalations develops over time. The ratio may change from moment to moment, depending on your oxygen and carbon dioxide levels. The Golden Ratio breathwalk is an easy way to synchronize breathing with exercise and tap the power of Nature's Secret Nutrient.

8. Breathing With Golden Awareness

Breathing. As we observed at the start of this chapter, it's our first act upon entering this world and our last upon leaving. While our breath (like our heartbeat) is the continuous pulse and soundtrack of our entire life, so often we breathe with zero conscious awareness. This, even though all movement, mindfulness, meditation, yoga, martial arts and athletic training systems are rooted in a working awareness of the breath. Breathing with awareness is like investing in a compounding health and longevity annuity. It also gently tunes you back into the natural rhythms of life—the wind in the trees, ocean waves and tides, moon phases. So become more aware of your breath's depth, breadth and quality. It is both the foundation of health and longevity and the fastest way to change or upgrade your energy and state of mind and body. As an added bonus, when you consciously enhance your breath with the Golden Ratio, you instantly access Nature's Secret Nutrient and its health bestowing powers. For example:

Too tired or fatigued? Try deepening and tuning your breath to the initial numbers from the Fibonacci Sequence, e.g., inhale to 2.. exhale to 3... Inhale with force and purpose; exhale like a powerful bellows on a fire. Try this energizing breath for 5 to 8 repetitions and observe how you feel.

Too wound-up, anxious or in need of greater calm and focus? With eyes closed, try deepening and tuning your breath to higher sequential Fibonacci numbers, e.g., inhale to 5..... exhale to 8........, or inhale to 8........ exhale to 13............. Keep the breath gently strong and steady; inhale peace and calm and exhale stress and tension. Try this relaxing breath for 8 to 13 repetitions and observe how you feel.

As with these and all Golden Ratio breathing exercises, play and experiment. The important thing is to simply start becoming more aware of the gift and potential of each breath. In the words of yogi master GM Khalsa, *Breath Is Life*. Your health, longevity and life will grow to the degree that you allow your breath to be conscious, full and free. *To Life!*

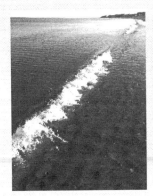
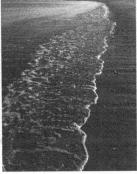

Go to our website at GoldenRatioLifestyle.com and click on Golden Ratio Breath Wave to learn how to synchronize your breath with that of the ebb and flow of the ocean. This multi-sensory exercise will gently entrain your physiology to Nature's Path of Least Resistance and Maximum Efficiency.

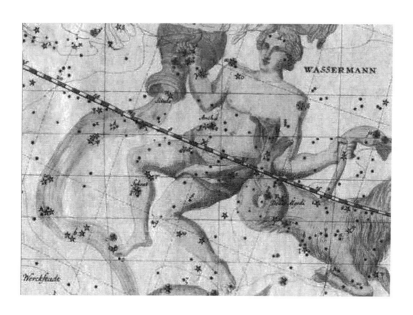

Aquarius the Water Bearer, pouring forth the liquid gift

of hydration and enlightenment from the heavens.

From a classic lithograph.

2.

WATER & HYDRATION

Water is the Driver of Nature.

Leonardo Da Vinci

Humans can only survive without water for a few days without increasingly compromised functioning and ultimately death. Throughout our evolution, we've had to either develop water conservation strategies or live with a water source close by. We didn't evolve like camels that can go several weeks without water or kangaroo rats that can go 3-5 years, so we need to have a constant intake of water in order to survive. Unless we can maintain our Golden Ratio fluid balance through regular water intake, our functioning will be compromised short-term, leading inevitably to compromised longevity long-term.

We can harness water's magical ability to act as a universal solvent not only to keep us hydrated, but also to transport nutrients for metabolic processes, for detoxification and temperature regulation. As most athletes know, even a 2% fluid loss can dramatically affect performance. We need nothing less than a radical paradigm shift in our appreciation of the importance of water's role, both in preventing chronic dehydration and in maintaining optimal health.

Dr. Batman to the Rescue

*Understanding dehydration will empower you to become much healthier
and you will be able to become your own healer.*

Fereydoon **Batman**ghelidj, M.D.

2

We know that in acute dehydration, our bodies will divert water away from organs and tissues like skin, muscle and the gut to vital organs like the brain, heart and kidneys in order to sustain life. If we broaden our vision and entertain the idea that there might be such a thing as chronic dehydration, then those same survival mechanisms may be activated, yet in slow motion—therefore going unnoticed. This was the revolutionary insight of Iranian physician Fereydoon **Batman**ghelidj, M.D. (1931–2004). Through his years of research, he hypothesized that most of the so-called chronic diseases of modern life were in actuality the body's attempt at "drought management." The disease manifestations are merely the body's attempt to stop dehydration by different adaptation mechanisms in different tissues. Dr. Batmanghelidj proposed the following list of functional ailments and pathologies directly related to dehydration:

allergies	*headaches*
asthma	*heartburn*
autoimmune diseases	*hormonal irregularities*
cancer initiation	*hot flashes*
cholesterol abnormalities	*hypertension*
chronic fatigue	*low back pain*
colitis	*kidney stones*
constipation	*mental and emotional problems*
coronary artery disease	*migraines*
diabetes	*obesity*
dry eyes	*osteoporosis*
dry skin	*pain of various causes*
fibromyalgia	*rheumatoid arthritis*
gout	

It might initially sound outlandish that chronic dehydration could be responsible for all of the above problems, yet theoretical mechanisms are offered in Dr. Batmanghelidj's many books, including *Your Body's Many Cries for Water*. One prominent example of chronic dehydration is in the case of "essential" hypertension—high blood pressure of unknown cause. Blood pressure is controlled by a symphony of neural and hormonal feedback mechanisms. Normally, blood pressure in the arterial system is high enough to perfuse the capillary beds all the way down to the cellular level. Adequate blood pressure is necessary for multiple vital reasons: to deliver oxygen and nutrients to the cells; to remove waste and simply to maintain consciousness, e.g., you'll often get light-headed if you stand up too fast because your brain isn't receiving enough blood. The body's intelligence regulates blood pressure to accommodate water fluctuations on a moment-to-moment basis.

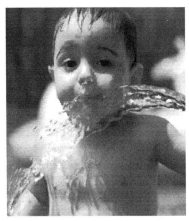

Water is the #2 driver in the Golden Ratio Lifestyle Diet.

Dehydration is usually thought of as resulting in low blood volume and low blood pressure—*hypo*tension. That may be the case in acute and sub-acute conditions of dehydration, but Dr. Batmanghelidj proposed an interesting theory of what happens to people in a chronically dehydrated state. The hypotension of acute dehydration is contrasted with the *hyper*tension (high blood pressure) of chronic dehydration. Although it may take months or years to arrive at a prune-like state, the water deficit is never replaced and the vascular system has no choice but to remain in overdrive for organ perfusion, thereby sustaining the high blood pressure. The treatment seems simple: recognize the state of chronic dehydration and give the patient water. This is just the opposite of what is normally done to patients with hypertension. They are prescribed diuretics and medicines that dilate the blood vessels. These treatments only exacerbate the dehydration, leaving the patient feeling drained and without energy. It's amazing that such a simple substance like water could be both the cause of disease and the cure, depending on the circumstances. This is a simple and profound example of how the power of water has been overlooked by mainstream medicine. Although this scenario doesn't take into account other factors involved in hypertension such as arterial stiffness, cardiac or kidney conditions or various endocrine effects, it may in fact explain the cause of "essential" hypertension in a significant number of people.

In drought management, your body will use various mechanisms to shunt water into the critical organs and tissues first, and then replenish the remaining tissues and organs in a hierarchical manner. The particular ailment that has manifested is only a compensatory mechanism for the underlying problem of dehydration. This is a revolutionary way of viewing our physiology and is Copernican in its impact on medical thinking, not to mention our health and longevity. Dr. Batmanghelidj says that doctors have mistakenly focused all of their attention on the *solute* (drugs

2

and medications) instead of the *solvent* (water). Again, this is a simple yet profound insight. The entire world-view of medicine considers the so-called diseases as actual entities in and of themselves, unaware that the causal mechanism might be something as simple as dehydration. Yet it makes perfect sense when you consider the fact that the exquisite Golden Ratio balance and efficiency of your entire physiology is thrown off when you're dehydrated, whether acutely or chronically. Knowing how the Golden Ratio manifests at different scales, we can surmise that the same process that is going on in acute dehydration might also be going on in the more extended time frame of chronic dehydration. Total body water and the intracellular/extracellular ratios become imbalanced when you're dehydrated. Adequate hydration is critical for a multitude of functions, including:

- Maintaining blood viscosity and clotting parameters: blood will abnormally clot if it gets too thick.
- Facilitating plasma transport of oxygen, CO_2, nutrients and waste products: water helps dilute the blood to make it easier to transport nutrients and waste.
- Hydrolyzing nutrients: breaking down nutrients for easy absorption by reacting with water.
- Maintaining vascular hydrostatic pressure: keeping blood pressure at the right level to perfuse all of the vital organs including the heart, brain and kidneys.
- Thermoregulation through perspiration, respiration and shunting of blood from extremities to core, or vice-versa: helps keep the body at the right temperature for optimal metabolism.
- Maintaining adequate urine flow—perfuses the kidneys with enough blood to generate adequate urine to remove waste products. Note: if your urine is darker than Chardonnay, you are very likely dehydrated.

The orthodox medical establishment has not yet embraced this hypothesis put forth by Dr. Batmanghelidj. However, this paradigm shift in medical thought aligns perfectly with the precepts of the Golden Ratio Lifestyle Diet. It's no accident that Water was determined to be the #2 driver in the Diet's hierarchy of needs, when you consider the full impact that adequate water has on health and longevity.

Hydration Rule #1: Drink *Before* You're Thirsty

The critical factor in the development of chronic dehydration is the remarkable fact that our thirst impulse doesn't accurately reflect our need for water. This is even truer as we age—an older individual's thirst reflex becomes extremely *dampened* and should not be relied upon to monitor fluid needs. We need to cultivate other strategies to preempt dehydration, such as evaluating our skin texture; seeing if we have dizziness on standing and of course, checking the color of our urine: unless your urine is very light yellow or clear, then you need to drink until it clears. Complicating matters is the fact that regular consumption of dehydrating beverages like tea, coffee and alcohol tend to make us run water deficits. We can temporarily have clear urine after drinking coffee or tea, yet later on our urine will become more concentrated and thus darker. The key here is that pure water alone is always the best hydrator. You can surmise that if you have any of the above noted ailments, you are probably dehydrated. Since our bodies are like sponges, the uptake of water into the deep intracellular compartments of our tissues can actually take days or even weeks to replenish—so regular, ample water consumption needs to become a way of life. We can begin approaching our ideal body composition and physiology by rehabituating ourselves to drink more water. See the Rx's at the end of this chapter to learn how to make the water that you drink easily and quickly absorbable. We can also build more water-containing tissue—muscle— while at the same time decreasing our body's percentage of fat. There are many easy and efficient methods available that accomplish both goals of increasing muscle mass while decreasing body-fat in chapter 4/Nutrition and chapter 6/Exercise.

Water and Golden Ratio Body Composition

Some people are afraid of heights. Not me, I'm afraid of widths.

Steven Wright, humorist

Let's imagine for a moment that your body was required to have a label that revealed your nutritional content. A typical nutritional analysis would include percentages of the three macronutrients: protein, fat and carbohydrates. This may be a fine way to look at the nutritional value of energy bars, but not practical for *Homo Sapiens*, or the new rapidly growing overweight species found in America, *Homo Fatruvius*. America has become a country with one of the most overfed, overweight yet undernourished populations in the world. Along with this increasing girth have come elevated rates of heart disease, cancer, arthritis, autoimmune disease and even Alzheimer's disease. How would we be able to determine the correct values to put on our own body's optimal nutritional label? Scientists have developed various techniques called Body Composition Analysis (BCA), to determine the amount of fat and fat-free mass. Total body fat is made up of subcutaneous fat (fat under the skin) and visceral fat

2

(fat around the organs). The remainder of our body is lean body mass, which is made up of muscle, bone and organ tissue. Several different measuring techniques have been developed to more precisely determine body composition. Thanks to Archimedes' principle, we can submerse a person in a tank of water and determine the amount of water displacement. This is known as Underwater Hydrostatic Weighing (UHW). Since the densities of fat and lean body tissue are different, percentages of body-fat and lean body mass can be precisely calculated. Another method—skin fold calipers—is much simpler. Skin-fold calipers are used to measure the thickness of subcutaneous fat at several different locations on the body: back, waist, arms, legs, etc. With these values, an estimate of percent body-fat and lean body mass can be made. One of the more recent developments is body composition analysis through the use of Bioelectrical Impedance Analysis (BIA). In this technique a weak electrical current is passed through the body. Since fat and muscle (lean body mass) conduct electricity at differing rates, the percentages of each can be determined. It's difficult to get a Golden Ratio handle on the ideal amount of fat you would want on your Body Composition Label, because typical recommendations for ideal body-fat percentages range from 8-19% for men (age 20-39) and 21-33% for women (age 20-39). Both ranges are really quite broad and don't give any indication of Golden Ratio dynamics. Perhaps there's another way of looking at Body Composition that would give us the precise information we need to align with the Golden Ratio's ideal template.

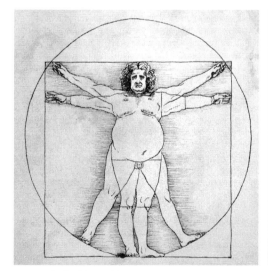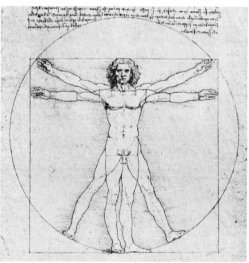

(*left*): Homo Fatruvius, with excessive body-fat percentage. (*right*): Homo Vitruvius, with idealized lean body mass and Golden Ratio water composition percentage. *Your waistline is your lifeline.* Jack LaLanne, *"The Godfather of Fitness."*

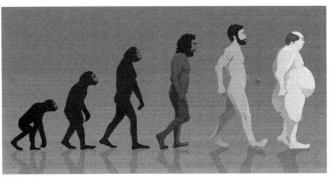

Human **de**-volution, with the advent of Homo-Fatruvius.

The BioDynamicsCorp.com website features data obtained from bioelectrical impedance testing, which reveals an interesting fact pointing directly to Golden Ratio relationships inherent in healthy body composition. If we instead look at body water percentage, we get some surprising results that can point the way to exactly where we want our body composition to be for maximal physiologic functioning. In the men's 25-34 age group, body water percentage measures 61.4%, within .4% of the more exact Golden Ratio percentage of 61.8%. This is uncanny, yet not surprising, since Golden Ratio relationships are infinitely ubiquitous throughout the human body. In this 25-34 age range the human male is at his prime, in terms of physiologic functioning and performance. The percent of body water measured for women was slightly lower, due to a natural gender difference in amount of body fat. Even though bioelectrical impedance testing is a modern technique of measuring body composition, there have been visionary artists that have masterfully captured different levels of body composition in their paintings. Prime examples of Golden Ratio body composition are strikingly demonstrated in Michelangelo's original *David* and in Leonardo Da Vinci's *Vitruvian Man*. In these masterpieces we can clearly see the sleek, muscular builds of prototypical human males in their prime. Michelangelo and Da Vinci demonstrated what ideal humans would look like with Golden Ratio proportions in both *structure* and in body composition, which represents *function*. We can surmise that these *Homo Vitruvians* would have had approximately 62% total body water content (see next page). As you can see, their total body fat is relatively low, probably in the 8-10% range. These masterpieces by Michelangelo and Da Vinci hold many secrets, ideal Golden Ratio body composition included.

Macro and Micro Golden Ratio Water Ratios

Since we know that the Golden Ratio appears at all levels of scale, we can predict that in addition to water being about 62% of ideal total body weight, Golden Water Ratios might be evident at the next lower scale in our bodies. This is indeed the case at the next level of our cellular water containing compartments. In the accompanying diagram, we can see the two main water categories of the body and their percentages

Idealized Golden Ratio Human Body Water Composition Label Facts	
Body Water %	
Men, ages 25-34	**62%**
Women, ages 25-34	**62% (-5 to -8%)**
Intracellular Water %	**62%**
Extracellular Water %	**38%**

What an ideal body water composition label would look like.

of 37% / 63%. These ratios are given for a healthy young male and are used to illustrate the general concepts pertaining to Golden Ratio water balance. Once again, we see the ubiquitous universal design constant of the Golden Ratio in the body's intracellular/ extracellular fluid compartment ratios. This 63% to 37% ratio is within 1% of the 62% to 38% Golden Ratio. We can only surmise that there must be an incredible physiologic advantage in maintaining these proportions in the internal aqueous environment of our body. The amazing water molecule itself is designed according to Golden Ratio harmonics and is truly Nature's Universal Solvent. This supreme Golden Ratio solvent gives us the quality of fluidity and solvency that we can utilize for optimizing our health and vitality. The golden key to accessing water's full power is to upgrade both the quality *and* the quantity of our daily water intake.

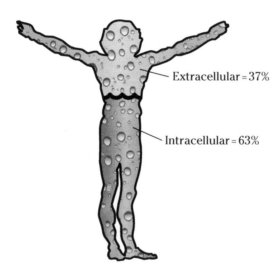

Intracellular 63% and Extracellular 37% water composition of the body closely approximates the 62/38% Golden Ratio.

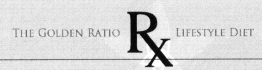

THE GOLDEN RATIO R_X LIFESTYLE DIET

WATER & HYDRATION

Pick one or more of the following Rx's to add to your daily health regimen.

1. W.A.M. (Water A.M.): 1 to 2 Tall Glasses of Water Upon Arising

Water is critical for the efficient functioning of your whole system. When you awaken in the morning, all of the metabolized toxins produced during sleep must be eliminated. This is a metabolic priority, which falls into the First 15% Percent of your body's daily requirements. The best way to facilitate the elimination of toxins is to drink one or two large glasses of pure water within 5 minutes of arising. This simple step in the first part of your day will improve your functioning all day long.

2. The Secret Password Revealing Your Daily Water Requirements: Chardonnay

It's often recommended to drink a certain number of glasses of water per day to maintain your hydration and replenish fluid losses through urine, breath, perspiration or stool. However, there is another, easier way to determine your daily water requirement in lieu of an absolute daily intake volume of water. This method takes into consideration individual variations such as gender, Body Mass Index (BMI) and activity level. By looking at actual physical signs, you can get customized, real-time feedback on whether you're hydrated or dehydrated. The most logical symptom to look at first is your sense of thirst. Yet you need to understand that your sense of thirst is often blunted and also has a phase delay from when your body is actually dehydrated to the time you're thirsty. One of the best ways to monitor your hydration (*input*) is by simply looking at your *output*: the **color of your urine**. Your kidneys filter your blood, getting rid of toxins and at the same balancing fluid levels, mineral levels and blood pressure. By gauging the color of your urine, you can quickly tell if you need to drink more water. The more dehydrated you are, the darker your urine will be. It can range from clear to various shades of yellow, with deep amber indicating more severe dehydration. Ideally, try to keep your urine in the range of clear to a light **Chardonnay**, or pale yellow. If your urine is darker, you need to drink until it clears. Remember that dark urine is your body's silent cry for water. You may not feel thirsty, but the darker your urine is, the more water you need to drink.

Note: Various substances including drugs, vitamins and certain medical conditions can also cause the urine to be various colors—red, bright yellow, orange, green, blue or brown. If you have any unusual color in your urine, you need to see your physician for evaluation. Also, if you have any heart, liver or kidney disease or hormonal abnormalities, you should be under the guidance of your physician to monitor your fluid intake, so as not to overload your system.

3. Water Thievery & Dehydrated Foods

Dehydrated food has only a fraction of the water volume of the original food, due to the water removed during drying. Depending on the amount of dehydrated food you're eating, you could be developing a sizeable water deficit. During digestion, a lot more water in the form of digestive juices is needed to process dehydrated, highly concentrated dried foods than if you ate the original food in its natural state. Imagine the difference between eating a juicy grape and a raisin and you'll get the point. Dried fruit is also far higher in sugar by weight versus fresh fruit, which can easily upset your body's insulin levels, simultaneously throwing off healthy blood sugar balance in addition to healthy hydration levels. This principle applies to *all* concentrated foods, including all food/meal bars. Obviously, eating food in its natural state lowers additional water deficits in your system. When you do eat dried foods, be sure to either soak them in water in advance to reconstitute them, or consume sufficient additional water to balance out the difference. This will help keep your body fine-tuned hydrodynamically.

4. Prune or Plum: The Skin Pinch Test

The hydration of your skin is another way to get information on how hydrated—or dehydrated—you are. We have seen that the sense of thirst is not the optimal way to gauge your hydration, since there is a lag time between being dehydrated and feeling thirsty. In many people, their sense of thirst is blunted, not actually registering how dehydrated they actually might be. We need as many dehydration cues as possible in order to remind us to drink. Another good way to monitor your hydration is via the skin pinch test. Here's how:

Simply pinch the skin on the back of your hand and see how rapidly it recoils back to its original state. If you're dehydrated it will look more like dough, slowly falling back to normal. This test can be confounded by loss of natural elastin in your skin. Elastin is the natural protein that gives your skin its elasticity, but is lost with the aging process or skin damage through too much sun exposure. You'll have to figure out if you're dehydrated or have skin damage or both. With a little practice you'll get the hang of it. Use the skin pinch test in conjunction with the sense of thirst, dizziness upon standing test and the urine color test to determine if you're dehydrated. Remember that rehydrating your entire system may not happen overnight. You may have to create a new habit of actually drinking before you're thirsty in order to reconstitute yourself from that dry prune back into a nice, juicy plum!

5. Water Quality Upgrade

It's extremely important that the water you drink is as pure as possible. Short of having access to fresh spring water, the best way to ensure that you have clean water is to either buy filtered water or do it yourself with a home filter. Your filter should remove both man-made and naturally occurring toxins, e.g., chlorine, fluoride, excess minerals, organic toxins, heavy metals, drugs, microbes, etc. Your filter should have at least a two-stage system that includes a carbon filter and a reverse osmosis filter.

Note: Glass storage bottles are recommended to avoid hormonally disrupting plastic toxins like phthalates and BPA. More sophisticated water purification systems include UV, ozonation, oxygenation, alkalinization and water structuring properties. This will give you clear, pure water and is recommended for those who want to avoid excess sodium in their diet. Note: while plastic is not recommended for water storage, safer plastics for water containers have one of the following recycling numbers on the bottom within a triangle: 1, 2, 4, 5; unsafe numbers are 3 and 6.

6. Water Absorption Enhancement

A quick way to enhance the absorption and assimilation of your drinking water is to add a small pinch of sea salt to an 8 oz. glass of water. This will optimize the water for quicker absorption and assimilation (not recommended for those who need to restrict sodium intake).

7. Yogi Pure Water

A quick way to oxygenate your water is by using an old yogic technique. Get two glasses, one full and one empty. Pour water from one glass to the other 5, 8 or 13 times to introduce oxygen into the water. As you pour the water from one glass to the other, try gradually increasing the distance between the glasses. Drink the water immediately while the oxygen is still in solution. This exercise helps your coordination as well. You might place your glass of pure water in direct sunlight for 5 to 8 minutes prior to this exercise, to activate the water with sunlight.

8. Nature's Perfect Golden Ratio Water

One of the best ways to get the ultimate in purified water is to drink fresh vegetable juices. Nature has already ultra-purified and super-charged the water in vegetables. As they grow, they slowly draw water, molecule by molecule, from the earth up their stalks, into the leaves and finally into the vegetables. This water is among the purest water you can get, yet is largely overlooked as a source of purified water. For more information on juicing, see Jay Kordich's 2007 edition of *The Juiceman's Power of Juicing: Delicious Juice Recipes for Energy, Health, Weight Loss, and Relief from Scores of Common Ailments.*

Here are the ingredients for a quick and nutritious juice recipe. Always use organic produce for your juice. Vegetable juice is preferable to fruit juice because it avoids the higher sugar content/glycemic index of fruit. Carrot juice has a relatively high glycemic index as well, so those with blood sugar problems should limit or avoid it. If you find the vegetable juices could use a little added sweetness, try adding ¼ to ½ of an apple, pear, a few strawberries or even a slice of beet, which has a surprisingly high level of natural sugar and sweetness.

1 carrot	**½ inch of ginger root**
3 stalks celery	**(optional; strong taste)**
½ head romaine lettuce	**handful of parsley**
¼ to ½ cucumber	

Even if you improve your diet radically and take all the right supplements, while you'll be getting some measure of preventive benefit, you still won't be doing enough to reverse existing damage. Add juicing to the mix, though, and you can actually begin to repair damage. ***Juicing is the key to reversing the progress of disease.***

Gary Null, Ph.D.

---

9. Keep Your Largest Organ Hydrated

When most people think about hydration, they automatically think about drinking enough water to keep internal fluid levels in a healthy range. Yet hydration of your largest organ—your skin—is also of vital importance. In addition to keeping it supple and youthful, external hydration of your skin also strengthens its role as temperature modulator and resilient barrier to environmental toxins. Select a high quality moisturizer without toxic ingredients, as creams and lotions can be absorbed directly into your blood. Try simple organic oils in your regimen of skin hydration, such as almond or olive. Ideally, your moisturizer should be pure enough to eat—if not, it doesn't belong on your skin (avoid mineral oil, a toxic petroleum by-product). Many toxic ingredients are easily identified by being multi-syllabic, hard-to-pronounce and/or have CAPITALS or numbers in their names, e.g., PEG-13. Visit the Skin Deep website at: www.cosmeticsdatabase.com to evaluate many cosmetic or personal care products or ingredients to check their safety.

Proper skin hydration seems like basic common sense, yet is often not common practice. It's no accident that Frenchwoman Jeanne Calment, at 122 the world's longest-lived documented person (thus far), hydrated her skin regularly with olive oil. Apply moisturizer as needed morning and evening—more frequently in drier climates and in wintertime.

10. Pucker Power Your H$_2$O

A quick way to alkalinize your water and thus restore an often out of healthy body acid/alkaline balance ratio is to simply squeeze the juice of ¼ or ½ a lemon into your water. You will quickly feel energized anytime you drink this simple yet magical potion.

11. The Dehydration Inflammation Connection

Anti-aging authority and dermatologist Nicholas Perricone, M.D. brings home the importance of proper hydration not only for the skin but for the body as a whole. His vital insight below makes the clear connection between dehydration and inflammation. In Dr. Perricone's view, chronic inflammation is a key factor in chronic cellular aging and disease. Essentially, proper hydration is a simple way to reduce premature aging (see pages 110-120 and 154 in chapter 4 for more on inflammation):

Logic tells us that when we have an unwanted fire, we throw water on it to put it out. Therefore it makes perfect sense that water would help quell the cellular inflammation that goes on in our bodies. In fact, this is true. Water will decrease inflammation in the body.

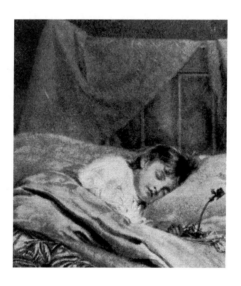

The Sleeping Innocence, from *Vivilore:*

The Pathway to Mental and Physical Perfection,

by Mary Reis Melendy, M.D.

3.

SLEEP, REST & RECOVERY

In the head of the interrogated prisoner, a haze begins to form.
His spirit is wearied to death, his legs are unsteady, and he has one
sole desire—to sleep... Anyone who has experienced this desire knows
that not even hunger and thirst are comparable with it.

Menachem Begin, former Israeli Prime Minister,
regarding his time as a prisoner of the KGB

Sleep Deprivation

As a result of his experiences under the extreme duress of sleep deprivation torture in a Russian prison, former Israeli Prime Minister Menachem Begin probably would have ranked his top three health drivers slightly differently than we did in the formulation of this book. Here is the contrast:

Menachem Begin's Probable Prioritization	The Authors' Prioritization
1. Air	1. Air
2. Sleep	2. Water
3. Water	**3. Sleep**

Although it would be extremely rare to die from sleep deprivation—like you certainly could from air or water deprivation—Menachem felt the extreme discomfort from

89

not being able to sleep. Such is the power of sleep on our physiology. Nicole Bieske, of Amnesty International Australia, corroborated Begin's thoughts on sleep by stating,

At the very least, sleep deprivation is cruel, inhumane and degrading. If used for prolonged periods of time it is torture.

If international authorities recognize the destructive effects of sleep deprivation, why would we want to subject ourselves to such easily preventable self-abuse? The speed of our lives has clearly accelerated to the point where most people are undergoing a societally induced sleep deprivation—or in other words, torture. A pernicious side effect of this slow and low-grade sleep torture is the disruption of our biorhythms. This leaves us vulnerable to many physiologic stresses including obesity, cardiovascular disease, hormonal problems and poor mental and emotional responsiveness, with attendant increased accident and poor performance risks. Healthy biorhythms are critical for maintaining a healthy quality of life and sleep is one biorhythm that we are all intimately familiar with. A century ago most Americans got around 9 hours of sleep per night. This was obviously before the modern era of 24/7 bombardment from all sides, including television, computers, cell phones, PDA's, etc. Today the average amount of sleep per night is around 7 hours, while a third of the population struggles to get by on less.

> *Sleep, the gentle tyrant: It can be delayed but not defeated.*
> **Wilse Webb, Ph.D., sleep researcher**

Based on lab experiments that allow people to find their natural, optimal amount of sleep, researchers found that many people's body clocks tend to require a little more than 8 hours of sound sleep every 24 hours. Maintaining optimal health and weight requires that we satisfy this 8 hours+ minimal requirement and preferably get closer to 9 hours of total sleep/rest within every 24-hour period. This could be broken up into 7 or 8 hours of sound sleep with a 1 to 2 hour rest or siesta break during the day. Since we know that the optimal physiologic blueprint of the human body is the Golden Ratio, then we can reconcile standard medical sleep recommendations with what would be in alignment with the 38:62 Golden Ratio. There are three easy ways to mathematically look at the Golden Ratio relationships of sleep:

- ❂ 15 hours awake out of a 24-hour day is equal to 0.625, which approximates the Golden Ratio of 0.618.

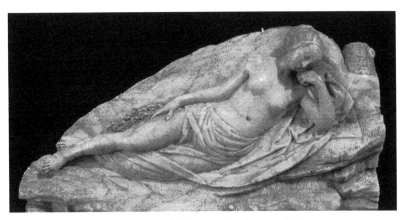

Restore your Golden Ratio sleep ratio to
approximately 9 hours of sleep/rest per every 24 hrs.

- 9 hours of sleep/rest out of a 24-hour day equals 0.375, which rounds
  up to the 0.38 smaller aspect of the Golden Ratio.
- 9 hours of sleep/rest to 15 hours awake equals 0.6, which approximates
  the Golden Ratio of 0.618.

Let's look at some of the aberrant physiology that can result from not satisfying our Golden Ratio sleep/rest requirements.

Obesity and Sleep Deprivation

Research shows that adequate sleep is crucial for maintaining healthy weight, especially over time. Dr. Sanjay Patel, Professor of Medicine at Case Western Reserve University, conducted a study of nearly 70,000 women, which followed the effects of sleep on weight over a sixteen-year period (1986-2002). The study's major findings include:

- Compared with sound sleepers, women who slept 5 or fewer hours
  per night were 32% more likely to experience major weight gain,
  defined as a gain of 33 lbs. or more.
- These same women were also 15% more likely to become obese,
  compared with women who got at least 7 hours sleep per night.
- The findings were unrelated to light sleepers who ate too much
  or exercised too little.
- The study results are said to apply equally to men and women.

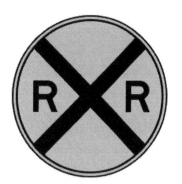

3

As at Railroad (RR) Crossings, it's best to stop and be sure you have enough R&R (Rest & Recovery) before proceeding to the next health & longevity drivers. For example, it's better not to exercise if you're sleep-deprived as injury, accident, immune system stress and poor digestion are likely results.

Some of the mechanisms of how sleep deprivation could lead to weight gain include:

- Altered hormone secretion, leading to increased hunger through altered leptin and gherelin secretion.
- Increased fatigue, leading to diminished/poor quality or no exercise the following day.
- Changes in a person's basal metabolic rate (BMR), a measure of the number of calories burned at rest.
- Sub-optimal digestion and diminished nutrient absorption, leading to increased food intake.

As a result of this research, new and innovative approaches to weight loss are sure to include therapies that better address synchronizing sleep/wake ratios with the Golden Ratio.

> *I have never taken any exercise except sleeping and resting.*
>
> **Mark Twain**

The Dark Knight and the Quality & Quantity of Sleep

The Dark Knight is not only a movie about a superhero's struggle against evil, it's also a reminder of the ideal sleeping conditions we should strive for in our bedroom at night. Maximum darkness (The Dark Night) is our best friend; the real evil is the unwanted light that disrupts our descent into—and dwelling in—restful sleep. The Golden Sleep Ratio refers to the *quantity* of sleep that allows one's circadian rhythms to harmonize and balance. This ratio is approximately 9 hours of sleep to 15 hours of waking. We also need to consider the *quality* of sleep/rest in order to optimize the beneficial effects of the Golden Sleep Ratio. We want to become aware of the difference between a Dark Night and a Light Night. Darkness is a relative term, since it's rare that people living in cities are spared from the constant barrage of light pollution.

According to the Tucson, Arizona-based International Dark-Sky Association (IDA), the sky glow of Los Angeles is visible from an airplane 200 miles away. In most of the world's large urban centers, stargazing is something that happens at a planetarium.

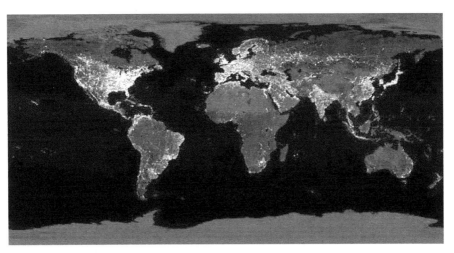

NASA composite night satellite photo of Earth, showing man's remarkably strong footprint of light. In large cities it can take extra diligence to insure a dark sleeping environment.

Indeed, when a 1994 earthquake knocked out the power in Los Angeles, many anxious residents called local emergency centers to report seeing a strange "giant, silvery cloud" in the dark sky. What they were really seeing—for the first time—was the Milky Way, long obliterated by the urban sky glow. Source: EnvironmentalHealthPerspectives.com

> *Darkness is as essential to our biological welfare, to our internal clockwork, as light itself.*
>
> **Verlyn Klinkenborg, *Our Vanishing Night*,**
> ***National Geographic* magazine, November 2008**

Even small amounts of light are able to suppress melatonin secretion—the pineal hormone of sleep—so it's imperative for good sleep hygiene to have our sleeping room as dark as possible. A truly good night's sleep is dependent on our brain's ability to secrete melatonin effectively and the circadian rhythm restoration that follows. Melatonin is released by the pineal gland in response to darkness and controls many neuroendocrine processes. Disruptions in normal brainwave activity and neuroendocrine secretions have been associated with numerous pathologies including breast and prostate cancer, cardiovascular disease, insomnia, depression and diabetes. In a striking paradigm shift around the possibility of considering carcinogens in a different "light," the International Agency for Research on Cancer has now classified "night-shift" work as a human carcinogen. This broadens our

3

Naps Cut Heart Attacks by 37%

Siesta in Healthy Adults and Coronary Mortality in the General Population— A study of 23,681 Greek adults over six years showed that those who napped at least three times a week for about a half an hour, had a 37% lower risk of dying from heart attacks than those who didn't nap (37% is virtually the smaller part of the 38/62 Golden Ratio). The study's senior author and researcher Dimitrios Trichopoulos, M.D. remarked,

My advice is if you can nap, do it. If you have a sofa in your office, if you can relax, do it.

---

perspective and lets us think of many commonly accepted behaviors as carcinogens in the same light as viruses and toxic substances.

Even during the lighter phases of the lunar cycle we can still protect ourselves, assuring a *dark night* by eliminating all light sources in our sleeping environment. With the use of adequate curtains and eye shades we can avoid unwanted stimulation of our retinas. Be aware of light pollution from your electronic devices, including TVs, clock radios, computers and night-lights.

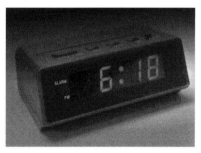

Even the seemingly small, faint light from clock radios and computers can disrupt melatonin secretion at night, thus interfering with sound sleep.

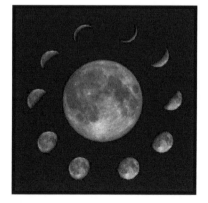

Moonlight through bedroom windows can disrupt your circadian rhythms.

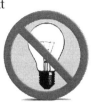

Depression, Weight Gain Can Result From Even Dim Light During Sleep

Sleeping with the light on could leave you feeling low the next day, researchers from Ohio State University have warned. They say that a night-light—however dim—may affect the structure of the brain, raising the odds of depression. The eerie glow emitted by a TV or the seemingly reassuring presence of a night-light could be enough to impact mental health, weight gain and have serious implications on overall health.

Key Message: Secure total darkness for your sleeping environment, to maintain optimal melatonin secretion for supporting and protecting your health.

Source: www.dailymail.co.uk, 11/18/10.

Alphabet Sleep

In order to access our greatest healing potential and regeneration, it's imperative to regularly drop into as deep a state of sleep as possible for 8–9 hours optimally. Our deepest sleep correlates with the EEG (electroencephalogram) frequency range known as Delta. However, to get to Delta we must drift down through several other restful, yet lighter states of sleep and rest known as Theta and Alpha. Not surprisingly, Nature has structured our brainwaves in categories that correspond to Fibonacci/ Golden Ratio numerical divisions, as we'll explore on the next page.

REM (Rapid Eye Movement) is also a prime component of healthy sleep. REM donates sleep zones which occur in increasingly longer waves over a full night's sleep. REM is crucial for healing, regeneration, learning, memory, problem solving and integration. In healthy Golden Ratio sleep of 8–9 hours a night, REM waves occur about 5 times (every 90–110 minutes) with the longer waves towards the *end* of the total sleep cycle. In addition, up to 80% of growth hormone—our body's prime catalyst for healing, regeneration and youthfulness—is secreted during sleep. So whenever you cut short your night's sleep, you exponentially reduce REM sleep along with growth hormone secretion. This is why it's so crucial to maintain a healthy base of sleep in the Golden Ratio range of 8–9 hours a night, making up any deficit through naps/rest periods during the day.

The four basic frequency ranges in human brain waves are measured in cycles per second, or hertz (Hz), and correspond to Fibonacci/Golden Ratio numerical divisions:

- Delta (0.5–5 Hz) is most prominent during deep sleep and is also associated with the secretion of growth hormone, healing and regeneration.

- Theta (5–8 Hz) is the level of sleep or very deep meditation, in which many creative ideas originate. Theta also offers an expanded window into intuition and deep memory.

3

- Alpha (8–13 Hz) is the state where you are awake, yet quiet and deeply relaxed, as in meditation. It is also the "twilight sleep" zone you pass through just before falling asleep and just as you're waking up. Alpha is the magical "window state" for accessing latent intuition and also a most powerful state for creative visualization. Simply closing our eyes and then deepening and slowing our breath can quickly induce the Alpha state.

- Beta (13-34 Hz and above) occurs when our mind is alert and active, as in daily waking activity.

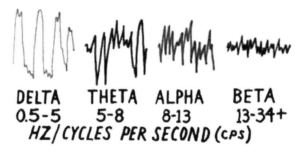

Brain waves in approximate Fibonacci intervals, as measured in Hz:
Delta, 0.5-5; Theta, 5-8 Hz; Alpha, 8-13; Beta, 13-34+.

The World's Fittest Man Got His Golden Ratio Sleep

Mark Allen won the Hawaiian Ironman Triathlon a record-tying 6 times. In 1997, the year after Allen won his 6th Ironman championship, *Outside* magazine named him "The World's Fittest Man" in a cover story. One of the key factors in Allen's training regime was his dedication to getting 9 hours of sleep every night, to sustain peak performance and optimize his recovery periods. Of course, 9 hours of sleep/rest every 24 hours is the Golden Ratio sleep zone ($15 \div 9 = 1.6$). Allen is also known to have benefited from strategic longer rest/recharge periods in the time leading up to his races, a protocol resonant with the Fibonacci Workout Wave (see chapter 6/Exercise). Mark Allen was keenly aware of the importance of the right ratio—and timing—of rest/recovery phases to the active phases of training, telling co-author Matthew Cross that,

95% of athletes go into races overtrained.

Winners Sleep, Losers Weep

Mark Allen is one of many athletes who practice sound sleeping habits for peak performance. In their *Business Insider* article *Sleep to Be An All-Star* (7/21/11), Steve Fabregas and Cheri Mah show that the average amount of sleep/rest enjoyed by

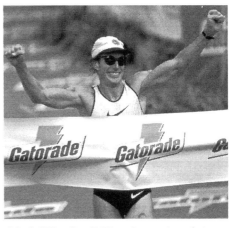

Mark "The Grip" Allen, Legendary 6-time World Ironman Triathlon Champion

champions from a wide range of sports approximated the golden sleep ratio of 9 hours out of 24. Mah is a professional sleep coach working with top athletes whose research applies just as strongly to the rest of us, whatever our fitness regimen. Some of Mah's food (or sleep) for thought:

- A 20-30 minute power nap improves alertness by 42%
- Chronic sleep loss can lead to a 30-40% reduction in glucose metabolism [the First 15% of energy generation]
- Well-rested tennis players got a 42% boost in hitting accuracy
- Sleep loss means an 11% reduction in time to exhaustion
- Sleep improves split-second decision making by 4.3%
- 2 days of sleep restriction can lead to a 3x increase in lapses of attention and reactivity
- A good night's sleep before the game = a winning game; a season of good sleep every night = a season of wins

Quotes from a few notable "sleep champions" offer added insight:

Sleep is just as important as diet and exercise [in reality and in the Golden Ratio Lifestyle Diet, it's actually a higher priority].

Grant Hill, professional basketball player, Phoenix Suns

Sleep is half my training.

Jarrod Shoemaker, Olympic triathlete/Duathlon World Champion

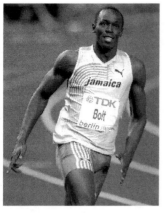

Usain Bolt of Jamaica, World and Olympic sprinting champion. Bolt's sound sleeping practice is a vital component to his record-shattering performances.

A well-rested body is a healthier, more efficient, more capable one. This could be the hardest thing to accomplish on my to-do list, but it always makes a difference.

Kerri Walsh, Olympic Beach Volleyball Champion

I think that napping every game day, whether you feel like it or not, not only has a positive effect on your performance but also a cumulative effect on your body throughout the season.

Steve Nash, professional basketball player, Phoenix Suns

Sleep is extremely important to me—I need to rest and recover in order for the training I do to be absorbed by my body.

Usain Bolt, sprinter; three-time World and Olympic gold medalist (100m, 200m, 4 x 100m relay)

Ample sleep/rest is a vital health and longevity driver which supports being at your best in sports, work and the whole of life. The following Rx's will help ensure that you're able to optimize the quantity *and* quality of your sleep and rest periods. Then you can awake fully recharged to meet your day like a champion.

Sleep is the golden chain that ties health and our bodies together.
Thomas Dekker, English dramatist during Elizabeth I's reign

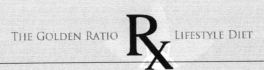

SLEEP, REST & RECOVERY

Pick one or more of the following Rx's to add to your daily health regimen.

1. Count Fibonacci Breaths for Enhanced Sleep and Meditation

Bruce Mandelbaum is a master acupuncturist, massage therapist and marathon runner from New York. Inspired by co-author Matthew Cross' book *The Millionaire's Map*,™ Bruce created the following easy method for easing into sleep and becoming mindful of the breath in meditation. You simply pay attention to each breath and count each full inhalation/exhalation to the Fibonacci Sequence: 1 breath, 1 breath, 2 breaths, 3 breaths, 5 breaths, 8 breaths, 13 breaths, 21 breaths… and so on. The key is to keep each breath deep and full. As Bruce notes,

You cannot be tense and contracted when your breath is full and deep.

You may find that when you go to sleep counting your breaths to the Sequence, you wake up more refreshed and rested (Bruce has yet to make it past breath 55 before he's sound asleep). Leonardo Fibonacci might have utilized Bruce's technique to count rabbits instead of sheep.

2. Chiaroscuro: Golden Ratio Biorhythm Resets

The word chiaroscuro (key-R-oh-skoo-row) describes the contrast of light and dark in painting and was originally developed by Golden Ratio genius Leonardo da Vinci. We could just as easily use it to describe our biorhythms. For optimal health and vitality, we want to ensure that our wake/sleep and light/dark cycle is better adjusted to the Golden Ratio. This helps support optimal health and vitality if we get it right. Likewise, the difference between a great painting and an average painting may rest in the fact of whether or not chiaroscuro wake/sleep and light/dark cycles are tuned to the Golden Ratio.

An artist has a palette full of colors to get the contrast just right, whereas we have several Golden Ratio adjustments to reset our wake/sleep and light/dark cycle in the more optimal proportions, e.g., 15 hrs. waking/9 hrs. sleep/rest.

3. Morning Adjustment: Sun Gazing

Light is the most potent *Zeitgeber*, or "time giver." Light is one key cue that our brain relies on to reset our biorhythms on a daily basis. Here's the easiest and most potent way to establish healthy biorhythms. Upon arising, preferably as soon as the sun rises, go outside and face the sun. With your eyes closed, move your head back and forth slowly, allowing the sun to bathe your eyelids. By doing this for 3-5 minutes, the sun will notify your brain's biological clock to begin its daytime activities. Your body's sleep hormone—melatonin—will be totally inhibited by the light. If you're up at dawn, just as the sun crests the horizon and before it's too bright, you can do the exercise with eyes open, for just a few minutes. Remember not to stare directly at the sun, but just be aware of it in the periphery of your visual field as you move your head from side to side. This same exercise can be used for jet-lag as well. People with Seasonal Affective Disorder (SAD) use full-spectrum lights, which are closest to natural sunlight, to accomplish melatonin inhibition. You may want to get these lights if you live in a cloudy area or have more wake/sleep problems in extreme latitudes or with seasonal changes. See Rx 13 in chapter 4/Nutrition for more information on full-spectrum lights.

4. Night Adjustment: Activate Melatonin

Try not to watch TV or be on your computer, cellphone/PDA for at least 1 hour before bedtime. When you're ready for bed, you have several choices to help your brain begin its descent into sleep through activating melatonin secretion. If you have no problem falling asleep, you're good to go, otherwise you may want to try some of the following suggestions.

1. Make sure that your room is as dark as possible. This will signal your nervous system to begin secreting melatonin, your sleep hormone. You can always use eyeshades if you can't get your room totally dark. Unplug clock radios and all other light sources.

2. Do the Fibonacci sleep breathing exercise as described in Rx 1.

3. Have a cup of herbal tea before bed. Remember to steep tea bag in a 1/2 cup of water or less, so you don't wake in the middle of the night with a full bladder. Good teas are Celestial Seasoning's Nighty Night, Sleepy Time or Chamomile.

4. Many people use over-the-counter melatonin (our natural sleep hormone) about 30 minutes before bed. Low dosages are better—anywhere from 0.5mg up to 3mg. Too high of a dosage can result in nightmares, so start on the low end. People with autoimmune problems or asthma should avoid melatonin since it has immune stimulating properties.

5. People with persistent sleep problems may need pharmacological assistance, as sleep deprivation may be more uncomfortable than extreme hunger or thirst.

In addition, all of the other drivers in the Golden Ratio Lifestyle Diet will cross-reinforce and help restore your Golden Ratio wake/sleep ratio to approximately 15 hours awake to 9 hours of sleep/rest, so try and incorporate as many as you can into your new lifestyle.

5. Fibonacci Power Naps

Afternoon naps can recharge your system and greatly increase your efficiency, enhance information uptake and processing and improve emotional health and immune function. The trick is to get just deep enough into the lighter stages of sleep to get some restful and regenerative effects, but not long enough to awaken with sleep inertia or grogginess. Numerous authoritative sleep studies show that the ideal length of a nap is from 5 to around 20 minutes. Here are some of the ideal lengths of naps that you may want to work into your schedule. These naps are calibrated to Fibonacci numbers that interestingly correspond to practical lengths of time for a nap. They are named after some of the more famous nappers. You may want to use an alarm to awaken you from your nap so as not to over-sleep; some people have the ability to program their internal clocks through autosuggestion.

- **The Fossett: 2-5 minutes**. Steve Fossett, (1944–2007) held world records for solo flight circumnavigation of the globe in a balloon and attributed his success to 2-3 minute power naps, of which he took 20-30 during his record-setting 67-hour journey.

- **The Einstein: 8 minutes**. Einstein was one of the preeminent Golden Ratio geniuses of the 20th century. He was also a frequent napper, who undoubtedly benefited from the increased creativity and mental acuity that naps bestow.

- **The Edison: 13 minutes**. Inventor of over 1000 different devices including the light bulb, phonograph and moving pictures, Thomas Edison took short naps daily to make up for the fact that he only slept 4-5 hours per night. Naps gave him the ability to walk a fine line between the worlds of unlimited imagination and waking reality, to bring his great insights back to waking consciousness.

- **The Bucky: 34 minutes**. According to *The Economist*, 2/15/07, Golden Ratio Genius Buckminster Fuller advocated taking 30-minute naps every six hours. He is reported to have abandoned the practice only because "his schedule conflicted with that of his business associates, who insisted on sleeping like other men."

6. Wake to the Golden Ratio with the Zen Alarm Clock

Wake-up gently in the morning with the Fibonacci awakening cycle instead of jolting yourself awake with a blaring alarm clock. Integral theorist Stephen McIntosh, founder of Now & Zen (www.Now-Zen.com) has designed beautifully crafted alarm clocks which gently awaken you with a series of tones that follow a decreasing Fibonacci Sequence. The effect on your nervous system is a very gentle stimulation, in sync with your innate Golden Ratio nature.

Your subconscious mind naturally recognizes the Fibonacci relationships of the tones and responds to the gentle arousal that feels as if Mother Nature herself were waking you.

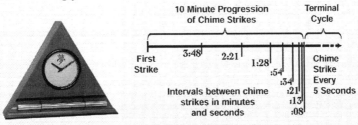

The Zen Alarm Clock gently awakens you to Fibonacci-spaced tones. Tones are calculated from 10 minutes downward to full awakening. Each tone marker is calculated in seconds and then multiplied by 0.618 to arrive at next lower tone.

7. Coffee, Tea or Sleep

Caffeine and related compounds (methylxanthines) are the active ingredients in coffee, tea, cola, energy drinks and energy bars and chocolate. What most people don't realize is that traces of caffeine can circulate in your system for many hours after you consume them. Caffeine is metabolized in your liver and has a half-life of around 5 hours, depending on liver activity. Contraceptive use, pregnancy, liver problems or medication use can extend 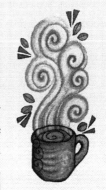 caffeine's half-life to 24-48 hours—or longer. This means that 5 hours after you drink a cup of coffee, half of the caffeine is still circulating in your system. In another 5 hours half of the half—or ¼ of the original amount—is still around. So, if you had an afternoon tea or coffee at tea-time—4 pm—you would still have some stimulant activity in your system when you went to bed, lasting through the night. Your ability to drop into deep sleep would be compromised and rejuvenation wouldn't be optimal. So, it's best to limit your caffeine consumption to the morning, so that your liver can metabolize most of it before you retire in the evening. Of course, an easy substitute for coffee or black tea is a cup of caffeine-free herbal tea, which can be enjoyed right before bed if desired.

8. More Advanced Sound Sleeping Tips

- Remove devices that produce light or electromagnetic fields: computers, clock radios, electric blankets, anything you'd plug into an electric outlet or is battery powered which can interfere with sound, healthy sleep. For those especially sensitive to electromagnetic fields, turn off the breaker switch that goes to your bedroom. This cuts off electricity to those pesky electrical outlets behind the headboard of your bed that could be interfering with sound sleep.

- Make sure that your mattress is made of organic material like cotton or similar natural material. Get rid of any petroleum derived or synthetic mattress that can short-circuit and unground the natural electromagnetic field of your body.

- For an ingenious bed-to-earth grounding system, see: www.sleepgrounded.com.

9. Sleep Apnea: The Intersection of Drivers #1 and #3, Air and Sleep

Sleep apnea occurs when breathing stops for 10 seconds or longer on multiple occasions through the night. This can happen hundreds of times during the night, leaving the person feeling totally depleted and fatigued the following day. Long-term, there is also an increased risk of cardiovascular disease and stroke. During the apneic episodes, oxygen levels in the blood fall and CO_2 levels rise, which then activate an alarm reaction in the brain. The person then usually has a startle reaction, regains their breath and then falls asleep again until the cycle repeats itself. In sleep labs, EEG recordings document the constant disruption of deep, restorative sleep phases in this condition. The most common type of sleep apnea is obstructive, which means that there is a biomechanical problem in the neck or throat: loose or collapsing pharyngeal tissue that is blocking the airway. Poor sleeping posture or positions—sleeping on your back, face-up, as opposed to on your side with a pillow between your knees—can also predispose one to snoring and sleep apnea. Many patients get relief from Continuous Positive Airway Pressure (CPAP) machines that hold the airways open while breathing. This malady highlights the importance of Air as the #1 driver in the Golden Ratio Lifestyle Diet. An alternative cure for sleep apnea is to institute the entire Diet, which will harness the synergistic healing power needed for regeneration and rejuvenation. Many times weight loss along with exercise and postural improvement can create more airway space, realign the airways and strengthen weak throat muscles, alleviating the problem.

10. The Human Star Sound Sleep Technique

This simple exercise takes just 5 minutes right before going to sleep. It's a powerful method which sets the stage for deep, refreshing sleep. The theory? When the 5 "star points" of our body (hands, feet and head) are relaxed, a wave of growing relaxation ripples back into our core. This theory has its roots in the practice of reflexology: our soles, palms and scalp/ears are said to each contain a fractal map of our whole body. When we massage each of these 5 "mini-maps" for even a few minutes, we initiate a chain relaxation reaction which leads us more effortlessly into sound sleep. Try it and see for yourself. This is also a wonderful gift to give someone or of course to receive. Here's how it works:

0. Get into bed when you're ready to go to sleep. Best not to get back out of bed after the exercise. Set your intention for a deeply refreshing night's sleep. Just after turning the lights out, sit up in bed and begin:

1. Massage the sole of your Left foot for 1 minute with both hands. Use a little oil or lotion if you like. Press and knead as firmly as comfortable; focus on loosening up any tension in the sole of your left foot.

1a. Repeat the above on your Right foot for 1 minute.

2. After your 1 minute sole massage on each foot, move to your head for 1 minute. Start by gently massaging your scalp with your fingertips, for about 20-30 seconds. Spend a few seconds gently massaging your ears. Then, move to your jaw muscles, Left hand on Left jaw, Right hand on Right jaw. Press into your jaw muscles with your fingers and thumbs as firmly as comfortable.

3. Now, spend 1 minute massaging your non-dominant hand with your dominant hand. Focus on the palm. Squeeze and massage your hand as firmly as comfortable.

5. Finish with 1 minute massaging your dominant hand with your non-dominant hand. Again, focus on the palm. Squeeze and massage your hand as firmly as comfortable.

8. Lie down now and take a few deep, relaxed Golden Breaths: inhale to the count to 5; exhale to the count of 8. Let yourself go, and sleep well…

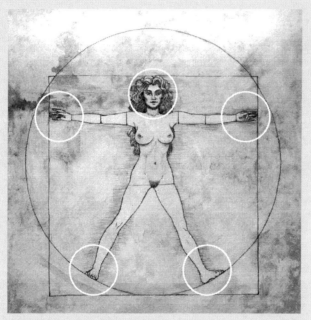

The Human Star Sound Sleep Technique reinforces our Golden Star geometry, gently setting the stage for a sound night's sleep.

11. Create a Softer Landing For Healthier Sleep

In an increasingly hectic 24/7 go-go-go world, many times the last light we see before going to sleep is the glow from our cell phone, PDA, computer or television screen. Often there is little or no quality time to more gently downshift from the fast-paced thinking, activities, distractions and electronic devices of our day. Yet a slower, non-electronic, more relaxing prelude is the vital First 15% to any night's healthy sleep. Here are a few simple, effective tips to make your pre-sleep time more of a relaxed transition. Modify as desired. For the next 3 weeks:

Bronze Level

• At least once a week, turn off ALL electronic devices 60 minutes before going to sleep—and don't access any until morning.

Silver Level

• At least twice a week, turn off ALL electronic devices 60 minutes before going to sleep—and don't access any until morning.

• At least twice a week, practice a calming, relaxing practice such as meditation, the Golden Doors of Your Day, etc., in the last hours before bed (see pages 258 and 261).

Gold Level

• 3 or more days a week, turn off ALL electronic devices 60 minutes before going to sleep—and don't access any until morning.

• 3 or more nights a week, practice a calming, relaxing activity such as meditation, the Golden Doors of Your Day, etc., in the last hours before bed (see pages 258 and 261).

• Once a week, use candlelight ONLY for the last hour prior to bed.

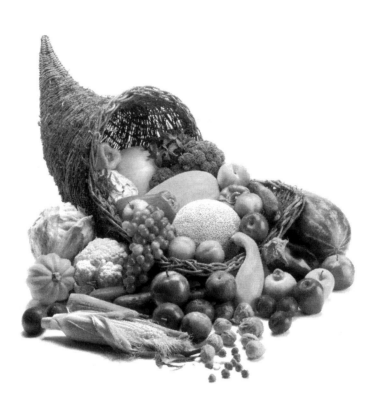

Legendary Cornucopia of infinite

abundance and sustenance, which always

unfolds in classic Golden Spiral form. ℃

4.

NUTRITION: FOOD & BEYOND

Your body has a BLUEPRINT, a SCHEMATIC of what perfect health is
and it is constantly trying to achieve this perfect health for you. All that
goes wrong is that you get in the way of this natural process.

Dr. Richard Schulze, N.D., Natural Healing Authority

Have you ever wondered what the goal of Nutrition is? If we answer the question by viewing it through the lens of the Golden Ratio, we could say that it is obtaining and maintaining that fine point of optimal sustenance—the point between being undernourished and over-nourished. In other words, we want to aim for the metabolic excellence of Da Vinci's evolved human—Homo Vitruvius—the place of ideal body composition and optimal physiologic function. That state of Golden Ratio balance isn't easy for most of the world's population to establish, as evidenced by the fact that in our world in 2009, 800 million people are starving, while another 1.3 billion are overweight or obese. A quick mathematical calculation reveals that 1.3 billion divided by 800 million is 1.62, the Golden Ratio. In Nature's perfection, she even keeps this example of biochemical imbalance in Divine Proportion. We're trying to find that Golden Ratio point of being neither undernourished nor over-nourished, where we're able to function at an extremely high level of efficiency and performance. We'll be looking at various approaches to health and Nutrition that are able to provide support by reaching all the way down to the genetic level. These approaches also appear to be able to control what may be one of the final common pathways to many disease processes—inflammation. As usual, the dietary protocols we advocate conform to the Golden Ratio, either directly or in spirit.

Golden Pro*portion*: Activating Nature's Secret Nutrient (NSN)

You're only as good as your last meal.

Barry Sears, Ph.D.

4

"Phenomenon" is a fitting description for the 40/30/30 "Zone" nutrition program promoted by Barry Sears, Ph.D. This dietary approach, extraordinarily popular among world-class athletes and movie stars, has turned dramatically away from the recommendations of the Standard American Diet (SAD) recommendations. The Zone emphasizes a 40/30/30 Carbohydrate-to-Protein-to-Fat (C:P:F) caloric intake ratio. The program is a phenomenon because after years of low-fat, high-complex carbohydrate mania, it offers a user-friendly eating plan for anyone who wants to achieve peak performance, maximum life span, increased energy, better mental focus, stable blood sugar, decreased food cravings and healthy weight loss. Through the Zone program, you can also avoid high blood pressure, high cholesterol and triglycerides and inflammation—which has been found to be at the root of many diseases. The Zone approach is also easy. You simply aim for a ratio of 40% of your calories coming from carbohydrates, 30% from protein and 30% from healthy fats and oils. What is especially important about this 40/30/30 food ratio is the degree to which it regulates insulin release. Insulin release is strongly activated by carbohydrates, while protein and fat cause moderate to minimal insulin release. If, due to their decreased ability to affect insulin release, we consider the percentages of proteins and fats together (30% + 30% = 60%), we discover a dietary ratio that approximates the 38:62 Golden Ratio:

40% (Carbohydrates) to 60% (30% Protein + 30% Fat)

This dietary Golden Ratio of 40:60 enables the carbohydrates, proteins and fats to transcend their normal nutritional potential. They are immediately and collectively transformed into Nature's Secret Nutrient, upon approaching Golden Ratio balance. This nutritional super-charging upgrade is no doubt the reason that the Zone approach is so effective in regulating metabolism and decreasing inflammation.

Stone-Age was the Zone-Age

In The *Omega Rx Zone*, Dr. Sears offers further commentary on the Zone diet, similar to the Paleolithic diet, which mirrors the natural diet of humans thousands of years ago:

When broken down into percentages of carbohydrates, protein and fat, it [the Paleolithic diet] comes to approximately 40% of carbohydrates, 30% of protein, and 30% of total fat.

Before the development of agriculture and industrialization, humans naturally ate a diet that essentially conformed to the Golden Ratio. The Paleolithic/Zone Diet reflects the body's maximum metabolic efficiency ratio for utilizing macronutrients. It's similar to achieving the optimal fuel/air mixture in a finely tuned engine, thereby maximizing efficiency and minimizing waste and wear. Why is this 40/60 Golden Ratio Pro*Portion* of nutrients so crucial in weight loss and health? A diet excessively high in carbohydrates (bread, pasta, grains, potatoes, fruit juices and sweets, etc.) over-stimulates your pancreas to secrete insulin, resulting in what is known as insulin resistance. Since your body uses insulin to transport sugar molecules into the cells, the cells will become progressively less sensitive to insulin's actions as the amount of carbohydrates in your diet increases. To compensate for the insensitivity, your pancreas begins to secrete more and more insulin. Your metabolism will switch from fat burning to fat storage. This can go on for years, resulting in what has been termed Syndrome X or the Metabolic Syndrome.

The Metabolic Syndrome consists of:

- Obesity (excessive fat, especially around the mid-section)
- High triglycerides and low HDL (good) cholesterol
- Insulin resistance with glucose intolerance
  (elevated insulin & blood sugar levels)
- Pro-thrombotic state (elevated blood clotting risk)
- Elevated blood pressure (130/85 mmHg or higher)
- Inflammation (elevated C-reactive protein; elevated silent inflammation index)

In many people, insulin resistance can be accompanied by reactive hypoglycemia. In this disorder, excess insulin is released into the blood after eating unopposed carbohydrates or sugary foods. The exaggerated levels of insulin released cause high blood sugar levels to rapidly fall, resulting in dizziness, sweating, weakness, irritability and foggy thinking. Typically, people respond by consuming more

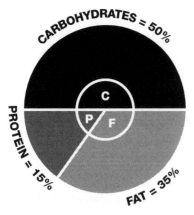

4

The **Standard American Diet (SAD)**. This off-ratio distribution of 50% (Carbs) to 50% (35% Fat + 15% Protein) is a major reason for the growing obesity and associated disease in much of the Western world. In addition to the off-ratio *quantity* of Carbs, Fats and Proteins consumed in the SAD, they are also most often of poor *quality*, e.g., fast foods, high animal fat, white flour and sugar, artificial ingredients, Genetically Modified Organisms (GMOs), pesticides, etc. The Golden Ratio Lifestyle Diet's nutritional approach restores healthy dietary quantities and qualities of nutrients consumed.

carbohydrates. However, this only leads to a continuous roller coaster ride of blood sugar peaks and valleys, which simultaneously puts a huge strain on your nervous and endocrine systems to compensate for the metabolic stress. Over months and years of out-of-pro*portion* carbohydrate consumption, insulin resistance may worsen and blood sugar levels may rise, leading to diabetes. A person with diabetes is usually advised to follow standard medical dietary recommendations. This includes eating according to a diet pyramid with abundant carbohydrates at the base. Insulin resistance only worsens as does its associated problems. Only by keeping your intake of carbohydrates in proper pro*portion* to the amount of protein and fat eaten, insulin resistance, inflammation and their negative effects can be avoided. Quality proteins and healthy fats are excellent at regulating the rise and fall of blood sugar levels and keeping insulin production well balanced. Once insulin control is established, other benefits, such as normalized blood pressure, lowered triglycerides and cholesterol levels, optimal weight levels and decreased inflammation in the body will naturally follow. For specific information about the types of foods included in the 40% carbohydrate, 30% protein and 30% fat categories, please refer to the Golden Ratio Lifestyle Diet Nutrition Decoder graph.

The Dangers of Abdominal Obesity

A study published in the April 2008 issue of *Circulation* by Zhang[et.al] showed that the death risk increased by abdominal adiposity [fat storage] was much greater in those who had cardiovascular disease and cancer. Men and women with largest abdominal adiposity [fat storage] were 79% more likely to die from all causes... and 63% more likely to die from cancer than those with smaller waists. The Golden Ratio appears in scientific studies more frequently than one might expect, albeit usually unrecognized.

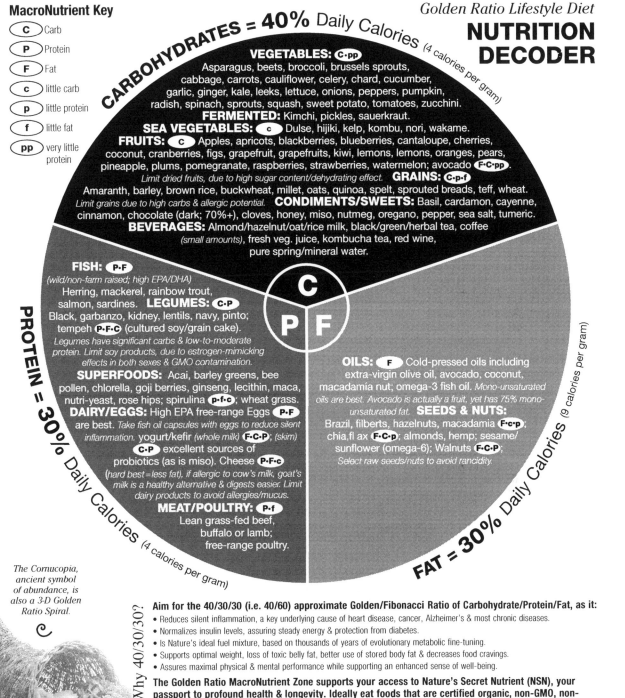

MacroNutrient Key

- (C) Carb
- (P) Protein
- (F) Fat
- (c) little carb
- (p) little protein
- (f) little fat
- (pp) very little protein

Golden Ratio Lifestyle Diet

NUTRITION DECODER

CARBOHYDRATES = 40% Daily Calories (4 calories per gram)

VEGETABLES: (C·pp)
Asparagus, beets, broccoli, brussels sprouts, cabbage, carrots, cauliflower, celery, chard, cucumber, garlic, ginger, kale, leeks, lettuce, onions, peppers, pumpkin, radish, spinach, sprouts, squash, sweet potato, tomatoes, zucchini.
FERMENTED: Kimchi, pickles, sauerkraut.
SEA VEGETABLES: (C) Dulse, hijiki, kelp, kombu, nori, wakame.
FRUITS: (C) Apples, apricots, blackberries, blueberries, cantaloupe, cherries, coconut, cranberries, figs, grapefruit, grapefruits, kiwi, lemons, lemons, oranges, pears, pineapple, plums, pomegranate, raspberries, strawberries, watermelon; avocado (F·C·pp).
Limit dried fruits, due to high sugar content/dehydrating effect. **GRAINS:** (C·p·f)
Amaranth, barley, brown rice, buckwheat, millet, oats, quinoa, spelt, sprouted breads, teff, wheat.
Limit grains due to high carbs & allergic potential. **CONDIMENTS/SWEETS:** Basil, cardamon, cayenne, cinnamon, chocolate (dark; 70%+), cloves, honey, miso, nutmeg, oregano, pepper, sea salt, tumeric.
BEVERAGES: Almond/hazelnut/oat/rice milk, black/green/herbal tea, coffee *(small amounts)*, fresh veg. juice, kombucha tea, red wine, pure spring/mineral water.

PROTEIN = 30% Daily Calories (4 calories per gram)

FISH: (P·F)
(wild/non-farm raised; high EPA/DHA)
Herring, mackerel, rainbow trout, salmon, sardines. **LEGUMES:** (C·P)
Black, garbanzo, kidney, lentils, navy, pinto; tempeh (P·F·C) (cultured soy/grain cake).
Legumes have significant carbs & low-to-moderate protein. Limit soy products, due to estrogen-mimicking effects in both sexes & GMO contamination.
SUPERFOODS: Acai, barley greens, bee pollen, chlorella, goji berries, ginseng, lecithin, maca, nutri-yeast, rose hips; spirulina (p·f·c); wheat grass.
DAIRY/EGGS: High EPA free-range Eggs (P·F) are best. *Take fish oil capsules with eggs to reduce silent inflammation.* yogurt/kefir *(whole milk)* (F·C·P); *(skim)* (C·P) excellent sources of probiotics (as is miso). Cheese (P·F·c)
(hard best=less fat), if allergic to cow's milk, goat's milk is a healthy alternative & digests easier. Limit dairy products to avoid allergies/mucus.
MEAT/POULTRY: (P·f)
Lean grass-fed beef, buffalo or lamb; free-range poultry.

FAT = 30% Daily Calories (9 calories per gram)

OILS: (F) Cold-pressed oils including extra-virgin olive oil, avocado, coconut, macadamia nut; omega-3 fish oil. *Mono-unsaturated oils are best. Avocado is actually a fruit, yet has 75% mono-unsaturated fat.* **SEEDS & NUTS:**
Brazil, filberts, hazelnuts, macadamia (F·c·p); chia, flax (F·C·p); almonds, hemp; sesame/sunflower (omega-6); Walnuts (F·C·P);
Select raw seeds/nuts to avoid rancidity.

(C)
(P) (F)

The Cornucopia, ancient symbol of abundance, is also a 3-D Golden Ratio Spiral.

Why 40/30/30?

Aim for the 40/30/30 (i.e. 40/60) approximate Golden/Fibonacci Ratio of Carbohydrate/Protein/Fat, as it:
- Reduces silent inflammation, a key underlying cause of heart disease, cancer, Alzheimer's & most chronic diseases.
- Normalizes insulin levels, assuring steady energy & protection from diabetes.
- Is Nature's ideal fuel mixture, based on thousands of years of evolutionary metabolic fine-tuning.
- Supports optimal weight, loss of toxic belly fat, better use of stored body fat & decreases food cravings.
- Assures maximal physical & mental performance while supporting an enhanced sense of well-being.

The Golden Ratio MacroNutrient Zone supports your access to Nature's Secret Nutrient (NSN), your passport to profound health & longevity. Ideally eat foods that are certified organic, non-GMO, non-irradiated & non or minimally processed; eat locally grown vegetables/fruits, off the vine as possible.

TIPS

- Many foods fit in multiple categories & are placed here in their dominant category, e.g., many nuts & seeds are good sources of both protein *and* fat. This chart is a general, ideal overview; it invites individual modification/expansion.
- Fill your plate about 1/3 with protein & 2/3 with colorful, non-starchy vegetables & a judicious amount of grains, breads & pastas (infrequently & in small amounts). Add small amounts of oil, seeds, nuts or condiments.
- For optimal digestion & absorption, eat consciously, in a relaxed manner. • Chew well, eating only to about 2/3 full (about what would 2/3 fill both hands cupped together). • Eat proteins first & then pause a few minutes.
- Rotate foods—only eat same food every 3rd to 4th day, to avoid allergies. • You'll get ample fiber eating from this list.
- Reduce consumption of meat/animal products, as the slimmest, longest-lived people eat small amounts, infrequently. This practice is also a major planetary health booster—environmental, compassionate/ethical, economic.
- Due to increasing seafood toxicity (heavy metals, PCB's, radioactivity, etc.), taking chelating compounds with fish/sea vegetables gives extra protection. Good oral chelators are vitamin-C, garlic, chlorella, EDTA, zeolite.
- Your metabolism is unique; customize above recommendations to support individual requirements & satisfaction.
- Combine these dietary recommendations with other Golden Ratio Lifestyle Diet drivers for optimal health & longevity.

The 40/30/30 macronutrient ratio is based on the work of Zone Nutrition pioneer Dr. Barry Sears.

4

Golden Ratio Lifestyle App:
Why An Apple a Day Keeps the Doctor Away

The apple is Nature's prototypical Golden Ratio fruit, with a pentagonal seed array, five-petaled blossoms and a 1:61 Golden Ratio of insoluble to soluble fiber (see chapter 7). Apples also have an unidentified, mysterious "X" factor that puts them above all other fruits in the prevention of lung cancer and asthma. Researchers are aware that antioxidant and anti-inflammatory effects of apple phytonutrients are involved, but this doesn't fully explain why apples shine above all other fruits in this area. Perhaps, since apples are one of Nature's prime examples of Golden Ratio balance, they contain high levels of Nature's Secret Nutrient (NSN), endowing them with their phenomenal health-giving benefits.

The Amazing Health Benefits of Apples

- Apple consumption is associated with a decreased risk of cancer, heart disease, asthma, diabetes and obesity
- The phytonutrients in one apple have the equivalent antioxidant activity of 1,500 mg of vitamin C
- The antioxidant protection afforded by eating an apple lasts only about 24 hours; hence, eating "an apple a day" keeps your antioxidant levels replenished and lowers your risk of the above-mentioned diseases
- Apple peels have a significantly higher antioxidant activity than the flesh, so eat the whole apple, raw and unprocessed; chew well to maximize nutrient uptake (make sure your apple is organic so it's pesticide-free)
- Cholesterol and triglyceride levels can be lowered simply by eating apples; as apple pectin binds cholesterol-derived bile acids in the gut
- Antioxidant potency varies greatly between types of apples—darker red apples contain more anthocyanin antioxidants
- Eating an apple 15-20 minutes before a meal can significantly decrease your appetite
- Apples favorably alter intestinal bacteria and apple extracts have even been shown to inhibit cholera bacteria
- Apple consumption reduces C-Reactive Protein (CRP), a blood marker of inflammation, a leading cause of many diseases including heart disease
- Of course, Apple Inc. (Macintosh Computers, iPod®, iPhone®, iPad®) and Apple Corps (The Beatles' record company) are both enormously popular, culture-shifting organizations named after the humble and health-bestowing superfruit with a Golden Star seed pattern at its core

Once you know what to look for, the Golden Ratio and its derivatives seem to pop up in areas of special importance. In this study, we see that in men and women with cardiovascular disease and cancer, those with the greatest abdominal obesity were 79% more likely to die from all causes. With a little easy mathematics, we know that the square root of the small Golden Ratio (0.618) is 0.786, which rounds to 0.79, or 79%. So, 79% is a Golden Ratio derivative.

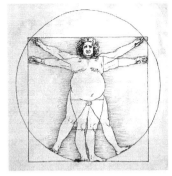

Homo Fatruvius, with extreme out-of-ratio belly fat.

Extra abdominal fat can also throw off spinal health and biomechanics by pulling your lumbar spine forward, causing an accentuated lumbar curvature (lordosis). This can stress not only your low back, but disrupt the alignment of your entire spine and predisposes you to back strain and possibly ruptured discs. The most common spinal levels for ruptured discs are at L4-L5 and L5-S1. The L5-S1 level is at the exact spinal Golden Ratio dividing point at the lumbar-sacral junction (see spinal diagram, ch. 5/Posture). The lower lumbar area is also directly opposite the navel, which is the main vertical Golden Ratio dividing point of your entire body. We also see that the same group of men and women from the above study were 63% more likely to die from cancer than those with the smallest/normal ratio waists. With a slight stretch, we see that 63% is very close to the Golden Ratio cut point of 62%.

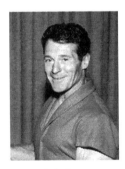

Jack LaLanne, fitness pioneer.

The Golden Ratio is commonly expressed as a 62% to 38% ratio. So, we have two Golden Ratio elements surfacing in this study on abdominal obesity. When multiple Golden Ratio elements appear in a study, it is usually a good idea to pay close attention, as some important information is surfacing and clustering around a mean—a Golden Mean in this case. The dangers to health and longevity from abdominal obesity as demonstrated in this study and others cannot be underestimated. Essentially, the health and fitness of your waist is a fractal representative of your longevity. It's an inverse ratio: every excess inch of abdominal fat increases proportionately the odds of disease and premature death. To underscore this important message, we need only look to the wisdom of healthy lifestyle legend Jack LaLanne, who said:

Your Waistline is Your Lifeline.

Losing Weight and Gaining Health

Here's great news for those wanting to lose weight: Lowered insulin levels mean that your body won't store as much fat. This allows you to better access stored body fat for energy, as well as for warding off hunger. A Golden Pro*portion* intake of carbohydrates to protein and fat keeps your blood sugar and insulin levels on an even keel. You use stored fats for their intended purpose—expending physical and mental energy. In the words of Dr. Sears:

> *It is excessive levels of the hormone insulin that makes you fat and keeps you fat. How do you increase insulin levels? By eating too many fat-free carbohydrates or too many calories at any one meal. Americans do both. People tend to forget that the best way to fatten cattle is to raise their insulin levels by feeding them excessive amounts of low-fat grain. The best way to fatten humans is to raise their insulin levels by feeding them excessive amounts of low-fat grain, but now in the form of pasta and bagels.*

Eating in Divine Pro*portions* (40% carbohydrates to 60% fat + protein) is meant to become a permanent eating pattern. If you decide to try it, use the 21-Day Quick-Start Checklist at the back of this book to embed it in your behavior. Be sure to celebrate your progress on the Fibonacci days and remember to build up some escape velocity to get beyond the usual bog-down around day 13. Always remain sensitive to which foods and how much you eat. Become attuned to the pro*portions* of food you take into your body during a meal.

Inflammation: The Silent Health Threat

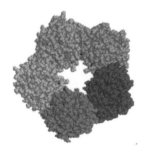

C-Reactive Protein (CRP) has a distinct pentagonal Golden Ratio shape and is a sensitive blood marker for inflammation and heart disease.

In Dr. Sears' book *Omega Rx Zone* he upgrades *The Zone* approach by the addition of high doses of pharmaceutical grade fish oil to the diet, to control the ratios of hormonally important fats called eicosenoids. These eicosenoids profoundly influence inflammation in your body. This eicosenoid balance completes the one-two punch along with the Zone Diet for controlling insulin. This combination is a superior way to achieve high-level health and performance and treat chronic diseases. Interestingly, the best way to measure eicosenoid balance is with a blood test. The ideal ratio of bad to good eicosenoids (arachadonic acid/EPA) is around 1.5. This is the ratio of numbers early in the Fibonacci Sequence—3:2—moving towards the Golden Ratio of 1.618. Again, from Dr. Sears,

In the final analysis, it's all about your genes, especially how an anti-inflammatory diet, like the Zone Diet, can turn off inflammatory genes and simultaneously turn on anti-inflammatory genes that promote cellular rejuvenation, repair and healing. Your ability to control inflammation becomes the molecular definition of wellness.

The Golden Ratio of Evolution: Omega-6:Omega-3 Balance

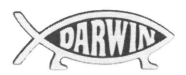

Darwin's evolutionary fish glyph takes on an entirely new meaning when one considers the impact of fish oils on human brain development and evolution.

Living in the Rift Valley of East Africa 100-200 thousand years ago, our Homo Sapiens ancestors' diet was composed of up to 12% lake fish and shellfish that had a polyunsaturated fatty acid—omega-6 and omega-3—content very close to that of the human brain. Those dietary conditions favored the evolutionary spurt of the human brain's neocortex that gave our ancestors the survival advantage needed to flourish. The quantum jump in brain evolution correlated with a diet consisting of an omega-6 to omega-3 ratio that ranged from 1–2:1, a range that Artemis P. Simopoulos, M.D. termed the "Ratio of Evolution." With our Golden Ratio lens, we can see that Dr. Simopoulos' fatty acid "ratio of evolution" encompasses the Golden Ratio of 1.618:1. Knowing that Nature always works with Golden Pro*portions* first in mind, we can refine the terminology, calling it the *Golden Ratio of Evolution.* This ratio was the most efficient physiologic path for evolutionary progress to occur. Over the millennia, our species evolution has gone through fits and starts that have had a high correlation to dietary conditions. Much of the world, including Western civilization, may currently be going through a period of *devolution* as a result of mass dietary ignorance and resulting poor dietary habits. In Western diets, the omega–6 to omega–3 ratio is around 16.7:1. This ratio is about 10 times greater than the ideal *Golden Ratio of Evolution*: 1.618:1. In some countries, such as India, the ratio is as high as 38:1. Not surprisingly, India has extremely high rates of cardiovascular disease and diabetes. Researchers Veronique Chajès and Philippe Bougnoux have discovered that an omega–6 to omega–3 ratio from between 1:1 to 2:1 has a protective effect against the development and growth of breast and colon cancers. Studies have also determined that a ratio of omega–6 to omega–3 of about 2.5:1 may protect against colorectal cancer. 2.5:1 is close to a Golden Ratio derivative, as 1.618 x 1.618 = 2.618.

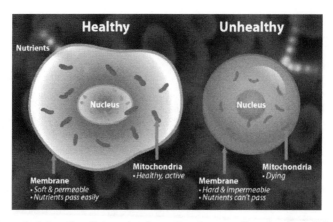

By optimizing the dietary intake ratio of omega-3 and omega-6 fats,
your cell membranes become softer and more permeable, improving
nutrient absorption, toxin elimination and cellular vitality.

4

Japanese researchers Tomohito Hamazaki and Harumi Okuyama have produced more evidence of a Golden Ratio connection regarding omega-6 to omega-3 ratios. Even though Japanese diets have a relatively favorable omega-6 to omega-3 ratio of 4:1, these researchers are recommending even lower omega–6 to omega–3 ratios in the range of 2.7–3.6:1. Again, these ratios are in line with Golden Ratio harmonics of 2.618:1 and 3.618:1 and are consistent with the overall efficiency principle of the Golden Ratio as Nature's Path of Least Resistance. Over-consumption of omega-6 fats in relation to omega-3 fats leads to an increase in inflammation and an increased tendency for blood clots associated heart attacks and strokes. Chronic inflammation also has negative effects on cellular membranes and also is associated with many chronic diseases including arthritis, diabetes, cancer and dementia. Peak living and performance coach Chris Johnson's cellular health membrane diagram above illustrates how shifting your essential fatty acid intake towards the Golden Ratio of Evolution's omega-3 to omega-6 balance helps make cellular membranes softer and more permeable. This improves intra and extracellular signaling, enhancing nutrient absorption and toxin elimination. As Johnson notes,

The key to optimal performance and health begins at the cellular level. By re-establishing a healthy balance of omega-3 and omega-6 fats—easily achieved by adding fish oil and ground flax seed to your diet—you can dramatically improve the health of every one of your 100 trillion cells. Since your body turns over 3-4 trillion cells every day, everyone has a great opportunity to rapidly upgrade their health by restoring healthy omega-3 and 6 fat ratios.

Iron Man's Secret: Tapping the Power of Green

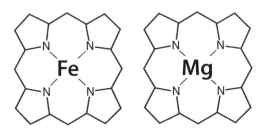

Both hemoglobin (blood's red pigment, left) and chlorophyll (plant's green pigment, right) are the O_2/CO_2 carrying molecules in humans and plants. Both are composed of 4 Golden Ratio-shaped pentagons (porphyrin ring). The main difference between the two is that hemoglobin has an iron molecule (Fe) at its center, while chlorophyll has a magnesium molecule (Mg) at its center.

Although not experimentally proven, many nutritionists theorize that by eating green leafy plants, our bodies transmute chlorophyll into hemoglobin, thereby boosting our blood's oxygen carrying capacity. Interestingly, whether it's Popeye and his can of spinach or the color of the Incredible Hulk, green is often associated with super strength. Drinking the Golden Ratio IronApe Green Smoothie (see Rx section, end of this chapter) is like getting a super energy-boosting natural blood transfusion. Perhaps this is also why Iron Man's alter-ego Tony Stark (Robert Downey, Jr.) can be seen drinking a green smoothie in the hit film *Iron Man*.

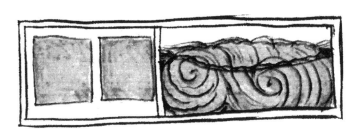

The green superfood Spirulina, from an illustration in the Florentine Codex (c. 1585), showing how the Aztecs harvested Spirulina off lakes by skimming the surface with ropes and then drying the algae into square cakes, to be eaten as a nourishing condiment. Spirulina, wheat and barley grasses, chlorella and common greens like kale and romaine lettuce are power-packed green sources of nutrition.

In general, all fish (especially salmon, mackerel and sardines), krill and plankton have high omega-3 levels and are recommended. Best to limit farm raised fish, as the fish are fed with grains which are omega-6's. Limit/avoid large fish like tuna, shark and swordfish due to their increased mercury content; avoid shellfish due to increased heavy metals/toxicity from bottom feeding. Avoid Pacific seafood due to probable radiation contamination from the ongoing and under-reported 2011 Fukishima, Japan nuclear distaster. If you buy canned fish, don't get it packed in omega-6 oils like sesame, sunflower or soy; choose water-packed instead. Taking fish oil or krill oil supplements is another solid option, e.g., Carlson's lemon flavored Norwegian cod liver oil is a good choice. All green vegetables like spinach and kale have good omega-3 to omega-6 ratios. Most nuts and seeds have high omega-6's, with the big exception of chia and flax seeds, which are very high in omega-3's (though not in the same metabolically active form as in seafood, krill or plankton). Grains are not your best choice for omega-3's and also should be kept to a minimum as they are less favorable carbohydrates due to their increased contribution to inflammation and being often allergenic. Fruits are basically negligible in their amount of fat, so best to minimize fruit sugar consumption due to their excessive carbohydrate load and adverse impact on insulin levels.

Raw, Green and Lean

*Nothing could be better than consuming greens and nothing
could be faster than consuming blended greens.*
Victoria Boutenko, author, ***Green for Life***

As we have seen in the previous section, The Golden Ratio of Evolution, the evolution of the human brain was driven by an increased dietary intake of omega-3 essential fats like EPA and DHA, resulting in a higher ratio of omega-3's to omega-6's that approached the Golden Ratio. Yet, since humans can't live on omega-3's alone, what else are we supposed to eat? One researcher, raw food proponent Victoria Boutenko, has theorized that since humans and chimpanzee's have around 99% of their DNA in common, humans might benefit from eating a diet similar to what chimps, who along with gorillas are known for their great strength, naturally eat in the wild. Interestingly, a chimp's diet has a natural Golden Ratio balance, with around 60% fruits and 40% green leafy plants, nuts, seeds, insects and occasionally a small amount of meat. This primitive, elemental diet supplies them with high amounts of enzymes, chlorophyll, vitamins and minerals. Boutenko noticed that a favorite chimp delicacy was a simple banana wrapped in a green leaf. Yet short of eating banana wraps, how could this chimp entrée be adapted to finicky humans? Her intuitive flash was to combine the ingredients into a blended green smoothie. By putting the ingredients into a blender, the combination would be much more palatable—as well as making it easier to predigest the fibrous greens. The total surface area of the food would also be vastly increased for more thorough and rapid absorption.

One of the most potent and easily available greens for the recipe is kale, which has one of the highest antioxidant potentials of any vegetable on the ORAC scale (Oxygen Radical Absorbance Capacity). This brassica/cruciferous family representative also has one of the highest nutritional values for the fewest calories of any vegetable known. In addition, kale normalizes bowel functioning, increases liver detoxification and reduces the incidence of many cancers. The smoothie recipe is almost too good to be true in that it also satisfies Golden Ratio health driver #2 for water/hydration. By consuming up to 32 oz. of water (or more) with the blended ingredients, chronic dehydration can easily be overcome in a short time. The large increase in fluid intake flushes the kidneys, relieves constipation and also improves skin tone and texture. Last but not least, the smoothie is incredibly quick to make, taking only minutes. You can take the extra leftover smoothie with you to work or to a workout. In her book, *Green for Life*, Boutenko documents some of her family's amazing healing stories as a result of adopting this simple smoothie into their diet. She personally lost over 180 pounds. In the Rx section of this chapter there is a supercharged version of Boutenko's original green smoothie called the Golden Ratio IronApe Green Smoothie. This Golden Ratio high-ORAC version unleashes the energy of King Kong, Iron Man and

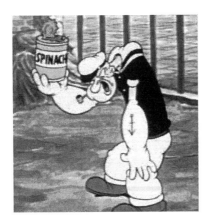

Early green food
champion Popeye.

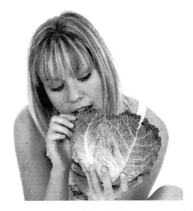

Raw kale has one of the highest antioxidant
potentials of any vegetable on the ORAC
scale (Oxygen Radical Absorbance Capacity,
a measure of antioxidant potential).

Popeye combined by kicking the original ingredients several notches up the evolutionary scale: more towards the carb/protein/fat ratios and antioxidant levels that our Zone/Paleolithic ancestors would have approved of. Remember that the evolution of our physiology was tuned and refined over millions of years, and that agriculture was introduced only about 10,000 years ago in our current history. The modern era of processed-for-profit, de-natured, nutritionally deficient and chemically/genetically violated foods has only occurred over the last 150 years or so. It is illogical, if not insane, to think that we can disregard millions of years of our natural evolution on whole, healthy foods and still be optimally healthy and enjoy maximum longevity.

The Golden Ratio Longevity Code and Caloric Reduction

4

Research from the Washington University School of Medicine in St. Louis indicates that caloric reduction can significantly lengthen life expectancy, reduce incidence of disease, increase overall health and lead to sustained optimal weight. As reported by Rob Stein in the *Washington Post* on April 20, 2004:

Small groups of people who are drastically restricting how much they eat in the hope of slowing the aging process have produced the strongest support yet for the tantalizing theory that very low-calorie diets can extend the human life span. The first study of people who voluntarily imposed draconian diets on themselves found that their cholesterol levels, blood pressure and other major risk factors for heart disease— the biggest killer—plummeted, along with risk factors for diabetes and possibly other leading causes of death such as cancer and Alzheimer's.

While it has long been known that eating well and staying trim helps people live healthier lives and avoid premature death, evidence has been accumulating that following extremely low-calorie diets for many years may do something more— significantly extend longevity beyond current norms. 'It is a very important paper,' said Roy L. Walford M.D., Biospherian and professor emeritus at the UCLA School of Medicine and a leading proponent of the theory. 'You may well be able to choose between [caloric restriction] and that double-bypass cardiac surgery you are not looking forward to.'

One member of the Caloric Restriction Society who inspired the above study, Dean Pomerleau, 39, decreased his intake of calories from around 3,000 to 1,900 daily. In other words, he allowed himself approximately 63%—close to the 62% Golden Ratio—of his normal daily calories. To reap the benefits of caloric reduction without

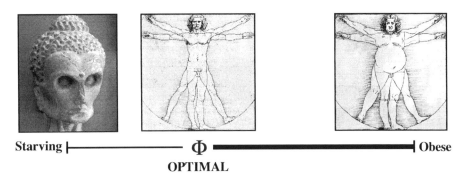

Starving |————————————— Φ ■■■■■■■■■■■■■■| Obese

OPTIMAL

This statue of a calorically challenged and pre-enlightened Buddha (*left,* 2nd century, C.E.) demonstrates the result of an ascetic approach towards life and diet. Extremely restrictive diets or eating disorders result in neither good health nor do they put an end to human suffering. The *Vitruvian Man (center)*, the ideal human prototype, shows the possibility of what can result from following a supremely balanced lifestyle and diet. The Golden Ratio Lifestyle Diet is not extreme in restriction nor indulgence and results in optimal health and an ideal muscle/fat ratio. The *Fatruvian* Man (*right*) is the epitome of an indulgent lifestyle and diet, similar to the condition of a large percentage of the population in most western countries. The extreme of obesity is just as unhealthy as being too thin.

going to extremes, one could mirror the formulae of these life-enhancement pioneers. To easily calculate your target daily Golden Ratio-adjusted intake of calories, simply multiply your current total daily calories by 0.618, e.g. 3000 x 0.618 = 1854. It's important to remember that the Golden Ratio Lifestyle Diet is about bringing one's dietary habits into balance and harmony. It has absolutely nothing to do with the draconian, extreme measures typical of many weight loss diets or extreme caloric restriction. In the following section we will see how an innovative doctor unknowingly used the Golden Ratio to integrate sensible caloric reduction into his weight loss program in an ingenious, manageable and low-stress way.

Reducing Calories May Protect Your Brain From Alzheimer's Disease

Research in non-human primates at the Mt. Sinai School of Medicine in New York City has shown that a lower calorie diet triggers the production of an anti-aging protein, SIRT-1 (the "Skinny Gene") that protects the brain from Alzheimer's-like disease. This protein has been shown to curtail and reverse the production of plaque in the brain, a common attribute of the disease.

The Alternate-Day Diet: Sensible Caloric Reduction

As we have seen, Dr. Roy Walford's innovative discoveries in the area of caloric reduction have opened the door to a new era of health and longevity. However, not many people are able to put themselves through the rigors of daily caloric reduction without feeling deprived, tired or unable to comfortably function. Taking Dr. Walford's basic premise to a more practical level, James Johnson, M.D. discovered some fascinating research that allowed him to devise a more realistic approach to caloric reduction. He discovered an ingenious way to take caloric reduction from the deprivation level and make it tolerable—even fun—while maintaining its effectiveness. Earlier animal studies had shown that, by fasting the animals only on alternate days, they still experienced weight loss, increased health and longevity. Perhaps there was some way that he could apply these animal experiments to humans. Johnson noted,

I knew I wouldn't be able to fast on alternate days, but I thought I might be able to restrict my calorie intake enough every other day to reap the same health benefits as those mice. I decided to become my own guinea pig (or lab mouse) and began to restrict my calories to 20 percent of what I normally ate on alternate days. On nonrestrictive days I ate whatever and as much as I wanted.

This was the birth of what Johnson calls the Alternate-Day Diet. He found that by alternating eating normally one day, and then calorie reducing the next, he avoided the compulsions and cravings induced by other diets. After a while on most diets, one's metabolic rate and weight loss plummet while food cravings increase. Not so with the Alternate-Day Diet. Johnson lost 35 pounds by week 11 of his alternate-day regime and he says that he's been able to keep it off since then (2003). The secret to the tolerable and steady weight loss is activation of the SIRT-1 or "skinny gene" (SIR stands for "silent information regulator") and once activated has the ability to prevent oxidative damage, inhibit fat storage and decrease inflammation at the cellular level. What this means on a practical level is that in addition to keeping your metabolic rate elevated and losing weight, you are decreasing your chances of developing chronic degenerative conditions such as arthritis, allergies, asthma, cancer, infection, stroke, heart disease, etc. Johnson says that by instituting alternate-day caloric reduction, a built-in cellular stress

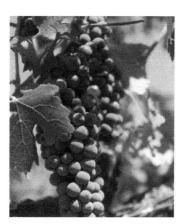

Grapes contain the nutrient Resveratrol, which slows the aging process by the same genetic mechanism as caloric reduction (activation of the SIRT-1 "skinny" gene).

response or "*hormesis*" is activated that in addition to facilitating weight loss, increases one's resistance to disease. He explains "*hormesis*" as follows:

> *The most widely accepted theory of why calorie restriction prevents disease and/ or delays the onset of age-related diseases is called "hormesis," which means that a harmful stress—one that might be fatal in large quantities—is beneficial in small amounts. Thus, if an animal is starved, it dies, but if its daily calorie intake is reduced to 60 percent of normal, it lives longer in very good health.*

Of particular interest is how Johnson's Alternate-Day Diet adheres to principles of the Golden Ratio, in that reducing calories to 60% of normal (averaged over a two day period) approximates a Golden Ratio calorie reduction. Johnson's practical caloric reduction breakthrough has taken the inspiration of Roy Walford, M.D. to a new level. This is a huge upgrade in our understanding of how to achieve and maintain vibrant health and maximum longevity. Using scientifically proven genetic and metabolic discoveries, you can now comfortably reduce your calories according to Golden Ratio principles and reap the benefits of weight loss, weight maintenance, disease prevention and increased longevity. Johnson has unknowingly harnessed Nature's Secret Nutrient with his Alternate Day Diet and has taken advantage of one of its many important properties: Nature's Secret Nutrient has zero calories!

A Profound New View of "Fullness"

The human stomach is shaped just like a Golden Spiral. Since the stomach structurally follows the pattern of the Golden Ratio, it stands to reason that it should

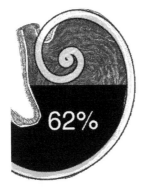

Golden Spiral-shaped stomach, at about 62% or 2/3 full.

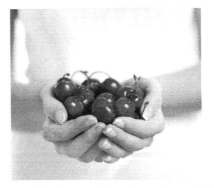

Filling both cupped hands to about 2/3 full approximates the natural Golden Ratio capacity of your stomach, supporting optimal meal portions and healthy digestion.

4

functionally follow it the as well. This would mean that the stomach is ideally meant to be no more than 62% full (and 38% empty) after a meal, for optimal digestive efficiency. Anything higher than 62% full will likely impede the healthy digestive process, in the same way an overloaded washing machine cannot properly wash clothes. The simplest way to assure you don't overeat at any meal is to use the finest meal portion measuring system ever invented: your hands. It turns out that there is a close correlation between the size of your stomach and the volume of both of your hands when cupped together. So, regardless of your plate size, only fill your plate with about as much food as would fill about 2/3 of your hands cupped together. The resulting portion will equal about 2/3 of the total volume of your stomach. If you eat in a relaxed manner, pause occasionally and chew well, you'll usually find this portion size amply satisfying. An all-too common challenge to healthy portion sizes and digestion is rushing our meals and eating amidst distraction or while multitasking, to the point where we've lost awareness of our body's natural satiety signaling system.

Relaxed, mindful eating is a great way to reactivate this system and support healthy digestion. In her article *Eating in the Slow Lane* from the October 2004 issue of *Alternative Medicine Magazine*, Judith S. Stern, Vice President of the American Obesity Association, notes that it takes about 20 minutes for the mind to get the message that the stomach is full:

> *If you eat too fast you outpace your body's natural signaling system. Studies show that if you draw out the meal, build in pauses, and allow for satiety signals to come into play* ***you will eat less***.

Stern's point is well taken. However, the ideal objective is to sense our natural Golden Ratio satiety signal: not eating until you are 100% full (no matter how slowly you might get there), but eating until you reach the Golden Pro*portion* of about 62% full. This profoundly redefines what "fullness" actually is. As Biospherian Roy Walford, M.D. recommended,

> *Optimal fullness equates to getting maximal nutrition with minimal calories.*

The message is simple: relax when eating. Enjoy your meals without distractions whenever possible. Don't drive, listen to the radio, watch television or talk on the phone when eating. Learn to pay better attention to your body's natural signals to pause and put down the fork from time to time. Finally, always give yourself permission to stop eating—even if there's food left on your plate. This will rarely happen if you follow the twin Golden Ratio Portion Guidelines: 1. Only fill your plate to the Golden Pro*portion* of about 2/3 and, 2. Only eat as much at one meal as would fill both hands cupped together to about 2/3 full. You'll feel better and support your efforts to reach and maintain your optimal weight. At the same time you'll awaken your ability to eat—and live—within the Golden Ratio zone.

CPR for a Healthy Heart: Golden Ratio Cholesterol Ratios

Heart disease is the number one killer in modern times. To counter this trend, the American Heart Association recommends that you lower your LDL level to under 100 mg/dl. Yet, by looking only at "absolute" single values such as isolated LDL levels, the enormous predictive power of ratios is lost. Luckily, certain ratios are still used by many physicians and labs, such as total cholesterol/LDL and total cholesterol/HDL. However, these ratios have not been referenced to the Golden Ratio in modern medical practice—until now. Nature has given us the true Golden Standard by which our physiology can be measured and optimized. It stands to reason that if we begin to learn and use this universal standard, our health and vitality can be dramatically improved. Analyzing basic data about cholesterol ratios reveals vital information on how your body processes and distributes fats and cholesterol in the blood. Whether your body is depositing more fats and cholesterol in your arteries—or is instead recycling and reprocessing them through your liver—becomes clear through this analysis. LDL transports cholesterol away from your liver and into your arteries. HDL is able to reverse that direction, carrying the cholesterol back to your liver, where it is then turned into bile and released into your intestines. It's easy to see if healthy Golden Ratios are displayed in the ratios of the different types of cholesterol in your blood. Total cholesterol is made up of four basic subtypes: LDL ("bad" cholesterol),

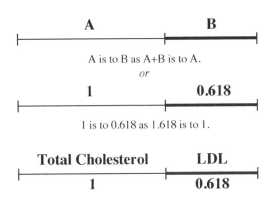

Your body's cholesterol ratios ideally should be in the Golden Ratio range 1.618...
The large section of the line is in ratio to the small section as the whole line is in ratio to the large section. When the ratio of total cholesterol to LDL ratio is in Golden Ratio, greater health is a natural result.

The hugely misunderstood cholesterol molecule: Cholesterol is a major building block of our cell membranes as well as being the mother of all steroid hormones, including vitamin-D, estrogen, testosterone, progesterone and cortisol.

4

HDL ("good" cholesterol), IDL and VLDL (small cholesterol sub-fractions). For practical purposes, only total cholesterol, LDL and HDL are usually reported when you get your blood test results. Golden Ratio philosopher Stephen McIntosh notes:

The Golden Ratio relationship is an expression of unity—a unity pattern—because each part is defined completely by its relation to the whole.

The unity pattern of cholesterol has a similar form. The whole is to the large part as the large part is to the small part. Total cholesterol is to LDL as LDL is to HDL (for practical purposes, VLDL and IDL sub-fractions won't be considered here). On your routine lab test, the cholesterol/LDL ratio is the easiest to calculate. Just divide your total cholesterol by your LDL and see how close you are to the Golden Ratio of 1.618. In our observations, this ratio is what is commonly found in most healthy people. If your ratio is close to 1.618, then by fractal inference, your HDL will be in a healthy range as well. If your cholesterol/LDL ratio is not close to 1.618, then you may want to begin incorporating key aspects of the Golden Ratio Lifestyle Diet into your daily routine.

Using Golden Ratios to estimate your ideal cholesterol levels may give you LDL recommendations that are higher than the American Heart Association recommends. Statin medications, like Lipitor, Crestor and Zocor, etc., are able to lower LDL levels in an exaggerated fashion. This treatment is currently in vogue; however, long-term deleterious side effects inevitably emerge, as they do with many (if not all) symptom-centric drugs/medications. Heart disease is multi-factorial and the final word is not in yet on the ultimate prevention and treatment. However, we believe that striving for Golden Ratio proportions within our cholesterol levels is a wise course of action, considering the multitude of deleterious side-effects possible with the use of pharmaceutical intervention. The more you can incorporate the Golden Ratio into your lifestyle, the sooner your blood values will begin to reflect more efficient, healthy ratios. This in turn will lower your risk for cardiovascular disease, stroke and diabetes. At the same time your energy, vitality and performance will dramatically improve.

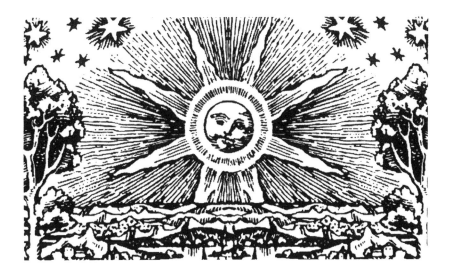

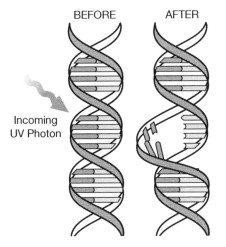

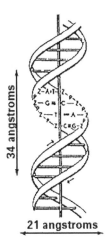

Excess UVA and UVB can damage DNA, producing an out-of-ratio molecule.

Normal DNA molecule with Golden Ratio proportions, 34 x 21 angstroms (34/21=1.61).

Solar Nutrition

Only mad dogs and Englishmen go out in the noon-day sun.

Rudyard Kipling

Paradoxically, the noonday sun has both health promoting and health destroying capabilities. The two edges, or what we might call the double-edged sword of the sun, are the back-to-back rays of ultraviolet light known as UVA and UVB. The range of wavelengths of UVA:UVB exhibits clear Golden Ratio harmonics:

UVA 320nm—400nm (with a range of 80nm)
UVB 290nm—320nm (with a range of 30nm)

The range of wavelengths of UVA is 80nm and the range of UVB is 30nm.

80:30 = 2.6

As we know, 1.618 is the Golden Ratio and one of the harmonics of this universal ratio is 2.6.

1.618 x 1.618 = 2.6

These two important UV wavelengths are necessary for our health—nutritionally, cosmetically and psychologically. The challenge is to bring the sun into our bodies in a healthful way, getting not too little yet not too much. The tanning effect of the sun is due to the immediate effects of UVA on melanin pigment release in the skin. UVB's tanning effects can take up to several days because the stimulatory effects on the skin's pigment forming cells—the melanocytes—take more time.

Each person needs to determine the ideal amount of sunlight to get, while avoiding the negative effects of over-sunning. UVB has been found to directly damage DNA, but at the same time is the critical wavelength of light that produces vitamin D. UVA gives us a beautiful healthy looking tan, yet prolonged exposure can result in the formation of damaging free radicals that can also damage DNA and collagen, causing skin aging and skin cancer. DNA structure is based on Golden Ratio proportions with a length/width ratio of 34:21 angstroms. As illustrated previously, DNA Golden Ratios can be disrupted due to excessive UV exposure. Although DNA has repair mechanisms, they are occasionally inefficient; thus, skin damage and skin cancers can result.

UV Distribution and the Golden Ratio

The tropics of Cancer and Capricorn—at 23.5° North and South latitudes—are two key latitude lines determined by the annual movements of the sun that demarcate the Earth's northern and southern tropical zones. These tropical zones happen to be located within 2° of Golden Ratio harmonic points of the earth's latitude lines. The Earth's Golden Ratio latitude lines are calculated as follows:

$$180° \times 0.618 = 111.24°$$
$$111.24° - 90° = 21.24° \text{ N \& S}$$

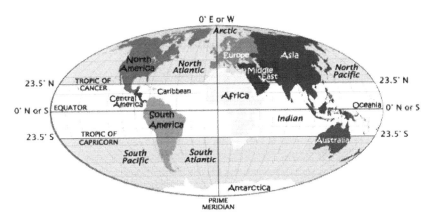

The tropics of Cancer and Capricorn are approximations of Golden Ratio divisions of the earth's latitude lines. These divisions also correspond to high levels of UV exposure. Ultraviolet rays are abundant in tropical regions and deficient in North America, Europe and Asia. Interestingly, the Golden Ratio symbol Φ (phi) is commonly used to designate geographic latitude.

As they say, *location is everything*. Such is the case with where you live and sunbathe in relation to the sun. As can be seen in the featured map of the globe, UVB distribution falls in line with the Earth's Golden Ratio-related latitude lines, the tropics of Cancer and Capricorn. Depending on the time of year and angle of the sun towards the earth, UV levels can vary widely. Sunbathing in the summer months can provide enough UVB to maintain adequate vitamin D conversion in the skin to raise levels to the healthy range. Since vitamin D is fat-soluble, your body can store it for months at a time. However, usually by January or February in the northern hemisphere and by June or July in the southern hemisphere, your Vitamin D stores are becoming depleted. This leaves your body more vulnerable to colds and various metabolic and immunologic problems, not to mention depressed psychological conditions such as SAD (Seasonal Affective Disorder). Only the southern part of the United States has any significant UVB during the winter, so most people living in more northern latitudes become deficient during winter months. UVB is necessary for the conversion of a cholesterol-like compound in the skin into vitamin D_3.

Vitamin D_3 is actually a steroid-like molecule with numerous functions in the body including the regulation of calcium levels and prevention of bone diseases ranging from rickets to osteoporosis. A connection between insufficient vitamin D levels and various forms of cancer, autoimmune diseases including MS, diabetes and hypertension has also been found. In addition to latitude, season, altitude, weather and length of exposure, the effects of both UVA and UVB are also dependent on age,

Deficient	Optimal	Treat Cancer	Excess
<50 ng/ml	50-65 ng/ml	65-90 ng/ml	>100 ng/ml

Vitamin D Levels

The best way to determine how much Vitamin D to take is by measuring our (25-Hydroxy) Vitamin D levels. Otherwise you can't know for sure if you're getting enough or too much. Vitamin D is measured in ng/ml (nanograms per milliliter). Source: www.mercola.com See Rx 11, page 149 for Vitamin D blood testing information.

4

skin color/amount of pigment, amount of skin exposed and application of sunscreens. Older people and dark skinned individuals tend to make less vitamin D per amount of time in the sun. Since we don't get tropical or subtropical sunshine in the U.S. mainland (with the exception of the southern U.S.) and in Europe, we need to bring the benefits of those climates to us in the form of adequate vitamin D through food or supplements to make up the difference. Even the best food sources like salmon, mackerel, sardines and tuna may not give you enough vitamin D. The most concentrated food source of vitamin D_3 is cod liver oil, but due to its often higher levels of vitamin A from brand variation, it's not advised to take too much.

Probably the best way to increase your vitamin D_3 is through a combination of sunlight, vitamin D_3 rich food, some cod liver oil and the balance through supplementation. Vitamin D_3 supplements come in various strengths, usually ranging from 100 IU's to 5,000 IU's. The best and only way to know if you're getting enough— yet not too much—is to monitor your blood level. We've featured here a chart from vitamin D expert Dr. Joseph Mercola from www.Mercola.com that shows his recommended vitamin D blood levels. His ranges are obtained from new clinical research and literature reviews that are somewhat higher than the more conservative levels recommended traditionally.

How do you get your vitamin D_3 levels into therapeutic range without toxicity becoming a problem? By utilizing a combination of sun, vitamin D_3 rich foods and vitamin D_3 supplements in the proper amounts. In summer months you may need less from your diet due to the increased UVB exposure, yet in winter, the reverse may be true. When using sun exposure to get vitamin D_3, remember that the sun is a double-edged sword with respect to UV rays: get just enough, yet not too much.

Golden Ratio 5-Sense Nutrition

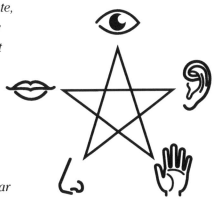

All human senses, including hearing, touch, taste, vision, smell and pain receptors, have not only spiral physiology, but also response curves that are logarithmic (having a Fibonacci structure). Cellular action membrane potentials, which are important for muscles and nervous system, have a voltage equal to the log of the ratio of the ion concentration outside the cell, to that of inside the cell. The brain and nervous systems are made from the same type of cellular building units and look similar microscopically, so the response curve of the central nervous system is probably also logarithmic.

Dr. Frederick A. Hottes, Anatomic & Clinical Pathologist

To close this chapter on Nutrition: Food & Beyond, let us briefly consider the nutritional quality of our 5 senses, our *sensory nutrients*. Our bodies are designed and operate according to the Golden Ratio. Every aspect of our structure, movement and input/output—including our senses—naturally reflects this principle of optimal efficiency and performance. Yet we don't often consider enhancing the nutritional value of what we see, hear, touch, smell and taste. Like air, water and sleep, each of our 5 primary senses could be classified as macro-macro nutrients, as we are continuously being nourished (or not) by our environment through them.

How can you improve the quality of your sensory diet? One way is to become more sensitive to opportunities to expand both the quality and range within each sense: less/more, cold/hot, light/dark, loud/quiet, etc. We often stay within narrow comfort zones in one or more senses, which can limit our perspective and opportunities for enhanced life nourishment. For example, most people regularly bathe at the same water temperature. They thus miss the proven range-expanding health benefits of integrating alternating cold/hot water therapy into their bathing diet (described in chapter 7). Many people are deficient in quality daily sound nutrition, whether it be the sounds of Nature, inspiring or soothing music or the simple absence of sound altogether. Continuing this theme, our total senses can be nourished and sharpened by occasionally giving one of our 5 main senses a short break. For example, wearing

> ## Taste the Colors of Nutrition
>
> Visual Nutrition includes the multiple benefits received from the broad palette of colors available in our food selection. We all know the pleasure and visual nourishment that comes from a colorful, attractive meal prepared with an artist's touch. Bestselling author Dr. Mehmet Oz highlights a key visual nutritional aspect of this point in the June, 2010 *Natural Awakenings* magazine:
>
> *Foods with bright, rich colors are packed with flavonoids and carotenoides, powerful compounds that bind with damaging free radicals in your body, lowering inflammation. Eat nine fistfuls of colorful fruits and vegetables each day and you'll reap the benefits without having to give up other foods. Whenever I shop in the produce aisle, I'm reminded that these foods are often more powerful than the drugs sold in pharmacies.*

a blindfold in the familiar environment of your house for 15 minutes while going about your usual routine amplifies *all* of your other senses. Touch is another great example of sensory nutrition, being the first sense to develop in humans. Yet touch is not traditionally considered a "nutrient," even though newborn babies can die when touch deprived—or survive, grow and thrive when touch is provided in healthy ratios. Touch malnutrition at *any* age is implicated in a wide array of physical, psychological and social health conditions. A 1997 *Life* magazine article, *The Magic of Touch,* by George Howe Colt explored the vital role of touch in human health:

> *...we instinctively know that touch is a primal need, as necessary for growth as food, clothing or shelter. Michelangelo knew this: when he painted God extending a hand toward Adam on the ceiling of the Sistine Chapel, he chose touch to depict the gift of life. From the nuzzles and caresses between mother and infant that form the foundation of the self, to the holding of hands between a son and his dying father that allows a final letting go, touch is our most intimate and powerful form of communication.*

Colt reported on psychologist Dr. Tiffany Field's research at Miami's Touch Research Institute (TRI), the world's only scientific center devoted to exploring the health effects of touch. TRI's numerous studies show the healing power of touch through massage to have positive effects on every condition studied, including: hyperactivity, diabetes, migraines, asthma, colic, immune system function, concentration, anxiety, depression and burn treatment. Colt highlights the direct connection between massage and increased nutrient uptake and absorption, noting that Hippocrates, the father of modern medicine, was a champion of massage:

Stronger, sustained touch can have even greater effect. Massage enhances immune function and lowers levels of the stress hormones cortisol and norepinephrine and may increase lymph flow. Massage also stimulates the vagus, one of 12 cranial nerves that influence various bodily functions. One branch of the vagus travels to the Gastrointestinal tract, where it facilitates the release of food-absorption hormones like insulin and glucose. That's one reason the massaged premature babies in TRI studies gain weight faster [up to 47%]. 'They aren't eating any more formula than non-massaged babies,' says Field, 'but their food absorption is more efficient.'

Contrasted with other countries, Dr. Field notes how "touch-phobic" America has become, pointing out that cultures showing more physical affection towards infants and children tend to have lower rates of adult violence:

'America is suffering from an epidemic of skin hunger,' says Field, who talks of a 'dose of touch' as if it were a vitamin… …TRI set up a study in which volunteers over age 60 were given three weeks of massage and then were trained to massage toddlers at the preschool. Giving massages proved even more beneficial than getting them. The elders exhibited less depression, lower stress hormones and less loneliness. They had fewer doctor visits, drank less coffee and made more social phone calls.

There is also a hidden, nourishing power in a closer touch/sensory connection with our food, with no utensils in the way. Yet most western cultures frown on this in adults, while children enjoy eating with their hands with healthy, carefree abandon. To this point, yoga pioneer Yogi Bhajan, whose Humanology philosophy views diet and lifestyle as one, suggested that if you eat with your hands and fingers, you can avoid 50% of neurosis. The main take-away is that most people are touch-deprived in their daily lives and thus out-of-ratio in a key sensory nutrient. This points to the concept that being "out of touch" with your environment and the people in it (physically and in other ways) can lead to being out of touch with oneself. Eventually this can lead to being out of touch with the fullness of life. We delve into the Golden Ratio aspects of sight and sound in more detail in *The Divine Code of Da Vinci, Fibonacci, Einstein & YOU*. Be sensitive to your own unique 5-Sense nutrient RDA's (Recommended Daily Allowances), address deficiencies or sub-standard quality and create new, positive habits to upgrade each sense's nutritive value.

The Power of 5-Sense Nutrition:
Decoding Michelangelo's 500 Year-old Secret

Your mother told you to chew your food well before swallowing. She was right. This simple advice was meant to make sure you didn't choke and to insure that you'd extract more of the nutrients from your food than if you swallowed your food whole. The adage to chew such that you "drink your foods and chew your liquids" is sound digestion wisdom 101. Similarly, each of our other senses has both a gross level of sustenance and a subtler, though less frequently accessed level of sustenance.

Looking at our sense of sight, we can use a part of Michelangelo's famous Sistine Chapel painting to illustrate this point. For 500 years, everyone took the section of God bestowing life to Adam at face biblical value—until 1990, when Frank Meshberger, M.D. activated his deeper sense of sight/insight and saw something even more incredible. The ellipsoid shape in which God rests actually bears an uncanny resemblance to a human brain, complete with amazingly accurate anatomic detail. For comparison, see our version of Michelangelo's painting overlaid with an anatomic drawing of a human brain. You can clearly see the uncanny correlation of the brain's prominent lobes—frontal, temporal, occipital and cerebellar and an emerging spinal cord—to Michelangelo's masterpiece.

Dr. Meshberger didn't just look at the artwork, he really saw with his depth of vision what Michelangelo had embedded in his painting in plain sight. Why was Michelangelo

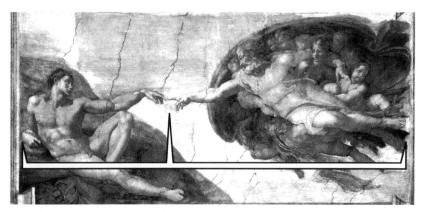

Michelangelo's *Creation of Adam* (1512), showing God giving Adam the touch of life
at the precise 38/62 Golden Ratio point between them. From the ceiling of the Sistine Chapel
in Vatican City, Rome. Look closely. What other intriguing detail can be clearly found
within this famous painting? Turn to page 138 to discover the amazing answer,
which eluded the world for 500+ years.

so secretive in his depictions? As it turns out, like his contemporary and rival Leonardo Da Vinci, he had a clear ulterior motive. Since the Catholic Church forbade grave robbing and dissection of cadavers, Michelangelo had to hide his anatomical research and the knowledge thus obtained to avoid persecution or even death. The simplest and most ingenious way to document his discoveries was to secretly embed the information within his paintings. Luckily for him and for us, the Church never found out. These secrets lay dormant for 500 years, until Dr. Meshberger had the depth of vision to see what had literally been right in front of everyone for centuries. Likewise, we can enliven all of our 5-Senses by simply slowing down and really beginning to see, hear, taste, smell and feel on a deeper and more profound level.

A great common example of this principle is a rose. At first glance, most just see the basic shape, color, petals, stem, leaves and thorns. Yet if we look deeper, with a relaxed eye for patterns, we see the universal imprint of the Golden Ratio: the multiple, elegant Golden Spirals formed by the petals in the face of every rose. Turning the rose around, we see the Golden Star pentagram, formed by the leaves behind the face of the rose. Looking deeper for patterns in anything, be it person, place or thing is a powerful way to activate a key facet of your innate genius: Pattern Recognition. The rewards of looking deeper in all of our senses can be nothing less than what Adam received from God—in addition to Eve, of course!

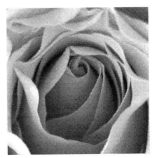 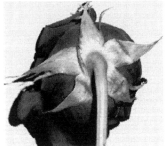

Every rose contains a double imprint of the Golden Ratio, hidden in plain sight: petals embedded in Golden Spirals on the front and a five-pointed Golden Star on the back.

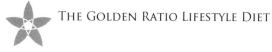

4

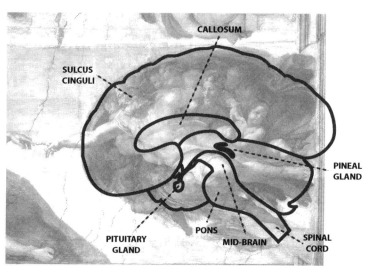

Michelangelo's *Creation of Adam* with superimposed anatomic drawing of a human brain and spinal cord. For more fascinating detail, see Dr. Meshberger's original 1990 article, *Explaining The Hidden Meaning Of Michelangelo's Creation of Adam*. See: www.wellcorps.com/Explaining-The-Hidden-Meaning-Of-Michelangelos-Creation-of-Adam.html

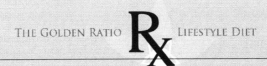

THE GOLDEN RATIO **Rx** LIFESTYLE DIET

NUTRITION: FOOD & BEYOND

Pick one or more of the following Rx's to add to your daily health regimen.

4

1. Breakfast First: Fuel Your Body Shortly After Arising

If you consider your entire nutritional intake in a day, breakfast would instantly fall into the front end of the First 15% of your day. A quality breakfast is clearly the most important meal of the day, because it gives your body the needed nourishment after a night of fasting. You know how your performance and state of mind can suffer if you skip breakfast. Unneeded stress is put on your adrenal glands, causing them to produce excess cortisol—the stress hormone—to stimulate your liver to keep blood sugar levels up. As timing is everything in greasing the wheels of metabolism, making breakfast a top priority makes your whole system more efficient and productive throughout your day. A healthy breakfast is also the smart way to achieve and maintain optimum weight. In a study by Dr. Daniela Jakubowicz, an endocrinologist at the Hospital de Clinicas Caracas in Venezuela and professor at Virginia Commonwealth University in Richmond, Virginia, obese women who had a healthy breakfast front-loaded with a larger percentage of their total daily calories lost four times as much weight than those who skipped breakfast. The message of this study and others like it is clear: a healthy breakfast—the First 15% of your day—is a vital key to optimum weight and health in general.

2. Eat Your Protein First in Every Meal

Eat your protein in the First 15% Percent of your meal, so that your stomach acids can get the first undiluted shot at the protein. Then, allow a few minutes after you finish your protein before you begin eating the rest of your meal. If you mix eating other foods together with your protein, chances are good that your digestion will be compromised and you won't break down and absorb the nutrients as well. This principle is even more important as you age, as digestive enzyme secretion decreases.

3. Quantity and Quality of Food Intake

By eating according to the 40% Carb, 30% Protein, 30% Fat ratio, you can incorporate the power of the Golden Ratio into your diet. Dr. Barry Sears gives a non-mathematical way of figuring out how much Carb/Protein/Fat to eat to maintain a healthy 40/30/30 Golden Ratio range:

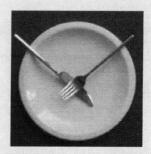

For reducing overall portions without paying attention to ratios, eat only what fits on the larger Golden Ratio section (about 2/3).

Short version:

Eat as much protein as the palm of your hand, as many non-starchy raw vegetables as you can stand for the vitamins, enough carbohydrates to maintain mental clarity (because the brain runs on glucose) and enough monounsaturated oils to keep feelings of hunger away.

Long version:

Never eat any more low-fat protein than you can fit on the palm of your hand. Let the volume of the low-fat protein you are going to eat determine the volume of the carbohydrates you can eat at the same time. If you're eating [unfavorable] carbohydrates (refined grains, starches, pasta, bread, etc.), then you can have the same volume portion as the low-fat protein that you're eating. If you're eating favorable carbohydrates (fruits and vegetables), then you can eat double the volume of the low-fat protein portion... use primarily monounsaturated fat—whether it's the teaspoon of olive oil that you cook your vegetables in or the avocado slices or handful of slivered almonds that you put on top of your salads... But the amount of monounsaturated fat I am talking about would be considered a dash.

All calories are not created equal. Always seek the highest quality calories.

Good Protein Choices: lean cuts of meat, turkey, egg whites, low-fat dairy, tofu, tempeh (cultured soy/grain cake), fish, skinless chicken.

Favorable Carbohydrates: most vegetables; most fruits; limit concentrated fruits like bananas, dates, figs and raisins (always drink additional water when consuming dried foods due to their dehydrating effect); limited amount of whole grains like oatmeal, quinoa, amaranth, buckwheat, millet.

Unfavorable Carbohydrates: refined grains and starches like pasta, bread, bagels, cereals; potatoes and corn; excess concentrated and/or dehydrated fruits like raisins, dates and figs.

Good Fats: olive oil, almonds, avocados, fish oils, flax seeds, hemp seeds.

Bad Fats: fatty red meat, egg yolks, organ meats, processed foods rich in trans fats, fatty animal products such as butter, high fat cheese, etc.

Avoid man-made/packaged foods. Best to eat minimally or non-processed, organic foods. See our full-page Golden Ratio Lifestyle Diet Nutrition Decoder featured earlier in this chapter.

> *If man made it, don't eat it.*
> **Jack LaLanne, "The Godfather of Fitness."**

4. Frequency of Food Intake

Although the practice of caloric reduction is not currently popular in our culture, we have figured out a simple way to make this valuable practice easier to swallow. By regulating the *quality* and *quantity* of your food intake, plus adjusting the *frequency* of your meals, you can creatively reduce your caloric intake, in an enjoyable and effective manner.

You might begin by eating about 62% or 2/3 of your usual calories one day per week. In one year's time, this could easily add up to 10 to 20 pounds of relatively painless weight loss, depending on your daily caloric intake. At only two days per week, this could add up to 20 to 40 pounds of weight loss.

4

5. The Golden Ratio IronApe Green Smoothie

This is a supercharged version of author Victoria Boutenko's original green smoothie, which only called for kale and fruit. This Golden Ratio high-ORAC (antioxidant) smoothie unleashes the energy of King Kong, Iron Man, The Incredible Hulk and Popeye combined, by kicking Boutenko's original ingredients several notches up the evolutionary scale, more towards Golden Ratio Carb/Protein/Fat ratios and

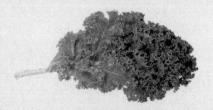

Organic Kale, the green superfood which has one of the highest and healthiest nutrition-to-calories ratio by weight of any food.

antioxidant levels. Note: It is highly recommended to invest in and use a high-power blender such as a BlendTec® or VitaMix®, to truly break open the plant cells, releasing their nutrients and liquefying the ingredients. Regular blenders just aren't powerful enough to get the job done well.

32 oz. water

3-4 kale leaves, chopped

½ to 1 banana

½ apple

5 strawberries (substitute or add blueberries, raspberries, etc.)

Recommended supercharging and carb/protein/fat balancers:

1 tbsp. green powder (try Dr. Schulze's SuperFood: www.herbdoc.com)

1 tbsp. protein powder (try hypoallergenic sprouted rice protein powder: SunWarrior.com)

2 tbsp. flax seeds, freshly ground

1 tsp. acai berry powder (Sambazon.com)

½ tsp. buffered vitamin C powder

Small piece raw ginger root or ½ tsp. ginger root powder

Super Beet Power Boost: For an extra stamina boost, add an organic red beet. A glass of red beet juice a day has been shown to increase stamina by an amazing 16%, according to a study led by Professor Andy Jones of England's University of Exeter's School of Sport and Health Sciences.

Blend on high speed 30–60 seconds, until smooth. Drink 1 or 2 cups; refrigerate the remainder and drink throughout the day. Add additional water as needed.

- Bananas, apples, carrots and beets are very high in carbohydrates (sugar) and can imbalance carb/protein/fat ratios, as well as over-stimulate insulin.

- Organic ingredients are highly recommended, as conventional kale, apples, strawberries, etc., are likely to contain toxic pesticide residues.

- Kale has a relatively high amount of oxalates and thus should be avoided or kept to a minimum if you are predisposed to kidney or gall stones. Raw kale consumption can also possibly inhibit thyroid function in some people, so if you consume kale regularly it's a good idea to have your physician monitor your thyroid periodically.

- For those who either don't like the taste of kale or need to avoid it for medical reasons, a good green substitute is romaine lettuce, which is neutral in taste and naturally low in oxalates and thyroid inhibitors.

- Caution is advised when first experimenting with this recipe as it can precipitate detoxification reactions. Newcomers to green foods might want to drink small amounts at first, until you get used to the potency.

6. Select Nutrient Dense Foods via the ANDI Scale

The ANDI Scale (Aggregate Nutrient Density Index) is a food nutrient scoring system developed by Dr. Joel Fuhrman, Chief Medical Officer of EatRight America, a non-profit organization devoted to transforming people's health. The ANDI Scale integrates measurements of key micronutrients, e.g., vitamins, minerals and carotenoids, and gives foods with high ORAC scores (anti-oxidant potential index) extra weighting. The result is an easy-to-follow healthy/ superfoods selection system. Dr. Fuhrman has treated more than 10,000 patients in 15 years, proving that a properly nourished body can conquer food cravings, seek its ideal weight, reverse chronic conditions, have more energy and result in brighter, healthier kids. The Eat Right America website points out that the USDA estimates less than 5% of Americans get the nutrients they need on a daily basis; America is predominantly overfed and undernourished.

To learn more and see the complete ANDI Scale, visit www.EatRightAmerica. com. Ideally, eat your fruits and vegetables raw or at most lightly steamed, as cooking always reduces or destroys their vital nutrients and enzymes.

ANDI Scale (Aggregate Nutrient Density Index)
Top 22 Super Foods Score (higher = better)

1.	**Kale, watercress, collard, mustard, turnip greens**	**1000**	
2.	**Bok choy**	**824**	
3.	**Spinach**	**739**	
4.	**Brussels sprouts**	**672**	
5.	**Swiss chard**	**670**	
6.	Arugula	559	
7.	Radish	554	
8.	Cabbage	481	
9.	Bean sprouts	444	
10.	Red peppers	420	
11.	Romaine lettuce	389	
12.	Broccoli	376	
13.	Tomatoes, tomato products	190-300	
14.	Cauliflower	295	
15.	Green peppers	258	
16.	Asparagus	234	
17.	Strawberries	212	
18.	Pomegranate juice	193	
19.	Blackberries	178	
20.	Plums	157	
21.	Raspberries	145	
22.	Blueberries	130	

7. Eat Foods High in Antioxidants (High ORAC Rating)

ORAC is an anagram for Oxygen Radical Absorbance Capacity, a measure of the antioxidant potential of foods. Eating these super-charged foods prevents "cellular rusting" and can result in dramatic improvements in immune function, overall health and longevity. Following is a sample list of foods with the highest ORAC (antioxidant) scores, excerpted from the USDA's 2007 study of ORAC levels of selected foods. ORAC values are determined based on a 100 gram (3.5 ounces) sample of each food. The first test of its type, the ORAC scale measures both time and degree of free-radical inhibition, to +/- 5% accuracy.

High ORAC/Anti-Oxidant Foods

Food	ORAC Rating	Food	ORAC Rating
Cloves, ground	**314,446**	Cranberry, raw	9584
Cinnamon, ground	**267,536**	Artichoke, boiled	9416
Oregano, dried	**200,129**	Red Beans	8459
Turmeric, ground	**159,277**	Plum, black diamond	7581
Rosehips	**96,150**	Blueberry, raw	6552
Cocoa powder,		Prune	6552
unsweetened	80,933	Blackberry	5347
Cumin seed	76,800	Raspberry	4882
Parsley, dried	74,349	Sweet cherry	4873
Nutmeg	69,640	Red Delicious apple	4275
Basil, dried	67,553	Granny Smith apple	3898
Curry powder	48,504	Russet potato	1680
Pecan, 1 oz	17,940		

As you can see, spices and fruits are among the highest in antioxidant potential and should be regularly consumed to enhance health and well-being. For a complete list of high ORAC foods, visit http://tinyurl.com/yrmfse.

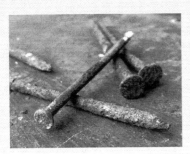 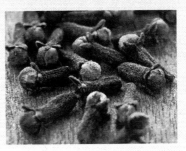

Rusty nails (*left*) are a good visual example of the power of oxidation. Cloves (*right*) have the highest ORAC/antioxidant rating of any food and thus can inhibit *cellular rusting*. A basic homeopathic tenet is *like treats like*. Is it just a coincidence that cloves, in both their reddish color and shape, are so similar in appearance to rusty nails, yet so different in anti-oxidant potential? By increasing our consumption of high-ORAC foods like cloves, it stands to reason that we can slow down internal oxidation, improve our health and extend our longevity. **Rx:** Try adding a few cloves to tea, hot chocolate or coffee to partake of their benefits.

8. Avoiding Pesticides

Toxic pesticides are an increasing threat to our environment, health and longevity, wreaking havoc on our immune/ecosystems, our hormones and genetic blueprint. The common sense rule-of-thumb is so simple: Buy organic foods whenever possible. Organic foods are free of all synthetic, violating lethal chemicals: fertilizers, soil conditioners, artificial flavors, colors, pesticides, preservatives, etc.

Following here are the "Dirty Dozen" (highest in toxic pesticides when conventionally grown); always buy these Organic whenever possible:

1.	Celery	7.	Bell Peppers
2.	Peaches	8.	Spinach
3.	Strawberries	9.	Kale
4.	Apples	10.	Cherries
5.	Blueberries	11.	Potatoes
6.	Nectarines	12.	Grapes

When not possible to buy Organic, use the following list from the Environmental Working Group (www.FoodNews.org) to limit your exposure to toxic pesticides by selecting these conventionally-grown foods from their "Clean 15" list (be sure to use a natural pesticide removal solution to wash your non-organic fruit or vegetables):

The "Clean 15" (when conventionally grown): Lowest in Pesticides:

1.	Onions	9.	Cabbage
2.	Avocado	10.	Eggplant
3.	Sweet Corn	11.	Cantaloupe
4.	Pineapple	12.	Watermelon
5.	Mangos	13.	Grapefruit
6.	Sweet Peas	14.	Sweet Potato
7.	Asparagus	15.	Honeydew Melon
8.	Kiwi		

9. Alternate Day Caloric Reduction for Weight Loss and Longevity

Easy:

Alternating days 1 and 2 allows around 1 lb. weight loss/week.

Day 1: eat normally

Day 2: skip one meal, or only eat **62%** (a little less than 2/3)
of normal amount at each meal.

Advanced:

Alternating days 1 and 2 allows around 2 lb. weight loss/week.

Day 1: eat normally

Day 2: skip 2 meals or only eat about **38%** (a little more than 1/3)
of normal amount at each meal.

Super-advanced:

Dr. Johnson's Level: alternating days 1 and 2 allows greatest weight loss,
gene-regulation and longevity, yet is also the most challenging level.

Day 1: eat normally

Day 2: eat 20% (about 1/5) of your normal calories to obtain the full
spectrum of caloric reduction benefits.

See *The Alternate Day Diet*, by James P. Johnson, M.D.

10. Water: Solid, Liquid and Gas

It is common knowledge that water exists in three different states: solid (ice),
liquid and gas. Although you might not think that food is as dynamic as water,
it actually is, also being able to exist in three phases: solid food, liquid (chewed
food) and gas (flatulence). We want to decrease the tendency towards the third
phase—gas production—by making sure we chew and digest our food as well
as possible. In addition to the chewing phase, the First 15% of your digestive
process actually includes the sight, smell and taste of your food. These sensory
inputs activate digestion by stimulating brain centers that cause the release
of digestive enzymes in your mouth, stomach, small intestines, pancreas,
liver and gallbladder. The actual chewing process is essential for increasing

4

the surface area of food as much as possible, thereby exposing it to maximal digestive enzyme action. The better you chew your food, the easier it is to digest. Jay Kordich (*the Juice Man*) once said that by chewing your food well, you become a human juice machine. So, make sure that you chew your food to liquid before swallowing. The amount of food that you actually absorb is directly proportional to how well it is digested, so remember: don't bite off more than you can chew.

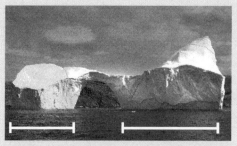

The 3 states of water. This picture of an iceberg shows how water exists in three phases: solid (ice), liquid (water) and gas (clouds/water vapor). Note how the two above-water sections of the iceberg are in Golden Ratio to one another.

11. Everyone Can Benefit from a Plan Bee

Bees have been friends of mankind and life on Earth since the beginning, as seen in their miraculous pollination work and the well-known benefits of bee products, including honey, pollen, propolis, royal jelly and beeswax. Yet the bee's role as a secret Golden Ratio agent has remained hidden in plain sight. From their navigation through their honeycombs to the idealized

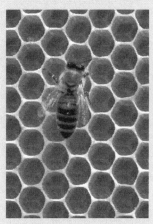

A honeybee, Golden Ratio special agent at work.

code governing their ancestry—both of which mirror the Fibonacci Sequence—to their flight in endlessly dancing Golden Spirals, every bee instinctively follows Nature's Path of Least Resistance and Maximum Performance. This is coincident with the remarkable fact that honey is the only food that does not spoil, even after thousands of years. Partaking of bees' generously given health and longevity boosting gifts is thus another recommended easy (and delicious) way to access the Golden Ratio. With concentrated bee superfoods such as pollen, propolis and royal jelly, it's best to start with small doses to allow your system to acclimate. Use raw, uncooked sources to preserve the vital live enzymes. Eating organic foods greatly reduces yours—and the bees—exposure to toxic chemical pesticides. Toxic farming practices, along with increasing exposure to Genetically Modified Organisms (GMOs) and electro-smog, are some of the newly identified factors likely contributing to the alarming worldwide mass die-off of bees, also known as Colony Collapse Disorder (CCD).

12. Blood Tests for Homo Vitruvians

Here are a few blood tests that may help you determine if your metabolism is evolving towards Golden Ratio balance. These are just a few of the many nutritional biochemistry related tests that are available, to help you get started. You will need to consult with your physician or nutritionist to get the proper understanding of the results in relation to your particular concerns.

- **CBC/Chemistry Profile:** general comprehensive blood screen
- **Thyroid, including TSH, free T3, T4, reverse T3, thyroid antibodies:** metabolic rate screen
- **C-Reactive Protein/CRP (high sensitivity):** non-specific measure of inflammation
- **Fibrinogen:** blood clotting factor that reveals heart attack and stroke risk.
- **Fasting insulin, Hemoglobin A1C and blood sugar:** check for diabetes and metabolic syndrome
- **Vitamin D (25-OH):** a multi-factorial essential vitamin/hormone; blood test at: http://tinyurl.com/6naey42
- **Homocysteine:** risk factor for heart disease or stroke
- **Omega Score™:** Unique measure of inflammation which can provide potentially predictive data on heart disease, stroke and other conditions/ chronic diseases. Blood test at: http:/tinyurl.com/7p9d6gg
  See Rx #16 for more detail

These are just a few important tests that can quickly reveal factors of significant impact to your health, if abnormal/out-of-ratio. Please use this list only as an adjunct to what your physician may recommend for you.

These tests are available through the Life Extension Foundation, which has health advisors on staff to review your test results with you; or, you can review the tests with your personal physician. Call **1-800-544-4440** and mention discount code LA, or visit: **www.LEF.org/LA**

13. 5-Sense Nutritional Enhancement

Here's an easy way to begin to enhance the quality of your daily sensory diet. Consider each of your 5 senses in turn and strive to expand the ratio of its positive potential. Jot down your favorite examples for each sense below. When complete, copy your top selections onto a Post-It note or 3 x 5 index card and carry it with you or place it where you'll see it daily. Lift the positive aspect of each sense by increasing the (Golden) ratio of time spent enjoying your selected sensory nutrient boosters.

 Sights/Visual: Uplifting, expansive? Inspiring photos/pictures in sight? Harmonious, clutter-free living/working environments?

Favorite Sights _____

_____

Sounds/Auditory: Soothing, affirming, inspiring? Includes healthy ratios of silence?

Favorite Sounds _____

_____

Touch/Kinesthetic: Healthy and regular?

Favorite Touches _____

_____

Smells: Pleasing, harmonious, inviting?

Favorite Smells/Scents _____

_____

Tastes: Delicious? Includes healthy ratios of the 4 primary tastes: sweet, salty, sour and bitter?

Favorite Tastes _____

_____

4

Utilizing your 5 senses to enhance imagination is also a proven factor in tapping its power for health and longevity. The intriguing age-reversal and DNA potentiation work of Harvard psychotherapist Ellen Langer and Japanese geneticist Kazeo Murakami (see chapters 9 and 10) underscores this point. While it may seem like science fiction that focused imagination triggers the release of literal fountain-of-youth hormones and other beneficial neurochemicals, it is scientific fact. One could say that this practice stimulates a powerful form of internal "self-nutrition." Utilizing your 5 senses to enhance self-guided visualizations of yourself at your best—in vibrant health and happiness—is a powerful, free tool for supporting optimal health and longevity.

Now that you've listed your 5 sense nutritional factors, you can use them to enhance your imagination exercises, e.g., in the Golden Prime Zone Holodeck Meditation (Rx 1, chapter 10). Everyone requires their own unique Golden Ratio balance of sensory nutrition for health and happiness. Tapping the increased nourishment opportunities via upgrading our sensory nutrition quality offers exciting health and longevity benefits.

14. Full Spectrum Lighting

A strongly suggested upgrade to conventional indoor lighting is full-spectrum light bulbs, which most closely approximate natural sunlight. Conventional incandescent and fluorescent bulbs project an uneven and unhealthy light which can cause effects ranging from irritability to lethargy and eyestrain, and can contribute to Seasonal Affective Disorder (SAD).

Full spectrum lighting promotes less eyestrain, shows more natural colors and is effective in treating SAD during the winter months in northern climates. The lights are available in both conventional and fluorescent bulbs at most larger hardware stores.

15. Calorie Decoder (for the mathematically inclined)

There's one vital piece of information that you need to know in order to make the 40/30/30 Zone/Golden Ratio calorie ratios make sense and be truly workable. This is essential information to know to decode labels and figure out correct meal proportions and types of foods to include in your menus. There's a caloric inequality between protein, fat and carbohydrates of which most people are unaware. Each gram of these three classes of macronutrients produces differing amounts of calories.

Macronutrient	Calories per gram
Protein	4
Fat	9
Carbohydrate	4

As you can see, all classes of macronutrients are not equal in the number of calories they produce per gram. Each gram of fat can produce 2.25 times as many calories as each gram of protein or carbohydrate. Here's an example from www.caloriesperhour.com/tutorial_gram.php that shows how to calculate calories per gram.

Imagine a food containing 10 grams of protein, 10 grams of fat, and 10 grams of carbohydrates. That would total 170 calories:

$$(10 \text{ g Protein} \times 4) + (10 \text{ g Fat} \times 9) + (10 \text{ g Carbs} \times 4) = 170$$

In this imaginary food 40 calories come from protein, 90 calories come from fat, and 40 calories come from carbohydrates.

As you can see, fat is the real Trojan Horse that sneaks extra calories into your diet. That's the first part of the decoding. The next step is to figure out the ratios of carbs/protein/fat to see how closely they conform to Dr. Sears' Zone 40/30/30 or approximate Golden 40/60 Ratio.

From the above imaginary example:

40/170 = 23.5% from Carbohydrates
40/170 = 23.5% from Protein
90/170 = 53% from Fat

This imaginary food has the following ratios:

23.5% Carbs / 23.5% Protein / 53% Fat

These ratios are too high in fat and too low in carbohydrates and protein and don't even come close to the 40/30/30 ratios. This method of calculation is too convoluted of a process for most people, so that's why Dr. Sears developed simple methods like the ones described in the Rx #3—**Quantity and Quality of Food Intake**—in order to get your Golden Nutritional Ratios balanced.

16. Cutting Edge Blood Testing for Health and Longevity

A landmark 2010 study in the *Journal of the American Medical Association* (JAMA) established a link between patients with high Red Blood Cell (RBC) levels of the Omega-3 fatty acids, EPA and DHA, with a decreased rate of telomere shortening. Telomeres (the protective shoelace-like aglets on the end of chromosomes; see ch. 10/Longevity) that are too short prevent cell division and lead to aging and ultimately death. RBC levels of EPA and DHA are known

4

as the Omega Index and appear to be not only a significant biomarker of aging, but also an independent risk factor for sudden cardiac death. This test is far more sensitive than the routinely tested risk factors of total cholesterol, HDL, LDL, triglycerides and C-Reactive Protein (CRP). This ground-breaking test is now available without a doctor's prescription at: http://tinyurl.com/7p9d6gg or call Life Extension Foundation at **1-800-544-4440** and mention Discount Code LA. The test evaluates your Omega Score™ by measuring the following:

- Omega-3 Whole Blood Score, Equivalence Score,
  EPA/DHA Equivalence Score and Red Blood Cell Equivalence Score
- Complete breakdown of fatty acids by weight, including the AA/EPA
  ratio and the Omega-3/Omega-6 ratio

Interestingly, both the AA/EPA and Omega-6/Omega-3 ratios should approach the Golden Ratio of 1.6:1 for ideal health and longevity. The typical western diet is overloaded with grains (Omega-6) and can result in ratios of over 15:1, 20:1 or even higher. Japanese people are amongst the longest lived in the world, have the lowest rates of heart disease and depression and have AA/EPA ratios ranging from 1.5:1 to 3:1. You can mimic the physiologically balanced diet of our neo-Paleolithic ancestors by eating a diet where caloric percentages of carbohydrate, protein and fat are consumed in a 40:30:30 ratio (or 40:60 ratio). Since eating a perfectly balanced diet can be difficult to do in our fast-paced culture, fish oils can be supplemented to shift the ratios more towards 1.6:1. The Omega Score™ blood test clearly reveals the success of supplementation with fish oils by revealing the AA/EPA ratios. These tests of silent inflammation are a great motivational tool to begin implementing various aspects of the Golden Ratio Lifestyle Diet and thus access Nature's Secret Nutrient.

17. Gluten: Not Always In The Breakfast Of Champions

Gluten can glue you up. As new undisputed world #1 men's tennis player (2011) Novak Djokovic of Serbia and other top athletes and celebrities such as Oprah Winfrey have discovered, eliminating gluten from the diet can result in greater energy, performance and overall health. Within six months of discovering he was allergic to gluten and removing it from his diet, Novak rocketed to the top of the tennis world, beating former nemesis Roger Federer and Rafael Nadal multiple times in the process. Novak engineered one of the finest men's single seasons in tennis' open era history, winning three of the four Grand Slam tournaments (Australian Open, Wimbledon, U.S. Open) and compiling a stunning 64-2 win/loss record as of mid September, 2011. He attributes much of his newfound lean fitness, energy, increased speed and focus to removing all gluten-containing foods from his diet. Many people have varying degrees of often hidden gluten sensitivity. Gluten is the glue-like component of the protein found in many common foods (such as breads,

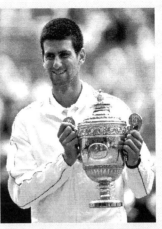

Gluten-free World #1 Tennis Champion Novak Djokovic, shown here with the 2011 Wimbledon trophy.

pasta, bagels) from grains like wheat, rye and barley (grains such as quinoa, buckwheat, amaranth and millet are gluten-free). In gluten sensitive people, it can cause inflammation, poor digestion, reduced performance and fatigue, weight gain and an array of other health ailments. If you think you have gluten sensitivity, your health professional can recommend various blood/allergy tests to help determine if a gluten-free regime is for you.

18. Dine Like Da Vinci

How we eat has a meaningful effect on *what* we eat. From Michael J. Gelb's masterwork, *How to Think Like Leonardo da Vinci*:

> *Don't eat, dine. "Grabbing a bite" while "eating on the run" usually leads to poor dietary choices and subsequent indigestion. Instead, discipline yourself to sit down and enjoy every meal. Create, as the maestro did, an aesthetically pleasing environment: a nice place setting with flowers and an artful presentation of even the simplest foods. A pleasant atmosphere and an unhurried pace improves your digestion, equanimity and the quality of your life.*

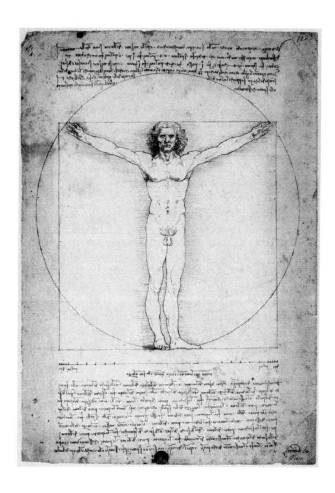

Leonardo Da Vinci's *Vitruvian Man*,

exhibiting naturally buoyant Golden Ratio posture.

5.

POSTURE:
GOLDEN RATIO STRUCTURE

A good stance and posture reflect a proper state of mind.
Morihei Ueishiba, founder of Aikido

It's unlikely that a fish swimming in the ocean ever considers the fact that it's wet. Similarly, we live and move under the influence of a gravitational field that has become so second nature, we forget that it even exists. Yet the sense of gravity that has become mostly unconscious still exerts its constant downward force upon us, 24/7. This relentless force field eventually takes its toll on our posture. Posture is that counterbalancing force that allows us to stand upright within gravity's field. If we have perfect posture there's no problem, but for most humans this isn't the case. Diminished health and longevity are of course the logical results of poor posture. The tendency to lose our vertical alignment puts abnormal stresses on muscles, joints, cartilage, discs and nerves, resulting in back pain, achy arthritis, compromised breathing and organ function.

The vertebrae that make up our spine attained their current Golden Ratio relationships through the evolutionary process, in order to be able to harmonize with the gravitational field while upright. The beautiful Golden Ratio-encoded S-curve of the human spine is the result of evolution's continual improvement and adaptation,

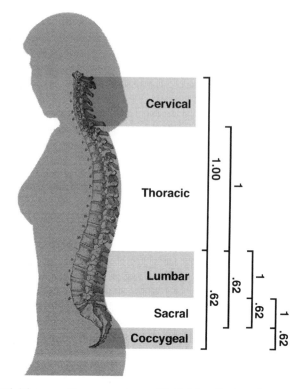

The beautiful S-curved human spine, with Golden Ratio relationships.

as our species gained upright posture. The awareness and maintenance of an optimal spinal S-curve allows us to best work with gravity, instead of against it. Only through regaining awareness of what our ideal relationship is to gravity can we begin to restore good posture. Adequate hydration (chapter 2/Water) also plays a hidden yet vital role in healthy posture and its maintenance over time: it's no accident that fallen leaves curl up in a reverse Golden Spiral as they dehydrate.

Our Golden Ratio Body Symmetry

Structurally and functionally all the bones in your body—arms and legs, fingers and toes—closely approximate the Golden Ratio in their relationships to one another. Your skull and pelvic bones reflect the Golden Ratio, as does the curve of your spine. The distance from your navel to your feet and from your navel to the top of your head tends toward the Golden Ratio. All of the bones in your body, indeed all of the parts of your body—muscles, tendons, ligaments and organs—reflect the Golden Ratio, in literally infinite examples.

158

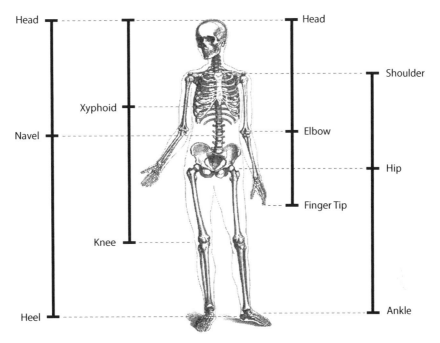

Some classic Golden Ratios of the human body.

> *Phidias, the Greek sculptor, revealed the Golden Ratio in his work—for example, in such proportions as the relation of the width of the head to the width of the throat, the width of the forearm to the wrist, the width of the calf to the ankle, and so on.*
>
> **James Wyckoff, *Pyramid Energy***

Whenever you discover an expression of the Golden Ratio in anything, you can be sure it's embedded at both micro and macro levels. For example, each bone in your finger is in Golden Ratio to the adjacent bones in that finger. And the length of that finger is in Golden Ratio to the length of your hand. As the length of your hand is in Golden Ratio to the length of your forearm, it should come as no surprise that the length of your arm is in Golden Ratio to the length of your entire body... and so on. Another fascinating manifestation of the Golden Ratio in our bodies is in the actual shape of some of our bones. For example, you can clearly see the shape of the Golden Spiral in the pelvic and temporal bones. The cervical, thoracic and lumbar vertebrae exhibit a smooth transition in size that reflects the Golden Ratio. When you curl your hand into a fist, it always takes the shape of the Golden Spiral.

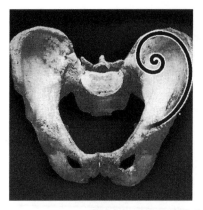 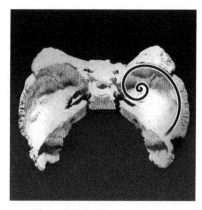

Pelvic; temporal and sphenoid bones (skull),
with embedded Golden Spiral structure.

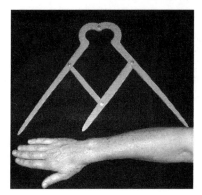 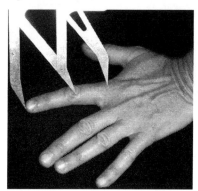

Golden Ratios in the forearm, hand and fingers.

> *Man is all symmetry, full of proportions, one limb to another, and all to all the world besides. Each part may call the farthest brother, for head with foot hath private amity, and both with moons and tides.*
> **George Herbert, English priest and poet**

The anatomical Golden Ratio points of the body's length are in dynamic flux during human development, from our beginnings as a Golden Spiral-shaped embryo to full-grown adulthood. In infants, the Golden Ratio points are at the level of the heart or at the genitals, depending upon which direction (head or feet) one measures from. As the body grows and develops, the Golden Ratio point is seen to shift to the level of the navel in the adult. Actual navel measurements are not always exactly at the 0.618 ratio point and can vary within individuals according to Fibonacci Sequence ratios. Since there are always variations in human proportions, some people's navels will

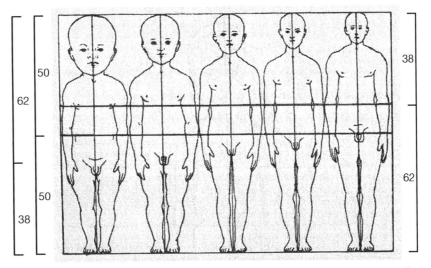

Dynamic flux of the Golden Ratio points of the human body, from infant to adult. The navel's position changes from the 50:50 point in the infant to the 38:62 Golden Ratio point in the adult, while the position of the genitals changes from 38:62 in the infant to 50:50 in the adult.

5

be at the 0.618 cut point whereas others may be slightly off. For example, some people may have a 2/3 (0.66), a 3/5 (0.6) or a 5/8 (0.625) ratio. This variability is known as *dancing around the [Golden] Mean*.

Golden Ratio Postural Alignment

The major Golden Ratio division of your body in the vertical plane is at the level of the navel. This ideal upper body-to-lower body ratio is important to maintain throughout life. The most common cause of loss of Divine Proportion in our stature is due to poor postural habits. A slumping posture and rounded shoulders result in a loss of vertical height in your spine. The natural, gentle S-shaped curve of your spine can become deformed with an accentuation or loss of curvature in the cervical, thoracic or lumbar regions. Poor postural habits are commonly seen and become fixed in the way that many people sit at their desks or computers, or work on their PDA's or cellphones when standing.

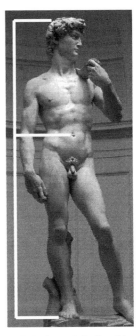

Michelangelo's *David*, exhibiting his flawless Golden Ratio body symmetry.

161

Over time, the slumping position becomes integrated into permanent structure with tight muscles pulling the spine, shoulders, arms, legs and pelvis out of natural alignment. This of course results in an avalanche of undesirable domino effects. In addition to eventual harmful wear on the vertebral disks and the spine as a whole, internal organs have less space in which to move and their healthy physiological function is inhibited. Blood flow is decreased in compromised areas, and headaches, tight shoulders and sore back muscles are just some of the more obvious symptoms. Poor digestion and elimination are also common symptoms when internal organs are cramped.

When poor postural habits combine with the aging process and hormonal decline, osteoporosis may result. Osteoporosis further accentuates loss of height in the spine, due to vertebral collapse and increased curvature of the spine.

The Golden Posture/Attitude Link

Good posture not only projects a favorable image to others, it also self-reflects, giving you more confidence in your own thoughts. In a study on the link between posture and attitude, people who were told to sit up straight were more likely to believe thoughts they wrote down about their qualifications for a job. Yet those who were slumped over their desks were less likely to accept these written-down feelings about their qualifications. According to Richard Petty, co-author of the study and professor of psychology at Ohio State University:

> *Most of us were taught that sitting up straight gives a good impression to other people... but it turns out that our posture can also affect how we think about ourselves. If you sit up [or stand up] straight, you end up convincing yourself by the posture you're in... sitting up straight is something you can train yourself to do, and it has psychological benefits... people assume their confidence is coming from their own thoughts. They don't realize their posture is affecting how much they believe in what they're thinking...*

This study reveals an intriguing insight into the body-mind connection of healthy posture, and as we have seen previously, better posture is always more reflective of Golden Proportion.

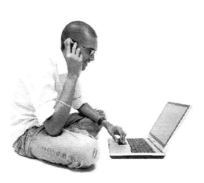

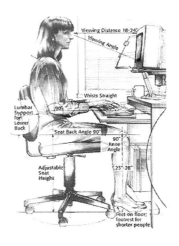

(left): This all-too-common foward-leaning example of poor posture pulls one out of postural alignment. *(right)*: Ergonomically correct desk posture for sitting. While good sitting posture is important, a growing body of research reveals that sitting for too long poses serious additional dangers to health and longevity. See Rx #8 at the end of this chapter for more details and targeted healthy sitting suggestions.

5

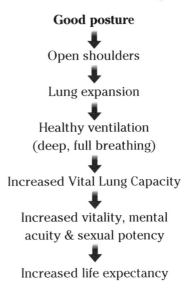

Posture's Effect on Health & Longevity

Posture initiates the following continuous causal chain:

Poor posture	**Good posture**
⬇	⬇
Rounded shoulders	Open shoulders
⬇	⬇
Lung compression	Lung expansion
⬇	⬇
Hypoventilation (restricted breathing)	Healthy ventilation (deep, full breathing)
⬇	⬇
Decreased Vital Lung Capacity	Increased Vital Lung Capacity
⬇	⬇
Decreased vitality, mental acuity & sexual potency	Increased vitality, mental acuity & sexual potency
⬇	⬇
Decreased life expectancy	Increased life expectancy

WARNING: Years of poor postural habits combined with osteoporosis results in back pain, loss of height and poor overall health.

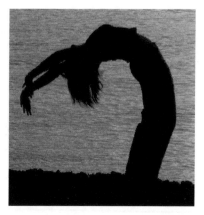

Beautiful Golden Spiral back bend. Safe, gentle back bending can help reverse the effects of poor posture.

5

This process only worsens the deviation from the Golden Proportion between the upper and lower body. The further from Golden Proportion one's posture becomes, the less efficient is one's mobility and physiological functioning.

Loss of natural Golden Proportions in how we carry ourselves has a powerful "butterfly effect" on our entire state of health, and thus our *quality*—and *quantity*—of life. Restoring postural Golden Proportions first requires awareness of its vital importance. Greater health and longevity are directly connected to this simple awareness and practice. Some easy ways to do this are to get in the habit of regular "check-in scans" regarding how you're sitting, standing or moving in any moment. For example, right this moment, how are you sitting as you read these words? Is your spine upright and flexible, with your head gently "floating" on top of your neck? Are your breaths full and deep? If not, gently correct whatever feels "out of proportion" in your body right now.

Taking advantage of therapies that reverse the daily stresses on the spine are an excellent practice. Any regular, balanced exercise regimen, such as stretching, yoga, Pilates, or Spiral~Chi's Evolutionary Movements are essential to regaining and maintaining proper spinal dynamics and good posture. Strength training builds your core, prevents osteoporosis and counters the effects of aging. Gravity inversion devices are also an effective way to gently traction your spine and relieve pressure on intervertebral discs. Make sure that your nutritional status is optimal, paying particular attention to mineral intake. Consult with your doctor to see if bioidentical hormonal therapy may be of value for you in preventing osteoporosis.

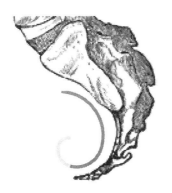

Origin of so-called *coiled serpent* Kundalini/Life Energy at the base of the spine mirrors a Golden/ Fibonacci Spiral, beginning at the 1st chakra level of the coccyx/sacrum.

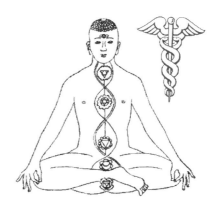

The seven primary energy centers or *Chakras* exhibit Golden Ratio symmetry. Note how the rising Kundalini/Life Energy spiral also mirrors the Caduceus.

5

As Thomas Edison said,

The doctor of the future will give no medicine, but will interest his patients in the care of the human frame, in diet and in the causes and prevention of disease.

Spirituality and the Spine

Sir John Woodroffe, a.k.a. Arthur Avalon, wrote in his classic book *The Serpent Power: The Secrets of Tantric and Shaktic Yoga*, that the body's primal Kundalini/life energy, also referred to as "serpent power," is coiled up three and one-half times at the base of the spine. When the Kundalini/life force is activated, it moves up the spine and is associated with varying degrees of psycho-spiritual development. As this subtle energy moves up the spine, it sequentially activates the body's seven subtle energy centers, known in Eastern traditions as the chakras (Sanskrit for "wheel," literally a "wheel of light"). The chakras have a correspondence with various endocrine glands (testes/ovaries, adrenals, pancreas, thymus, thyroid, pituitary, hypothalamus and pineal) and nerve plexi (sacral, lumbar, solar, cardiac, etc.). The ultimate result of the Kundalini rising up the spine and into the seventh chakra is variously known as spiritual enlightenment, nirvana, samadhi or bliss.

The seat of this infinite power is always referenced as being at the base of the spine, which is composed of the coccyx and sacrum. Traditional anthropologists view the coccyx, otherwise known as the tailbone, as a vestigial tail remnant with little or no value. Yet could the coccyx and sacrum have a powerful, yet hidden function? Among other things, tail-bearing animals use their tails to maintain balance during movement. Humans have adapted to being tail-less by developing large gluteal muscles, which act as torso stabilizers during movement. The coccyx is composed of three to five fused vertebrae attached to the sacrum by fibro-cartilaginous ligaments. The sacrum is a triangular-shaped bone composed of 5 fused vertebrae. When you view the sacro-coxygeal segment from the side, its distinct Golden Spiral shape is visible. It looks like a curled fetus, a shrimp or even a cuckoo's beak—coccyx translates as "cuckoo's beak" in Greek. It is also interesting that the translation of the word sacrum is "sacred bone." The ancients obviously knew that inherent in the structure and function of the sacred sacral bone was potential Divinity. Could it be that the mysterious coiled serpent power that has been revered by yogis throughout the ages is identical with what we know as the Golden Spiral? The Golden Spiral and Ratio don't limit themselves to the base of our spines, as they can be seen throughout the spine, as in the ratios of the cervical, thoracic, lumbar, sacral and coxygeal segments to one another.

5

> *The ideal posture we seek results from consistently optimizing our strength-to-flexibility ratio, to support coming ever closer to our own perfect body balance. This balance is always being challenged by gravity, which we must diligently learn to work with if we are to succeed. Lifting upward towards the sky, we must be like the young sapling; tall, straight, and flexible, able to bend with the strong wind, yet not break.*
>
> **Robert Kaehler, Master Body Balance**
> **Coach and former U.S. Olympic rower**

The Caduceus and the Spine

A symbol universally associated with medicine and healing is the Caduceus (cad-DO-shis), the winged staff of Hermes, the ancient Greek "Messenger of the Gods." The Caduceus features two serpents intertwined around a pole or staff, with spread wings at the top. It bears an uncanny resemblance to images of Kundalini life force energy rising in serpentine fashion, wrapping around the spine; its spread wings corresponding to the unfurling of infinite awareness at the head, ready to take flight. The ancients clearly understood the vital importance of the healing and enlightening power associated with energy moving freely up the spine, preserving this knowledge for all with the eyes to see it in the Caduceus. The Golden Ratio appears to be embedded at many levels of the Kundalini/chakra system:

- The crossing points of the winding serpents on the Caduceus occur at the levels of the Golden Ratio–spaced chakras. For example, the fourth chakra, located at the level of the heart, marks the .38 Golden Ratio point between the navel chakra and the crown chakra.

- If you examine the numbers comprising the first three digits of the Golden Ratio, 6—1—8, some additional interesting correlations can be made with the Caduceus symbol. The number "1" corresponds to the central pole spine. The number "8" resembles the serpents wrapped around the pole/spine and the number "6" represents the Golden Spiral energy, coiled at the base of the spine.

Good posture smooths the pathway for the unimpeded transmission of neural impulses—Kundalini life force—up and down the spine. When these neural impulses rise to their full potential, you can be sure that spiritual, scientific and/or artistic creative insights will emerge. In any event, "Something Great" usually manifests, as DNA researcher Dr. Kazuo Murakami would say (see chapter 8/Happiness & Inner Peace).

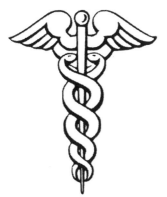

The Caduceus, classic symbol of medicine, healing and transformation has Golden Ratio elements.

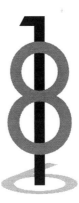

The first three numbers denoting the Golden Ratio, 6—1—8, are arranged symbolically to mirror the caduceus.

5

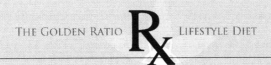

POSTURE:
GOLDEN RATIO STRUCTURE

Pick one or more of the following Rx's to add to your daily health regimen.

1. Support Your Feet: The First 15% of Healthy Posture

A. Since your feet are the First 15% Percent of your upright posture, it's imperative that your feet are properly aligned when contacting the ground, whether standing or moving. This assures that as the impact forces move up your body no added or abnormal stresses will be placed on your other joints, e.g., knees, hips, pelvis, spine, shoulders and cranium. When sitting in a chair, consider your pelvis as the base and align your sitting bones side-to-side and front-to-back. This will allow you to sit without back pain and avoid crunched, crimped back, neck and shoulders. Even a few degrees of misalignment in the beginning at the foot level can produce problems downstream, or upstream—the spine in this case. The same principles apply when walking, running or engaging in any sport.

Think FAB: *Foundation, Alignment, Buoyancy.* Foundation = level contact with the ground; Alignment = feet properly aligned front-to-back, supporting the First 15% alignment of Hips/Heart/Head; Buoyancy = Keeping a buoyant attitude of relaxed shoulders and a buoyant, lifting head. Your FABulous alignment will be reflected in your overall health and performance. Injury and wear and tear on your body can be greatly reduced or even prevented by this simple correct initial orientation.

B. Because our feet are the foundation of our entire skeletal system and thus healthy posture, it makes sense to upgrade this critical First 15% posture factor whenever we can. In his bestselling book *Born to Run*, author Christopher McDougall makes a convincing case for avoiding shoes whenever possible. His book profiles Mexico's Tarahumara Indians, who race barefoot or in thin sandals. Running shoes—and most modern shoes, for that matter—prevent the full range of healthy foot motion. Indeed, many shoes are like straightjackets for the feet. Ironically, conventional running shoes can actually cause harm, due to their higher heel design, which actually encourages heel striking and the accompanying heavy shock to the body with every step. When barefoot, feet naturally land more towards the front of the foot. This is much healthier as it best engages the natural spring function of the arch. This means far less shock or "collision force," as Harvard University evolutionary biologist Daniel Lieberman says, in support of McDougal's work. As a practical matter, two ends of the foundational foot care spectrum are suggested:

1. Natural, full freedom of motion. Walk or run barefoot on grass or sand for full freedom of motion, minimal stress on the feet and body and natural development of all the muscles, ligaments and bones of the feet. Being barefoot on the ground also naturally discharges built-up static electricity in the body and supports feeling more "grounded" (also great to do for a few minutes after a long flight). Next best: wear minimalist shoes or sandals, which allow maximum freedom of movement while offering protection from hard surfaces, glass, etc.

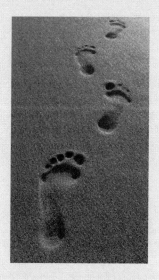

2. When wearing shoes, use optimal support for proper foundational feet alignment. This can be done with a quality support insert, such as Superfeet® insoles, which mold to the shape of your foot. Good insoles can support maximum freedom of motion of the feet while in shoes, lowering the risk of misalignment, fatigue and injury.

By balancing and thus expanding our range between these two extremes, we can enjoy enhanced foot and total skeletal alignment posture and health.

2. Hips-Heart-Head: Give Your Spine a 3H Lift

An easy to remember way to assure that your spine is aligned is the Yogic method known as the 3H Technique: Hips, Heart and Head. When your hips, heart and head are aligned, your total posture is naturally carried along into Golden Ratio alignment. This works equally well whether you're sitting or standing. Imagine a big blue (or your favorite color) helium balloon above your head. Now imagine that this balloon is gently attached to your neck and head by a harness, with just enough lift to almost—yet not quite—lift you off your feet. Imagine how your Hips, Heart and Head are gently pulled into vertical alignment, and feel the lift of your whole spine and body. Try it now. This instant and easily remembered 3H practice is great to do throughout your day and is especially valuable before, during and after exercise. Source: Master Yogi GM Khalsa, www.BreathIsLife.com

3. Restoring Your Spine's Divine Proportions

There are many highly effective methods, tools and devices to strengthen your core spinal muscles, regain and maintain healthy spinal flexibility and restore your natural Golden Ratio postural proportions. The following are a few of the author's favorites; the first was developed by co-author Robert Friedman, M.D.

- Spiral-Chi Evolutionary Movement is an innovative movement system that utilizes spinal wave motions and spiral movements to restore Golden Ratio proportions in the body. DVD available on Amazon.

- The MedX Core Spinal Fitness System™ is the world's most advanced spinal rehabilitation and core muscle strengthening equipment. It was designed by Nautilus®/Golden Ratio inventor Arthur Jones and is used by doctors and chiropractors worldwide. Profound benefits are reported from sessions lasting just 20 minutes, once or twice a month. www.CoreSpinalFitness.com

- The Body Bridge is a semicircular shaped apparatus on which you lay in order to decompress your spine and increase spinal length. By gently arching your body face-up over the Body Bridge for 3 to 5 minutes, your spine gently relaxes and decompresses. Your internal organs relax and your lungs and heart are given more space to move. www.BodyBridge.com

- The Elaine Petrone Miracle Ball Method™ uses a pair of soft, 4" air-filled balls to roll on and decompress your back. The balls are easy and fun to use and are a proven system for relieving pain and stress. www.ElainePetrone.com

- The MA Roller is a simple, do-it-yourself back massage device that stimulates acupressure points as you roll over it. It also lengthens your spine, helping restore your spine's Golden Proportions. This low-tech device has a comfortable spinal contour and is one of the quickest ways to get rid of tight spots in your back. www.TheMaRoller.com

- Exercising on a Swiss or Yoga Ball is another wonderfully simple, yet effective method for gently stretching and restoring your spine's Golden Proportions.

- Yoga, Chiropractic, Rolfing, Pilates, Alexander Technique, Feldenkrais Method and other effective body structure restoration systems.

- Two used tennis balls tied tightly together in a sock makes a great low-tech, high value spinal therapy tool. Lying down (ideally on a carpet) place such that each tennis ball is on either side of the spine starting at the base. Feel the gentle pressure of the balls and breathe into the release of tension for a few minutes. Move the balls a few inches up the spine and repeat. Continue until you reach the back of the neck. This tool is also great for travel.

- Limit added spinal disk compression by avoiding backpack use or carrying bags on your shoulders. Even moderately weighted bags can compress disks and throw off healthy posture. This especially applies to children, whose developing spines can be adversely affected by overloaded backpacks.

Remember to breathe deeply and slowly while engaging the above methods and tools. Always consult your health practitioner or physician prior to trying any of these suggested therapies.

4. Go Upside Down, Expand Your Perspective and Lengthen Your Spine

Dan Brown, bestselling author of *The Da Vinci Code*, further expands his perspective and creativity when writing by hanging upside down every hour for a few minutes, as a part of his hourly writing breaks. Should you decide to turn your world upside-down, we recommend the DEX II Spinal Decompression and Extension System, one of the most comfortable and supportive do-it-yourself gravity traction devices available. By safely supporting you by your pelvis (vs. your ankles, as in other devices), your spine gently lengthens, as it is gently tractioned by gravity. The DEX II is one of the quickest ways to give your spine a Golden Ratio tune-up. Recommended hang time is anywhere from 30 seconds up to 5 minutes. *Inversion therapy is not for everyone, as there are certain contraindications. Check with your physician before using inversion therapy.* The DEX II is available at www.EnergyCenter.com.

5. Aligning Your Spine with Nature's Path of Least Resistance

Aligning your spine with the plumb line of gravity is the best way to ensure that all of your nerves are able to function optimally, without any short-circuits or compressions. This is an awareness exercise that you can do all day long. Whether you're sitting, standing or walking, you can harmonize your posture by maintaining a buoyantly erect yet relaxed stance. A simple way to check your posture is by:

- turning sideways and looking in a mirror or glass reflection to see if your ankles, knees, hips, shoulders and ear are all in vertical alignment.
- looking in a mirror front-on to see if both eyes, shoulders, hands and hips are balanced on the horizontal plane. Pretend your body is a carpenter's level and you are trying to get the bubble to balance.

You can make subtle adjustments in your spine to balance both the sideways and front-on views of your posture, remembering that balance starts in your feet and moves up through your body. If you find that it's difficult to achieve perfect posture, you may want to begin a yoga practice as well as beginning some of the various back therapies we've recommended.

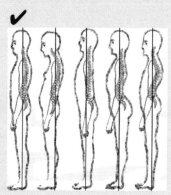

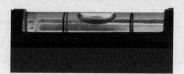

Side view posture check.
Don't slouch, and remember
to align your ankles, knees,
hips, shoulders and ear like
the example on the left.

Front view posture check.
Use the analogy of a
carpenter's level to balance
your ears, shoulders and
hips on the horizontal level.

6. iPhone/iPod/iPad *Upright*

The *Upright* is the world's first posture alert system. It's an iPhone/iPod/iPad App that lets you know whenever you slouch. The interactive program beeps, buzzes or flashes whenever your alignment goes out of vertical. Here's one of the comments from a user:

This application does exactly what it says it does. I work from home and sitting at a desk all day can wreck your back, but Upright certainly helps me to be aware of when I'm slouching. In fact, I didn't realize how bad my posture was until I bought it.

Upright is available online at: www.apple.com/iphone/appstore/

7. Golden Ratio Posture Check

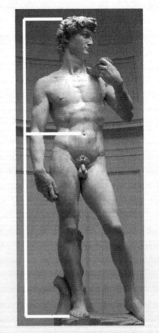

Become aware of the ratio of your upper to lower body. Take a tape measure and see what the distance is from the top of your head to your navel. Then measure the distance from the ground to your navel. The ideal ratio of your upper to your lower body should come close to 0.62. There are natural variations above and below 0.62, depending on your body type. Add a daily dose of postural awareness, exercise and stretching to your regimen to help restore your body to its natural Golden Proportions and healthy functioning.

8. Sitting Pretty: Avoiding Sitting Death Syndrome

Those who sit less live longer than those who sit more. A massive 13-year study of over 123,216 healthy men and women by the American Cancer Society (ACS) revealed sobering details about an element of daily life most people do in excess without thinking twice. As reported by CNN senior medical producer Danielle Dellorto (7/22/10) and reporter William Hudson (6/24/11):

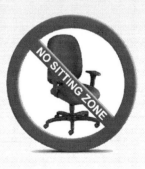

- Sitting for several hours each day does significant damage to human health—*which cannot be undone by exercising.*
- The percentage of women who sat for more than 6 hours a day who were more likely to die during the ACS study was about 40%; for men, about 20%.
- Even when people do significant and regular exercise, they still increase their risks of serious illness from hours of physical inactivity.

Hudson also points out that:

these findings are also consistent with lifestyles in so-called "Blue Zones," longevity hotspots places such as Okinawa, Japan, and Sardinia, Italy, where people live much longer on average than the rest of the developed world (see chapter 10 for more on Blue Zones). In addition to plant-based diets and strong communities, near-constant moderate physical activity is the norm in these areas. More Americans are adapting modern work environments to suit these physiological needs better by installing standing and adjustable desks that allow for switching between sitting and standing positions, and treadmill desks, which operate at low walking speeds.

Some suggested new habits to address the dangers of sitting for too long:

• Sit less—get out of your chair more often, every 20-30 minutes at a minimum, even for a short walk to get some fresh air, stretch and get your blood circulating better. This is especially important on planes, to reduce the risk of potentially deadly blood clots forming.

• In addition to sitting tall and bouyantly with good posture, gently rock or spiral from time to time (see the top of page 196 for a simple and effective Golden Spiral sitting exercise). Even a little movement is a good thing while sitting.

• Vary your sitting position from time to time. Experiment sitting cross-legged on the floor if possible (interestingly, the majority of the world's population does not sit in chairs and are healthier for it).

• Standing at your desk can also be a healthy alternative to sitting.

• As with breathing, the important thing is to sit consciously. Don't allow yourself to sit on autopilot.

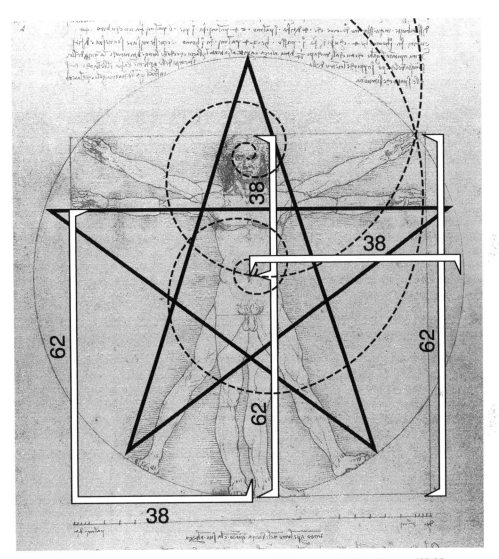

Da Vinci's *Vitruvian Man*, showing some of the many Golden Ratios (62:38 measurements) in the structure of the body. When posture is aligned and healthy our body's natural Golden Ratios are enhanced, as is our health and longevity.

5

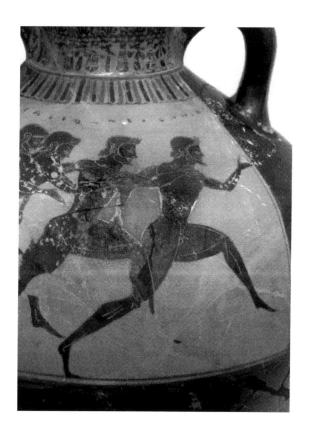

Greek vase with runners at the Panathenaic Games,

530 B.C. Phidippides (Φειδιππιδης), a hero of Ancient Greece,

is the key figure in a myth which inspired the modern

26.2 mile marathon; note that 26.2 is a Golden Ratio

multiple, as 1.618 x 1.618 x 10 = 26.2

6.

EXERCISE:
GOLDEN RATIO MOTION

Nature's Path of Least Resistance and
Maximum Performance follows the Golden Mean.
Dr. Ronald Sandler, Golden Ratio Peak Performance Pioneer

Exercise holds a unique place in the Golden Ratio Lifestyle Diet in that it unifies all of the other drivers into a powerful cross-reinforcing system of health and longevity. When you exercise you need to breathe as well as drink water and have adequate nutrients on board. You also have to be well rested and maintain good posture for a healthy workout. Ideally you will also break a sweat and get rid of some toxins, while at the same time releasing natural feel-good endorphins. Not only will your physical structure, personal power and attractiveness improve, you will also end up feeling happier, with a greater sense of inner purpose and peace. If you continue this process over many decades, you may very well end up living vibrantly to a ripe old age.

One of the hallmarks of the Golden Ratio is the principle of unification that arises when Golden Ratio relationships are established between the individual parts of any system of practice. In the case of the Golden Ratio Lifestyle Diet, a higher order of functioning emerges when all of the drivers are fine-tuned to the Golden Ratio. This especially applies to Golden Ratio Lifestyle Diet Driver #6, Exercise. Of all that has been written about exercise, very little has focused on the application of the Golden Ratio to working out. Research has shown that either too little or too much exercise is a risk factor for sudden cardiac death, but the billion-dollar question is: how much exercise is ideal for you? There must be a way to customize exercise to each individual's specific needs and requirements. That way is of course by applying the universal principle of the Golden Ratio to exercise. Let's begin by looking at the remarkable Golden Ratio anatomy and physiology of the heart.

Our Golden Ratio Designed Holographic Hearts

Blood does not flow in a straight line as it courses through our arteries and veins—it actually flows in a multitude of spirals and vortices. Likewise, our hearts don't move like linear up-and-down pistons as we might have thought. Instead, our hearts contract and relax in elegantly efficient Golden Spiral, corkscrew-like motions. The electrical signature of the heart directly reflects the Golden Ratio as well. Contraction and relaxation phases are in clear Golden Ratio. This can be easily seen on an electrocardiogram ECG, a.k.a. EKG. During the contraction phase, blood moves into your body and lungs. When your heart relaxes, blood moves from your body and lungs back to the heart. A dynamic interaction between lung and heart activity is required for efficient oxygenation and release of carbon dioxide to occur. At rest, the approximate ratio of respirations to heartbeats also reflects the Golden Ratio:

$$\textbf{(Respirations/Heartbeats) x 10 = 1.6}$$

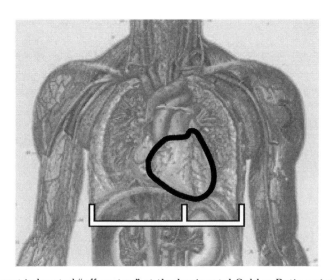

The human heart is located "off-center," at the horizontal Golden Ratio point of the chest.

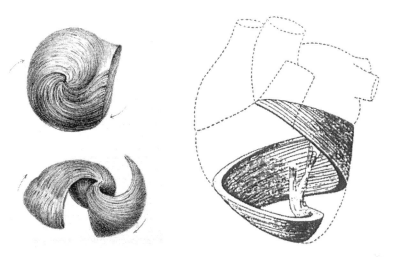

Our hearts are aligned structurally and functionally with the Golden Ratio.
Note the multiple Golden Spirals in our heart's design.

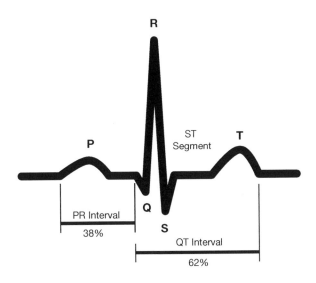

The electrocardiogram/ECG is an electrical snapshot of the contraction
and relaxation phases in a heartbeat. Many Golden Ratios between
waveform sections can be found within an idealized ECG, e.g.,
QT Interval (62%) / PR Interval (38%) = Φ (the Golden Ratio)

P wave: Atrial Depolarization; contraction of the atria (upper chambers
of the heart). QRS complex: Ventricular Depolarization; contraction of
the ventricles (the heart's large pumping muscles). T wave: Ventricular
Repolarization; the heart's state of filling and relaxation. ST segment:
Time between end of contraction and beginning of repolarization/relaxation.

181

For example, a person with a respiratory rate of 12 breaths/min. and a resting heart rate of 75 beats/min. will have this ratio:

$$(12 \div 75) \times 10 = 1.6$$

If you have ever hyperventilated or had a panic attack, you know how it feels to have your respirations and heart rate go out of Golden Ratio. Referring to recent research in neurocardiology, Joseph Chilton Pearce, in *The Biology of Transcendence*, notes that,

> *About sixty to sixty-five percent of all the cells in the heart are neural cells, which are precisely the same as in the brain, functioning in precisely the same way, monitoring and maintaining control of the entire mind/brain/body physical process as well as direct unmediated connections between the heart and the emotional, cognitive structures of the brain.*

Of course, the 60 to 65% of heart cells, which are neurons, makes one think again of the 62% Golden Ratio. In order for the heart to be the super-efficient, lifetime pump that it is, Nature had to engineer the Golden Ratio into both its anatomical and physiological design. The heart neurons have three main functions. First, they are responsible for the spark of life, which are the neuron's electrical pacemaker function. Second, the neurons conduct these electrical impulses throughout the heart, causing the heart to rhythmically contract and relax with miraculous precision over a lifetime. The third function, which Pearce describes, is the direct communication and ongoing dialogue between the heart and the emotional-cognitive brain. The unifying ability of the Golden Ratio integrates both head and heart through Divine Proportion into the holographic heart-mind.

6

Nature's Secret Nutrient (NSN) for Predictable Peak Performance

All athletes—from the elite level to the weekend warrior—are looking for that special nutrient that will give them the edge. For some athletes, that edge may be vitamins, minerals or herbs; for others it may be steroids, blood doping or other illegal adaptogenic substances. What few have realized, however, is that Nature's Secret Nutrient (NSN) is one of the most potent performance enhancers available. It's also legal—and free. The first to describe the workings of this special nutrient in the fitness and peak performance arenas was Dr. Ronald Sandler, a top podiatrist in Houston, Texas. In 1982, Dr. Sandler began his ground-breaking work on an ingenious exercise and training system based on the Golden Ratio. He subsequently perfected his system through decades of scientific studies, personal experience and real-world application with his patients and athletes from nearly every sport. For athletes, Dr. Sandler's system system shows you how to successfully plan ahead for peak athletic performance and avoid injury. Best of all, it applies equally well to both competitive and non-competitive athletes. Dr. Sandler discovered how to maximize the impact of any workout, regardless of intensity, without investing unnecessary effort and time—and without getting injured. As Dr. Sandler and the many athletes he's worked with have shown, the secret to injury-free exercise and peak performance lies within the simple yet profound application of the Golden Ratio. Every athlete—whether competitive or those simply wishing to stay fit—knows that some days you just don't have it, no matter how

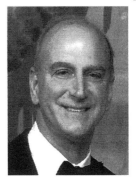

Dr. Ronald Sandler, Golden Ratio Peak Performance Pioneer.

consistently or how hard you might train. Yet on other days you feel an unexpected though welcome surge from within that enables you to turn in a great performance. How can one better understand those days of surprising, sustained energy and those of unexpected lethargy? The secret lies in honoring the ratios of proper exercise and rest periods required to balance and energize your total workout regimen. Dr. Sandler's system uses precise cycles or ratios of training and rest tuned to the Golden Ratio. This allows you to actually schedule and predict optimal results on the days you want them. See the Golden Ratio Workout Wave™ on page 185 for more detail. Dr. Sandler's approach has proven safe and remarkably effective for both beginners and seasoned athletes. He decodes both why peak performances occur and how to plan for them. He shows how you can achieve predictable quality results without injury, illness or burnout—all typical outcomes of many training systems. Following the old adage of "no pain, no gain" actually increases your susceptibility to injury and burnout. It sets you up to work against Nature's Path of Least Resistance, as opposed to having a strong, steady wind at your back. For the competitive athlete, confidence in one's ability to hit a peak on a crucial day comes not only from the knowledge that you've put in many hours of training, positive thinking and visualization. It also comes from strategically modifying your training schedule by aligning rest and activity periods to cycles mapped to the Golden Ratio.

Peak Performance on Demand

According to Dr. Sandler, to perform at your best you select a target date in the future, e.g., a race or other competition, when you want to experience peak performance. You then schedule backwards from that date, creating a springboard that positions you for peak performance on your chosen day. From his experience, Dr. Sandler suggests a three-month or longer cycle of training and rest for major events like marathons; a three-week cycle for smaller events such as shorter road races; and a three-day cycle just before your event for the final catapult effect. These suggestions assume that you have already built an initial training base, whether small or large. For optimal results all three cycles may be blended together; it depends on how much time remains before your event. Dr. Sandler's system can also be easily adapted to greatly minimize or even eliminate injury, and support peak performance on a regular basis for those athletes who compete frequently. Everyone's body has natural cycles of ups and downs. If you don't believe it, Dr. Sandler says, keep your own workout records for three to five months. Each day note how you feel about your physical stamina and strength. For example: Rate your day's workout on a scale from 1 to 10, where 10 is a great day; 5 is average; 1 is a day when you barely get through your workout. When you study your workout records, you'll recognize the natural rising and falling performance cycles typical of the Golden Ratio workout waves which naturally occur in your body. It's all part of our Divinely-tuned physiologic cycles. Learning to manage those cycles so that you can maintain energy and drive (and peak when you want to if you're competitive) is what Dr. Sandler's program supports. Again, the system results in two major benefits:

★ By training in accordance with the Golden Ratio you greatly reduce the potential for injury.

★ You can actually predict and schedule in advance—with 90% or better accuracy—when your peak day will be, weeks and even months ahead of your event. The predictive power of this universal principle applies to all sports at all levels, from weekend warrior to world champion.

The Fibonacci-based Elliott Wave cycle used by stock traders is the secret behind Dr. Sandler's magic formula. He translates Elliott Wave cycles and Fibonacci/Golden Ratios into days and types of training and rest. By simply learning to calculate and map your up and down periods, you can predict and control—to the day—when you will peak. For the average exerciser, this means you don't need to force yourself to exercise when overly tired, because you know you'll gain more from resting and allowing your body to regenerate. On rest days you could take a short easy walk to keep your body loose—but not a fast one that would create an aerobic training effect. Dr. Sandler's Golden Ratio-based theory suggests that performance moves in waves, which consist of sub-peaks, and that your overall up cycles are larger than your down cycles. This means that each complete cycle ends with your performance at a higher baseline than

GOLDEN RATIO WORKOUT WAVE™

The Golden Ratio Workout Wave is based on the work of sports performance pioneer Dr. Ronald Sandler. The original Elliott Wave, which inspired Dr. Sandler, was discovered by economist R.N. Elliott and further developed by macro-economist Robert Prechter, Jr. The Wave reflects the natural growth expansion/contraction cycles found throughout Nature, which mirror the Golden Ratio/Fibonacci Sequence. Dr. Sandler calls it using *Nature's Path of Least Resistance and Maximum Efficiency.* Tuning your workout and rest/recovery periods to the Wave offers these key benefits:

- The Wave provides a flexible method to harness our body's natural physiological performance cycles. Exercising on this Golden Ratio Wave of rising and falling intensities naturally increases performance capabilities and results, simultaneously reducing/eliminating overuse injuries. This also keeps workouts fresh and interesting, avoiding boredom and burnout.

- Builds in vital rest periods to support healthy recovery/recharge; also feels great to be working with your body's natural workout and recharge cycles.

- For competitive athletes, supports predictable peak performance on future selected competition days: puts the wind at your back when you need it most.

- For fitness and recreational exercisers, steadily builds energy and fitness in a safe and predictable way.

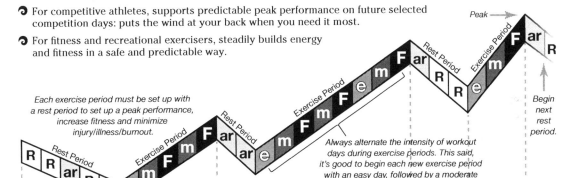

Each exercise period must be set up with a rest period to set up a peak performance, increase fitness and minimize injury/illness/burnout.

Always alternate the intensity of workout days during exercise periods. This said, it's good to begin each new exercise period with an easy day, followed by a moderate one, before going to full intensity days.

Peak ──►

Begin next rest period.

Days: 5   5   2   8   3   3

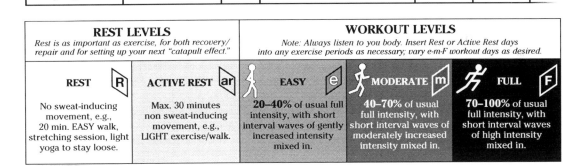

REST LEVELS		WORKOUT LEVELS		
Rest is as important as exercise, for both recovery/ repair and for setting up your next "catapult effect."		*Note: Always listen to you body. Insert Rest or Active Rest days into any exercise periods as necessary; vary e-m-F workout days as desired.*		
REST [R]	**ACTIVE REST** [ar]	**EASY** [e]	**MODERATE** [m]	**FULL** [F]
No sweat-inducing movement, e.g., 20 min. EASY walk, stretching session, light yoga to stay loose.	Max. 30 minutes non sweat-inducing movement, e.g., LIGHT exercise/walk.	**20–40%** of usual full intensity, with short interval waves of gently increased intensity mixed in.	**40–70%** of usual full intensity, with short interval waves of moderately increased intensity mixed in.	**70–100%** of usual full intensity, with short interval waves of high intensity mixed in.

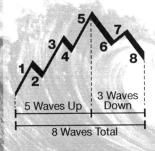

5 Waves Up   3 Waves Down

8 Waves Total

The Essential Elliott Wave
has an up wave and a down wave which are in 5:3 ratio to one another. In the up wave there are 3 waves up and 2 down; in the down wave there are 2 waves down and 1 up. These sequenced waves repeat infinitely.

- The rest/recovery periods or "down slopes" are the hidden, secret weapons that many people neglect, but without which you can't access Nature's "catapult effect" and rise to new levels of health, fitness and performance.

- The steepness of Wave segments are unrelated to the steepness or grade of the terrain upon which you're exercising. They simply illustrate a steady and consistent rise in your fitness level, especially over time.

- The Workout Wave can be scaled up to include weeks/months or down to a single workout, e.g., it transforms interval training sessions (see: Fibonacci Interval Training/FIT Rx's, end of this chapter).

- Always begin workouts with a gentle warm-up of approximately 13 minutes, followed by some short, easy stretches of maximum 2 seconds each.

- Follow the Golden Ratio Lifestyle Diet's Air-Water-Sleep-Nutrition-Posture-Exercise regimen. Best to skip a workout if *any* of the 5 preceding health drivers which support optimal exercise are insufficient. Light activity such as walking or gentle yoga is generally always OK.

- Utilizing the Fibonacci Sequence Numbers (1, 1, 2, 3, 5, 8, 13, 21...) for your rest/workout periods automatically builds in the 62/38 Golden Ratio, as the ratios *between* the Fibonacci numbers mirrors the Golden Ratio of 1.62:1. The rest period is generally the smaller of the rest and workout periods.

when you began—and your next upward cycle will start from that higher level. This illustrates a two steps forward, one step back principle of progressive improvement (in Fibonacci terms, five steps forward and three steps back). This builds a natural catapult/regenerative effect into your workout sessions.

Dave Scott and the Secret Power of Rest and Recovery

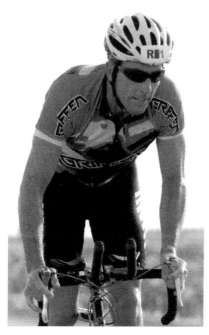

Dave "The Man" Scott, 6-time Ironman World Triathlon Champion.

Among his compelling research stories, Dr. Sandler describes how Dave Scott, six-time winner of the grueling Ironman Triathlon, unknowingly utilized the essential Fibonacci-based Golden Ratio training technique enroute to his 1986 and 1987 victories. The legendary Scott found himself forced to take many "rest" periods of three to five days, due to speaking engagements and other commitments, before the 1986 and 1987 races. Initially, Scott was concerned that these unplanned rest periods might negatively affect his performance. To his surprise however, the opposite proved to be the case:

The more time I missed the better I did. After about five days off I felt lethargic and stiff, but then I felt better in training than before.

In the 1986 Ironman, Scott turned in a course record. In 1987 he won again, in what he considered to be his best race—even though his time was five minutes slower than in 1986, due to much tougher conditions including severe headwinds. Scott's unintentional, Golden Ratio resting periods clearly played a strategic role in his triumphs. As an interesting footnote, Scott retired from competition in 1989 at age 35, around the time Dr. Sandler introduced him to the Golden Ratio training technique.

Five years later at age 40, Scott made a stunning comeback at the Ironman, coming out of retirement to celebrate becoming the first inductee into the Ironman Hall of Fame. His finishing time in that year, 1994, was good enough for second place, *eclipsing all six of his previous first-place finish times*. In 1996, at age 42, Scott came back again, this time placing fifth at the Ironman. Dave clocked his third-fastest personal best time—which again beat all six of his previous first-place finish times.

Dave Scott's Ironman Finish Times

Year	Age	Place	Time
1980	26	1	9:24:33
1982	28	1	9:08:23
1983	29	1	9:05:57
1984	30	1	8:54:20
1986	32	1	8:28:37
1987	33	1	8:34:13
1994	40	2*	**8:24:32**
1996	42	5	**8:28:31**

6-time Hawaiian World Ironman Triathlon Champion Dave Scott's 1st place finish times, along with his 2nd and 5th place times achieved seven and nine years after his last 1st place finish. Note how *both* of Scott's finish times at ages 40 (2nd place) and 42 (5th place) were faster than *all* six of his 1st place times in his prime—an astonishing feat. Scott was introduced to Dr. Ronald Sandler's Golden Ratio peak performance training system around 1990. Interestingly, during the period in which he won all six of his Hawaiian Ironman triathlons, Scott followed a 100% vegetarian (vegan) diet.
Scott (then aged 40) missed winning his 7th Ironman by just four minutes.

Variability Adds Efficiency

It is known that varying your training intensity is the best way to promote the health and efficiency of your cardiovascular system. For instance, you wouldn't want to exclusively use the traditional long-slow-distance (LSD) method as did Jim Fixx, author of *The Complete Book of Running*. In using the LSD method, Fixx likely decreased the efficiency of his cardiovascular system over time, which contributed to predisposing him to the sudden-death heart attack from which he died in his early forties (poor diet, stress, etc., were also likely contributing factors). It is far healthier to include some variability within the duration and intensity of your individual workouts, as well as between your workouts over time.

In running, this practice is known variously as fartlek training, tempo running, intervals or speed play, where you mix in sprints of various lengths and intensity during the course of a run. A good metaphor is the shifting of gears in a car's transmission. For maximum fuel efficiency and minimum wear, we upshift or downshift as appropriate, sometimes paying attention to the tachometer so we don't redline or over-rev the engine. While this process happens automatically in an automatic transmission, it's a good idea for us to take an involved, manual transmission approach during exercise. We can minimize the effects of overly red-lining our body and simultaneously enhance our performance by shifting or varying our gears during our exercise sessions. Being sensitive to your body's performance and needs increases your range and overall health, as opposed to exercising on autopilot.

Again, as with a car, exercise should always begin with an adequate warm-up phase, before shifting into the higher intensity workout phases. Ideally your warm-up should be of sufficient duration so that you break a light sweat, usually after about 13 minutes. This signals that your body has reached a safe operating temperature, which helps you get the most from your workout and avoid injury. Reversing this process by allowing an adequate cool-down time, gradually decreasing exercise intensity at the end of your workout, completes the easy up/workout/easy down optimum exercise cycle. This is why track athletes take an extra cool-down lap after their races. This practice also makes it far easier for your body to process excess adrenaline and neutralize accumulated lactic acid in the muscles. As with a car, we want to be sure to always warm up to more strenuous activity, while allowing an ample cool-down period of gradually decreasing activity afterwards.

6

Balancing Exercise and Rest: How Working Smarter vs. Harder Can Deliver a 50% Gain by Splitting Workout Sessions in Two

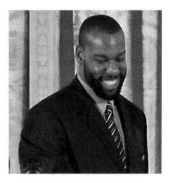

NBA basketball star Baron Davis, who demonstrated the great benefits of split workouts for peak performance and recovery.

When NBA superstar Baron Davis was with the New Orleans Hornets basketball team, he demonstrated the benefits of splitting workouts. Due to overtraining and resultant poor performance, Davis' $80 million contract was in jeopardy. Instead of continuing his downward spiral by working out for six hours straight as was his usual practice, Davis' lead trainer Dartgnan Stamps split his off-season daily training regimen into two separate sessions—one in the morning and the other that afternoon. In so doing, the men took advantage of a little-known concept in fitness dynamics.

By breaking his workout in two—with rest and refueling in between—Davis was able to substantially increase the impact of his training. He regained his superstar status and was then able to perform at his full potential. For the average person, this means that two separate

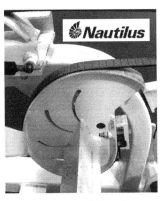

The secret of Nautilus exercise equipment: the variable resistance Golden Spiral cam.

20 minute sessions, with rest and refueling in between could be as beneficial as one continuous 60 minute workout. This simple yet powerful method of achieving more results with less effort was successful because of the increase of the *ratio* of rest to exercise.

Another example of benefits obtained from increasing the rest-to-exercise ratio is research conducted at the Human Energy Research Laboratory at the University of Pittsburgh. The study revealed the hidden advantages of multiple, shorter daily workouts. It showed that women who did two or three separate daily 15–20 minute workouts—instead of the typical longer 30–60 minute single workout—burned more fat and lost up to 25% more weight. They were also far more likely to stick with their exercise regimen over time. This research exploded the popular myth that one has to exercise for at least 20-30 minutes in order to receive an aerobic or fat burning benefit. Multiple exercise sessions, as short as even 10-15 minutes each, can provide greater benefits than longer single workout sessions.

In these examples, the subjects were honoring the crucial rest phase in relation to the exercise period and reaping the benefits. You can also strongly amplify the positive effects of your exercise by simply breaking it into two or more smaller sessions over the course of a day. This practice maximizes recovery and healing while simultaneously minimizing the chances of burnout and injury. When you know that two daily workouts as short as 10 minutes each can actually be equivalent to 30 minutes of total exercise, you're far more likely to get in that 10 minute walk or run in the morning and then again in the evening. An easy way to incorporate the Golden Ratio into a split workout would be to have a 13 (or 21) minute AM workout, followed by a 21 (or 34) minute PM workout. Depending on your goals and available time the duration of the ratios could be lengthened to different Fibonacci Ratios: 34/55, 55/89, etc.

Iron rusts from disuse; water loses its purity from stagnation...
even so does inaction sap the vigor of the mind.
Leonardo Da Vinci

The Power of High Intensity Training (HIT)

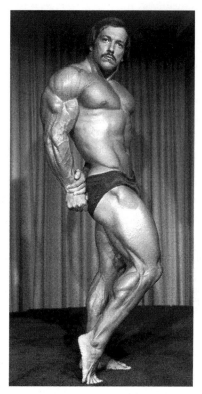

Casey Viator, youngest-ever
Mr. America (age 19) and High
Intensity Training (HIT) pioneer.

Golden Ratio Genius Arthur Jones is the pioneer behind the Nautilus exercise system. He harnessed Nature's Path of Least Resistance by mirroring the curves of the Fibonacci Spiral-shaped Nautilus shell in exercise equipment design. This innovation enabled full muscular activation at every degree of a joint's range of motion. Jones' genius didn't stop with just *designing* revolutionary exercise equipment; he also invented a super-efficient way of *using* the equipment: the HIT method (High Intensity Training). The HIT exercise method complemented his Nautilus exercise equipment, enabling him to produce some of the world's greatest body builders, including at age 19, the youngest-ever Mr. America, Casey Viator. Using the HIT method, Viator attained uncanny Golden Ratio-like measurements in his Greek-God-like appearance. The essence of the HIT method is to use maximal exertion with minimal repetitions, followed by longer than accustomed recuperation periods. Muscle fibers can thus be super-stimulated into maximal hypertrophy (growth) in a minimal amount of time.

The results obtained were simply phenomenal, as evidenced by the flurry of bodybuilding adherents to the HIT system. Another one of Jones' protégés was the amazing Mike Mentzer, a Mr. America and Mr. Olympia winner. Mentzer claimed that for optimal results in bodybuilding the workouts needed to be **brief, infrequent and intense**. His definitive work on the subject is *High-Intensity Training the Mike Mentzer Way*.

Intriguingly, the power of HIT workouts aren't limited only to anaerobic strength training and bodybuilding. They are easily adapted to *any* sport, including running, swimming, cycling and even calisthenics. The earliest application of a HIT-like workout in the cardio/aerobic training arena was fartlek or speed play interval training, originated in 1937 by Swedish running coach Gösta Holmér. Fartlek training alternates periods of jogging interspersed with sprinting in order to increase the runner's dynamism and efficiency. Fartlek training can be shifted into overdrive via HIT methods. Speed play would now become, as Mentzer would say, brief, infrequent and intense. A series of short all-out sprints, each separated by a variable recovery period would constitute the 2 to 3 times a week HIT workouts. The entire workout could be as short as 13-21 minutes, as opposed to traditional and tedious long-distance workouts. Research into HIT for runners is corroborating what Jones, Viator and Mentzer proved decades ago by bulk example: HIT methods are a super-efficient way to train and can be done in a fraction of the time required for traditional workouts. According to McMaster University kinesiology professor Martin Gibala,

> *Our study demonstrates that interval-based exercise is a very time-efficient training strategy. This type of training is very demanding and requires a high level of motivation. However, short bursts of intense exercise may be an effective option for individuals who cite 'lack of time' as a major impediment to fitness.*

In addition to dramatically reducing workout time, HIT methods also build lean body mass, increase metabolic rate and fat burning, and stimulates the release of growth hormone, which speeds healing, lifts the mood and prolongs youth. Increasing metabolic rate is the golden key to fat burning—and most amazingly, the weight loss that happens during the 24-48 hours *after* a workout. Paradoxically, the actual number of calories burned during a workout is insignificant compared to the number burned *after you're done working out...* even when you're sleeping! An easy way to see what HIT sprinting does for muscle building is to compare the physiques of sprinters, middle distance runners and long distance runners. Sprinters like world record holder Usain Bolt and former Olympic Champions Carl Lewis and Michael Johnson have highly developed, muscular bodies. Middle distance runners are more lithe and less muscled up, while long distance runners often have a thin, almost emaciated look. Not everyone has the time or desire to develop his or her muscles or endurance to the Olympic level. However, by taking the essence of HIT techniques and adapting them to a modern-day, busy lifestyle, one can reap incredible benefits with amazingly little time... and with just a little more effort/intensity for short bursts during exercise sessions.

Get Fit Fast With Fibonacci Interval Training (FIT)

The Golden Ratio Lifestyle Diet catapults the proven HIT method to the next level by applying Golden Ratio principles to HIT. This powerful upgrade creates the FIT system: Fibonacci Interval Training™. As we've seen in Dr. Ronald Sandler's Golden Ratio training breakthrough, he optimizes activity and rest periods according to Fibonacci Ratios. The Golden Ratio Workout Wave uses

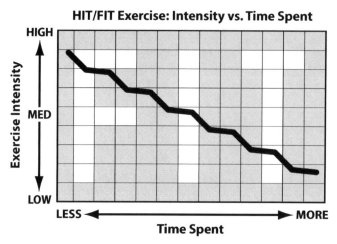

HIT/FIT Exercise: Intensity vs. Time Spent

From HIT (High Intensity Training) to FIT (Fibonacci Interval Training).
In HIT/FIT workouts, time spent exercising is inversely proportional to
exercise intensity. Translation: greater intensity delivers more benefit in
less time. When HIT is fused with FIT we get super-fit.

Fibonacci Ratios between activity and rest periods not only on a weekly and monthly basis, it also moves down to the next fractal levels and uses the ratios between each sprint and recovery period within single workout sessions. Here's a quick review of the beginning numbers of the Fibonacci Sequence:

6

0, 1, 1, 2, 3, 5, 8, 13, 21, 34, 55, 89, 144, 233, 377, 610…

For example, if your first sprint was 21 seconds your next one might be 34 seconds, followed by 55 seconds and then 89 seconds. You would also embed Fibonacci Ratios into your rest periods, such that if your first sprint was 21 seconds, you might rest for 34 or 55 seconds—or some Fibonacci harmonic, e.g., 89, 144 or 233 seconds… as long as you need for your heart rate to recover. This sets up your internal catapult for maximum energy in your next burst. This flexibility scales and individualizes the workout to whatever your endurance capacity is at the time. What's important to remember here is the 60/40 or 40/60 *ratio*, not necessarily the actual Fibonacci Sequence numbers. Remember that 60/40 is an easy-to-use approximation of the 62/38 Golden Ratio. While Fibonacci numbers are an easy way to practically work with the ratio during your workouts, you can also take any number and simply multiply it by 1.6 (or 0.6) to find your ratio. For example, if you ran for 10 seconds you could rest for 16 seconds (10 x 1.6 = 16). Other Fibonacci variables that can individualize your workouts are the number of sprints per set and the total number of sets per day, week and month. Remember that even intensity can be a variable in FIT workouts; you don't necessarily need to go all-out to reap the benefits of FIT workouts. If you are a beginner, out-of-shape or have a medical condition, you will first need to be evaluated by your physician with a maximal cardiac stress test, to ensure that your cardiovascular system is up to the task of the increased intensity that typifies the FIT method. You would then be cleared to establish a baseline of endurance before beginning your FIT workouts. This is best achieved, at least initially, with the guidance of a personal trainer. In the Rx section at the end of this chapter there are several examples of easy and advanced FIT protocols that can be applied to running, cycling, swimming or any other exercise you choose. The results will amaze you.

The Golden Olympic Training Ratio: *GOT Ratio?*

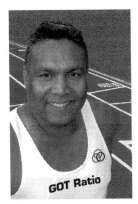

Dawn Saidur is a former world-class sprinter and the first person from Bangladesh to represent his country at the Olympics (1984, Los Angeles). Dawn now lives in Mamaroneck, NY, where he owns the popular Mozart Café. As a sports performance psychologist, he also trains a variety of competitive athletes. Dawn notes that the optimal training ratio or time spent on endurance, strength and flexibility, regardless of one's total weekly training hours, is not simply an even three-way split. Instead, this Golden Olympic Training Ratio turns out to be a 40/30/30 split, tailored to your sport.

Olympic sprinter Dawn Saidur, proponent of the Golden Ratio-based **G**olden **O**lympic **T**raining Ratio: *GOT Ratio?*

6

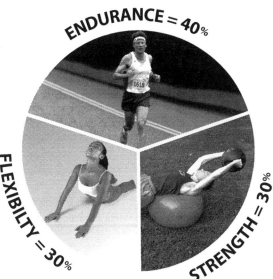

Example endurance-weighted **G**olden **O**lympic **T**raining Ratio of endurance, strength and flexibility; the larger segment is always weighted towards your chosen sport's focus.

Recall the Golden Ratio Nutrition Decoder from chapter 4/Nutrition: a 40:30:30 ratio can be reconfigured to be a 40:60 (30+30=60) ratio, which is a good approximation of the 38:62 Golden Ratio. 40:30:30 offers a dynamic balance of the three key cross-reinforcing exercise disciplines. The example graph on the previous page is weighted towards endurance: 40%. If you wanted to increase your strength for a specific sport, you'd simply switch the ratio positions of the disciplines, e.g., your strength training would move into the 40% ratio position. Accordingly, if you needed more flexibility, you would increase the flexibility-training ratio to 40%, and so on. Finding your personal Golden Olympic Training Ratio is a golden key to increasing the efficiency and enjoyment of whatever your sport or exercise regimen may be.

Golden Ratio-based Active Isolated Stretching (AIS)

An alternative method for rapidly and safely restoring our full Range Of Motion (ROM) was developed by peak performance pioneer Aaron L. Mattes. Mattes' clients have included football legend Johnny Unitas, world #1 ranked tennis players Pete Sampras and Andre Agassi, Olympians Carl Lewis and Michael Johnson, basketball greats Michael Jordan and Shaquille O'Neill and countless other collegiate and professional athletes. Mattes' Active Isolated Stretching (AIS) system restores flexibility to muscles, tendons and joints, increasing optimal movement potential. The goal is balanced holistic stretching, which restores optimal range of motion. Mattes discovered that our muscles can stretch 1.6 times (the Golden Ratio) their resting length before they will tear. This is yet another fascinating example of how the Golden Ratio is embedded in our physiology at all levels. Mattes' stretching method might be considered revolutionary, according to conventional wisdom. For example, he is a strong proponent of short, dynamic stretches vs. long, static stretches. Mattes says that the longest a stretch should be held for is *2 seconds*. 6-time Ironman World Champion triathlete and

Relaxed Muscle Length	**1.0**
Maximum Muscle Stretch Range	**1.6**

The Golden Ratio Muscle Stretch Range. As Aaron Mattes reports in his Active Isolating Stretching (AIS) system, our muscles will stretch 1.6 times—the Golden Ratio—their resting length before tearing. Mattes advises not holding any maximum stretch longer than 2 seconds; 6-time World Ironman Triathlon Champion Mark Allen suggests a half second or less.

Outside magazine's *World's Fittest Man* Mark Allen told co-author Matthew Cross that stretches should not exceed half a second. According to *Stretching USA*:

> *Over the past decades many experts have advocated prolonged stretches up to 60 seconds. For years, this prolonged static stretch technique was the gold standard. Prolonged static stretching actually decreases the blood flow within the tissue creating localized ischemia and lactic acid buildup. This potentiates irritation or injury of local muscular, tendinous, lymphatic as well as neural tissues, similar to the effects and consequences of trauma and overuse syndromes.*

The Mattes Method of Active Isolated Stretching (AIS) challenges long-standing beliefs popular in yoga and other traditional stretching systems. The age-old notion of holding stretches for prolonged periods needs critical reevaluation. Mattes' research clearly indicates that remaining in a pose for an extended amount of time may not be the optimal way to stretch. In addition to inhibiting protective stretch reflex mechanisms, holding postures and stretches too long can cause actual tissue suffocation, enabling lactic acid and other metabolites to build up to toxic levels. Long-held static stretches prevents the adequate blood circulation needed to oxygenate tissues and clear toxins. Muscular micro-tears are far more likely under these hypoxic (low oxygen) conditions. Newer approaches to stretching, such as Mattes' AIS system—with full stretches not exceeding 2 seconds—and the flowing movements of yoga, Spiral-Chi and similar dynamic movement systems are recommended. These can break the spell of other potentially damaging stretching methods.

6

Golden Ratio Movement

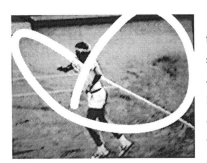

A great example of natural spiral movement: tennis great Bjorn Borg's forehand stroke.

Eastern mind-body disciplines such as yoga, tai-chi, karate and other martial arts are based on systems that integrate our spine, bones, muscles and organs with a much larger electromagnetic field. These disciplines teach you to be consciously aware of your body and its responses as you perform certain movements. Since your body's structure and form is designed according to the Golden Ratio, you will find that your body naturally functions best when moving according to the Golden Spiral. A simple exercise example follows:

Sitting with your spine erect and weight equally balanced on your sitz bones (your derriere's bony part), begin to move your pelvis in a gentle spiraling motion, starting in the center of an imaginary spiral and unwinding 3 times, tracing an expanding Golden Spiral. Then, spiral back to the center by reversing the exercise. These spirals can be traced in both clockwise and counterclockwise directions. Note that the Golden Spiral moves up through the spine and entire body, even though it's initiated in your pelvis. As you spiral back to center, the center of the spiral may even feel like a gentle still point.

When we move in Golden Spirals, we are moving along Nature's Path of Least Resistance and Maximum Performance. Let your body get a sense of this natural integration of form and function. Develop your ability to recognize spiral tendencies in your movements. This is the way Nature intended you to move. All of your joints are designed to move according to the Golden Ratio; whenever it's a conscious part of your exercise you send a message to your whole body to reactivate the Golden Ratio. Many people take up practices like yoga and tai-chi to address and reduce physical problems such as fatigue, stress, back pain, insomnia, etc. In addition to addressing these conditions, moving in Golden Spirals restores physical balance, coordination and timing. It reintegrates the physical structure of your body. This will positively transfer to any sport or movement routine you participate in. For example, a golf swing contains multi-dimensional spiral motions, as do the movements in many other sports, such as tennis strokes. Awareness of this simple fact may encourage you to emphasize smooth, natural spiral motions into your movements. This is how everything in Nature most efficiently moves. Once reactivated, the Golden Ratio will support your body in moving with minimal resistance and maximum efficiency, while greatly lessening the chance of injury.

6

The most perfect actions mirror the patterns found in Nature.
Morihei Ueshiba, founder of Aikido

Rob Moses and David Carradine: Spiral Fitness and the Human Gear

Sifu Rob Moses is the Kung Fu wizard behind the cutting-edge Spiral Fitness System, whose movements mirror the Golden Ratio geometry found in Nature. Through his system the original, more aggressive animal archetypes of Kung Fu have been transformed into more gentle and peaceful movements. Rob's best-known student was *Kung Fu's* David Carradine, who he trained for over 25 years. Together they worked on three movies: *Kung Fu, The Legend Continues* and Quentin Tarantino's *Kill Bill*

I & II. Moses took Nature's invisible Path of Least Resistance and manifested it in his PhysioStix—a Fibonacci-based fitness/workout stick—which he describes as follows:

Humankind has harnessed natural movement for exercise, healing and survival. Throughout history movement has evolved by emulating Nature. The Fibonacci Spiral represents a prime way Nature expands and contracts; it is Nature's formula for beauty and strength. The PhysioStix design is based on the Fibonacci Spiral/Golden Ratio in order to tap into this universal dynamic of movement-alchemy. Thus the PhysioStix is the simplest yet most advanced human gear in the history of the planet. It helps you activate your highest potential by enhancing your circulation, articulation and breathing. Movement becomes free flowing, like liquid. It offers a perpetual approach to the martial arts while minimizing bloodshed imagery. The shape itself is the perfect contour of sacred geometry and human expression. Spirals of intention flow freely to and fro, expanding and reducing internally and externally without ever crashing into a fracturing halt. This truth holds up at all velocities, allowing the practitioner to resonate at a frequency close to that of plant growth, shaping itself like infinite seashells expressible in all directions. These concepts are derived from a lifetime of studying the Art of Kung Fu. PhysioStixs are the result of many years of experimentation in combining these truths.

The evolution of the martial arts has taken a quantum leap with Sifu Rob Moses' Spiral Fitness system. The heretofore-invisible secret of martial arts—the Golden Spiral—has now become transformed into a visible guidance system, through which healing and transformative movements flow. The PhysioStix workout tool is designed with Nature's intelligence in mind and is a must addition for your Golden Ratio Workout toolbox. David Carradine was a leading proponent of the Spiral Fitness System and collaborated with Rob on the excellent Spiral Fitness DVD series.

6

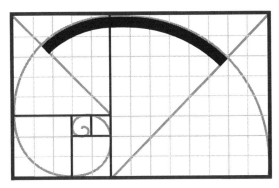
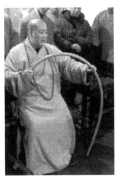
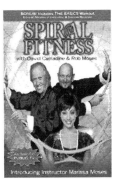

(*left*): The PhysioStix's design is a section of the Golden Spiral.
(*center*): Shaolin Monk with PhysioStix long version.
(*right*): *Spiral Fitness* DVD cover, showing actor David Carradine, Rob and Marissa Moses.

197

Balancing Blood Pressure the Golden Ratio Way

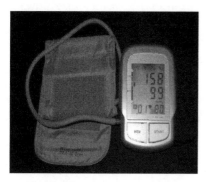

Blood pressure cuff showing hypertension with Golden Ratio compensation; systolic/diastolic ratio, 158/99 = 1.6

Since the invention of the blood pressure cuff 100 years ago, physicians have missed the observation that blood pressure readings often reflect the Golden Ratio. Our bodies have a finely tuned homeostatic mechanism that always tries to maintain the Golden Ratio with respect to systolic and diastolic blood pressure. For example, a so-called normal blood pressure has been typically reported as 120/80: a ratio of 1.5. Viewed through the lens of the Golden Ratio, a normal blood pressure reading would be 120/74: a ratio of 1.62. You could have other normal Golden Ratio readings, such as 113/70 or 116/73. Even if a person has high blood pressure, the wisdom of the body still tries to maintain the Golden Ratio. A blood pressure reading of 160/100, even though high, gives a ratio of 1.6, essentially the Golden Ratio 1.618... This Golden Ratio compensation keeps the physiology efficiently functioning through a wide range of bodily stressors, even though the long-term effects of hypertension still may occur. Once the Golden Ratio of systolic to diastolic blood pressure is lost, general adaptation is compromised and the individual may begin suffering a more rapid downward spiral in their health. In the future, blood pressure cuff designs may well have a window that calculates the ratio of systolic to diastolic pressure to inform the user how close to the more optimal Golden Ratio they are.

Maintaining Golden Ratio Blood Pressure Decreases Death Risk

In a ground-breaking scientific discovery, Austrian statistician Hanno Ulmer, Ph.D., and his research group confirmed our Golden Ratio hypothesis that having one's systolic:diastolic blood pressure in Golden Ratio is beneficial to one's health. They evaluated a large primary care-based patient cohort of 166,377 people and found that the systolic:diastolic blood pressure ratio was 1.618 in participants who *didn't* die during the 20 year study and 1.745 in people who did die during that same period. They concluded that,

> ...*blood pressure values in 'well' individuals, but not in those who are at risk of dying, exhibit the Golden Ratio.*

This is a staggering confirmation of the Golden Ratio's power in promoting one's health and longevity. We must always consider both quality and quantity when looking at physiological parameters, such as blood pressure. Maintaining quality is of course keeping the systolic and diastolic pressures in Golden Ratio. Maintaining quantity is making sure that blood pressure doesn't get too high, even though the systolic and diastolic pressures may be in Golden Ratio. For example, a blood pressure of 160/100 (ratio of 1.6), although typically considered high, is in Golden Ratio and will afford some level of protection against death as evidenced by Dr. Ulmer's study. However, a greater level of health and survivability could be obtained by having both an overall lower blood pressure in addition to being in Golden Ratio e.g., in the range of 120/75 (ratio of 1.6). The power of the Golden Ratio in looking at physiological parameters is being validated before our eyes. The Golden Ratio is unleashing nothing less than a Copernican revolution in medicine. How? By revealing a simple low-tech yet high-impact method to: 1. Re-conceptualize valuable diagnostic information about our bodily systems; 2. Allow us to harness its therapeutic power in rebalancing out-of-ratio physiology through application of the Golden Ratio Lifestyle Diet.

A New, Innovative Way to Check Your Blood Pressure

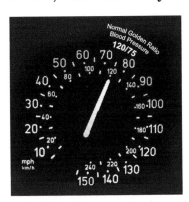

Golden Ratio Blood Pressure Gauge. The authors' utilization of km/h to mph on a speedometer illustrates the Golden Ratio proportions of systolic and diastolic blood pressure. A normal Golden Ratio blood pressure reading would be in the range of 120/75, a 1.6 ratio.

By using the universal Golden Ratio conversion system, you can quickly plot your blood pressure readings to see how close they are to the Golden Ratio. This scale is derived from an automobile speedometer, which conveniently shows miles per hour (mph) alongside kilometers per hour (km/h). The scale of the speedometer is such that the ratio of mph to km/h is very close to the Golden Ratio. Amazingly, this scale of proportions is able to be used not only as a speedometer, but also to evaluate blood pressure readings. For example, if you look at your speedometer you will notice that the following Golden Ratio readings are plain to see, and they resemble various possible blood pressure readings:

100 km/h: 60 mph... ratio of 1.6
120 km/h: 75 mph... ratio of 1.6
160 km/h: 100mph... ratio of 1.6

To see if your blood pressure readings are in Golden Ratio range, find your systolic reading (the higher of your two blood pressure numbers) on the kilometers/hour (km/h) line. Then look directly across at the miles/hour (mph) line and plot your diastolic reading (the lower of your two blood pressure numbers) in miles/hour (mph). If your systolic reading is directly across from your diastolic reading, then they are in Golden Ratio. Golden Ratio blood pressure evaluations always look at *quality* and *quantity*. Whether or not the systolic and diastolic readings are in Golden Ratio determines the quality of the reading. How high or low the readings are determines the *quantity*. In the speedometer examples listed above, 100/60 is considered low blood pressure, but still maintains a Golden Ratio. 120/75 is in the normal range and is also in Golden Ratio. 160/100 is considered high blood pressure, but still maintains its Golden Ratio. Even if a blood pressure reading is too high or too low—*quantity*—there is still a presumed physiologic advantage if the reading is in Golden Ratio—*quality*. If your blood pressure readings are either too high or too low and/or aren't directly across from one another on your speedometer, you should begin incorporating the Golden Ratio Lifestyle Diet recommendations into your life, in addition to consulting with your physician or health care professional.

Note: Explore the curious Golden Ratio link between miles and kilometers in our companion book *The Divine Code of Da Vinci, Fibonacci, Einstein and YOU.*

6

> *The impulse of all movement and all form is given by Phi Φ (the Golden Ratio).*
> **Schwaller de Lubicz, *The Temple of Man***

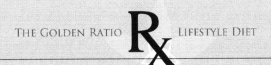

THE GOLDEN RATIO **Rx** LIFESTYLE DIET

EXERCISE:
GOLDEN RATIO MOTION

Pick one or more of the following Rx's to add to your daily health regimen.

1. Workout with Fibonacci's Fitness Code

A simple way to integrate the Golden Ratio into your exercise routine is to modify the number of repetitions per set of any exercise. By using adjacent Fibonacci numbers for the number of repetitions per set, you automatically build the power of the Golden Ratio into your workout. It may seem a little odd at first, doing for example 8 pushups followed by 13, rather than 10 followed by 10. Yet this simple change in your reps counting method can switch your body into reactivation of your latent Golden Ratio performance capabilities. Here are some example adjacent Fibonacci number pairs with which you can structure the number of repetitions in sequential sets:

2:3 3:2 3:5 5:3 5:8 8:5 8:13 13:8 13:21 21:13
21:34 34:21 34:55 55:34

You might also try dividing the ratios of your exercise and rest cycles into Fibonacci Ratios. For example: exercise for five minutes, then rest for three, or exercise for eight then rest for five, etc. When your sets correspond to Fibonacci numbers and thus Golden Ratios, you send a powerful message to your nervous system to synchronize with the Golden Ratio and thus activate your greater performance potentials.

2. Split Your Workouts For Better Results, Health and Easier Weight Loss

Split your daily workout into two sessions in Golden Ratio to obtain greater benefits for less effort. This practice will optimize the ratio of your exercise and recovery cycles. For example, workout for 21 minutes in the morning and 34 minutes in the afternoon. If you need longer workouts, try ratios such as 34:55 or 55:89. If you would like to do a shorter workout, try a 13:21 ratio or even an 8:13 ratio. Splitting your daily workout in two can increase the overall benefit of your total day's workout investment by up to 50%.

3. Easy FIT Training: Workout/Rest in Golden Ratio

Walk, jog or run 8 minutes and then rest 5. Repeat three times. You may increase the number of repetitions and intensity as your endurance and desire allow. Feel free to experiment with other Fibonacci ratios, such as: 3:2, 5:3, 13:8, etc. You can also "jump" ratios, e.g., 13:5, 21:8, etc. These Fibonacci workout/recovery ratios are an easy and fun way to tap the power of the Golden Ratio in your workouts. They also give your body ample time to clear lactic acid and recharge your cells.

6

4. Coach Fibonacci's More Advanced FIT Workouts

To easily experiment with the High Intensity Training (HIT) workout system fused with the power of the Fibonacci Sequence/Golden Ratio (FIT: Fibonacci Interval Training), try any of the suggested workout regimens which follow as a starting point. *NOTE: Always consult your health professional before trying this or any new exercise regimen. If you are a beginner, out-of-shape or have a medical condition, you will first need to be evaluated by your physician with a maximal cardiac stress test, to ensure that your cardiovascular system is safely ready for the increased intensity that typifies the FIT method.* It is then recommended that you establish a baseline of endurance with a personal trainer before beginning your FIT workouts. To begin, warm up at an easy pace for at least 13 minutes. Remember to maintain tall and buoyant posture. When you feel fully warmed up—indicated by a light sweat and a "green zone" sense of readiness—you're ready to begin your FIT workout. After your warm-up, the FIT system is divided into the following alternating cycles:

- Full Sprint/burst effort, near or at your safe maximum effort or pulse rate, followed by a...
- Rest/recovery phase, where you downshift to a relaxed, slow walking pace, during which time your pulse rate recovers from your maximum level.

To leverage the power of the Golden Ratio in your FIT workouts, you simply tune your alternating Sprint/Rest cycles to the Golden Ratio, via Fibonacci Sequence numbers. Here's a recap of the Fibonacci Sequence:

0, 1, 1, 2, 3, 5, 8, 13, 21, 34, 55, 89, 144, 233, 377, 610...

You can easily customize your FIT intervals ladder; following are three easy examples. Feel free to "jump" numbers up or down in the sequence as you like; Golden Ratio harmonics will remain in effect. Note: workout lengths do not include required warm-up and cool-down periods of at least 13 minutes each.

1. Moderate Intensity

Sample FIT Workout/Rest Sequence in SECONDS:
8-21, 8-21, 13-34, 21-55, 34-89, 21-55, 13-34, 8-21...

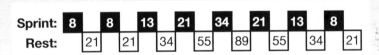

= 7 minute, 36 second workout

2. Advanced Intensity

Sample FIT Workout/Rest Sequence in SECONDS:
8-13, 8-13, 13-21, 21-34, 34-55, 21-34, 13-21, 8-13...

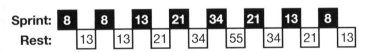

= 5 minute, 30 second workout

3. Competitive Intensity

Sample FIT Workout/Rest Sequence in MINUTES:

1-1, 1-1, 2-1, 3-2, 5-3, 2-1, 1-2, 1-2...

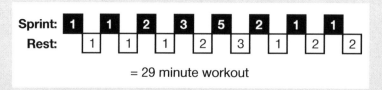

= 29 minute workout

4. Simplified Competitive Intensity: Equal Sprint/Rest

Sample FIT Workout/Rest Sequence in MINUTES:

1-1, 1-1, 2-2, 3-3, 5-5, 2-2, 1-1, 1-1...

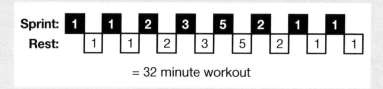

= 32 minute workout

5. FIT Workout Tips

Variations on the FIT theme are virtually infinite. Experiment with longer or shorter sprint/rest times, by selecting the next (or next-next) higher, and next (or next-next) lower Fibonacci numbers to define your sprint/rest cycles. To keep it simple, you can also train using *equal* sprint and rest intervals tuned to the Fibonacci Sequence numbers, as shown in example #4 above. Start easy and pay attention to your body's natural sprint/rest shift-point indicators. On some days you may need longer recovery cycles; other days less. Over several weeks, seek to build up to your safe maximum pulse rate intensity for your sprint segments, followed by ample rest/recovery segments. Vary the total intensity of your FIT workouts in waves over the course of a week and month. Remember HIT workout pioneer Mike Mentzer's advice to keep the workouts brief, intense and infrequent. Experiment with 1 or 2 FIT sessions per week and see how your body responds. Adjust the frequency and length of FIT workouts as desired. Add lower intensity workouts or do some cross training on other days of the week; just be sure to also take ample rest/recovery days as needed. An easy way to make sure you're not over trained is by taking your resting pulse in the morning before arising. If your pulse is 10 beats or more greater than normal, you need to back off until your body recovers.

Keep in mind that the real benefits of exercise are stronger in the hours and days after your workout, during your rest and recovery phase. While it of course provides us with great feelings of achievement, freedom and even transcendence, exercise (especially when rigorous and/or too frequent) is actually physically damaging to the body. In addition to causing micro muscle tears and increased wear, it also generates excessive free-radical activity, due to the higher oxidation rates generated during exercise. This is why it's vitally important to allow ample rest periods in any exercise regimen, to honor your body's need to properly heal, recover and come back even stronger. To offset the increased free radicals produced during exercise, try a Golden Ratio IronApe Green Smoothie (see chapter 4/ Nutrition, Rx section) after your workout, which facilitates post-workout recovery. Remember, as with food calories, *quality over quantity*. The secret to effective FIT workouts is the *quality* of your sprint cycles vs. *quantity*. The key is to make the intensity of your sprint segments harder than your usual maximum training intensity and make your rest segments amply restorative. At the end of each sprint cycle, transition slowly into the rest phase—come out of your sprint into a fast walk, followed by a slower, relaxed walk. During longer rest phases, you might even try briefly lying down with your feet up, after tapering down first with a few minutes of progressively slower walking.

From a Fibonacci Sequence perspective, every rest cycle is a natural catapult-loading phase for your next sprint cycle—when your rest cycle is properly timed in proper proportion to your sprint cycle. Tuning your FIT workouts to the Golden Ratio via Fibonacci Sequence numbers supports your natural alignment with Nature's Optimal Performance Code. This is also the secret formula for the elusive 2nd wind, 3rd wind, 4th wind… and so on. Lastly, there's no need to obsess with perfection when timing your sprint/rest cycles. While a watch or timer can be handy, try the low-tech/high-ease method of counting off the numbers to yourself during your sprint/rest cycles. Once the

Fibonacci Sequence Numbers are in your memory, it's easy and fun to keep track. So, what are you waiting for? On your mark... Ready, Set..... GO!

6. Easy Golden Spiral Movements

Try moving in a gentle Golden Spiral the next time you get out of bed, stand up from a chair, sit-up in the bathtub or get out of a car. With your spine relaxed, allow your body to gently spiral up as you rise. You'll feel less effort, more flow and put significantly less stress on your back when you move this way. Modifying your movements by simply incorporating the Golden Spiral into them can greatly enhance your movement, balance and breathing. At the same time, stiffness and rigidity in both body and mind is gently released.

7. Spiral~Chi Infinity Movements

In co-author Robert Friedman, M.D.'s *Spiral~Chi* DVD, he offers many ingenious, unique and easy-to-learn ways to integrate figure 8/spiral Golden Ratio-based movements into everyday exercises and stretches. You will be pleasantly surprised at your newly found flexibility, coordination and increased energy.

8. Lighten Your Load with Golden Ratio Weight Lifting

The next time you're lifting weights or are using a Nautilus,® Bowflex,® or other machine, try synchronizing your repetitions with Golden Ratio Breathing. Begin with a light weight or easy resistance until you get accustomed to the Ratio. As you *lift* the weight or move against the resistance, breathe out to a count of 5. As you *release* the weight or resistance, breathe in to a count of 3. Your motions should be slow and synchronized with your breath. For variability, experiment with different ratios, such as 2:3, 3:2, 3:5, 5:3, 5:8 or 8:5. Different ratios will give you different results. When you are working with the Golden Ratio, you can make amazing gains in a short amount of time.

9. Golden Ratio Blood Pressure Check

Divide your systolic by your diastolic blood pressure—your systolic is the higher one on top. For example, if your blood pressure reading is 120/75, this equals the Golden Ratio of 1.6. See how close your blood pressure ratio comes to the Golden Ratio of 1.6. The closer to the Golden Ratio, the more efficiently your cardiovascular system is operating. By implementing the recommendations in this book, you'll be able to optimize your blood pressure in the direction of the Golden Ratio and greater health and well-being.

10. The Golden Core Training Zone

The modern focus on Core Training reflects both the Golden Ratio and the First 15% principle. The Golden Ratio division point of the body—the navel region—is a most powerful First 15% starting point for building optimal fitness, posture, balance and strength. It's no accident that the martial arts place such emphasis on this region known as the hara, which is slightly below the navel. In addition, the solar plexus, the 2nd largest nerve center in the body (known as the "second brain") is slightly above the navel. This core postural/nerve/gravitational matrix that surrounds your navel—above, below, sides and back—also strengthens your balance, poise and focus. This translates to strengthening the same qualities in your mind, emotions and spirit as well. A few simple, effective methods for strengthening your Golden Core Zone:

- Forward and reverse sit-ups, especially on a Swiss/Yoga Ball; a diagonal/spiral twist enhances the core workout.
- Golden Breaths: Full Buddha-belly and then expand up into chest on inhale; then letting the breath go completely, navel pulled towards the spine on exhale. Strengthens the diaphragm and core muscles at the same time. See chapter 1/Air, Rx 1: Golden Breath Retraining.
- Yoga, Pilates, Jumping Rope, Hula-hoop, Pull-ups.
- Wobble Board—Standing and balancing on one for a few minutes a day activates & strengthens the core. Key: Better Balance = Greater Strength.
- Medicine Balls: www.Spri.com

- *ABCore* Medicine Ball Workout DVD, by co-author Matthew Cross; available 2012 at www.GoldenRatioLifestyle.com
- *Spiral-Chi* DVD, by co-author Robert Friedman, M.D.; buy on Amazon.
- Kettlebell workout: www.PowerByPavel.com
- Performance Coach Chris Johnson's excellent, easy-to-follow *Let's Get Moving* Exercise DVD, available at: www.OnTargetLiving.com

As with all suggested exercises in this book, consult a health professional before any new exercise regimen, go at your own pace and listen to your body.

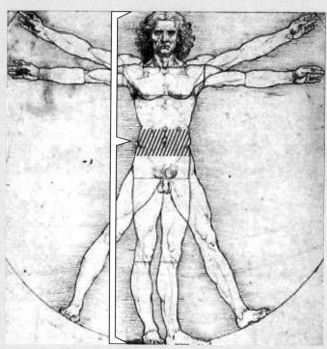

The Golden Core Training Zone, composed of navel, hara and solar plexus, centered around the upper Golden Ratio division point of the body.

11. Upgrade Your Brain & Body's Operating Ratio

One of the fascinating talents of Golden Ratio genius Leonardo Da Vinci was his ability to use both his left and right hands with near-equal skill. Yet most people are 100% right or left dominant and never question it; we've come to accept without question that one side does all. This is like using only a portion of your whole potential. Ambidexterity is not just a freak talent reserved for the lucky few. In fact, *not* cultivating your non-dominant hand/side wastes a huge opportunity to upgrade your brain synchronization, creativity and health. So invite your non-dominant side to the table and get your whole brain and body more in the game. Take some baby steps to move from a 100:0 Ratio of Right or Left side dominance towards a 60:40 approximate Golden Ratio. At first it may be challenging, yet like learning any valuable skill, the rewards are vast and growing.

Benefits
- More integrated whole-brain function
- Enhanced creativity and innovation
- Better body-balance, symmetry, proportion and movement
- Increased ability to adapt to physical and mental challenges

Exercises: practice switching to your non-dominant side while
- Brushing your teeth, combing hair
- Holding a fork, knife or glass
- Practicing sports, e.g., tennis, ping-pong, baseball, basketball, archery
- Opening doors, flipping switches
- Listening to your phone with your non-dominant ear
- Writing, drawing and painting

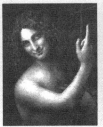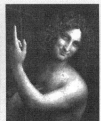

Leonardo da Vinci's *St. John the Baptist*, a.k.a. *St. John the Ambidextrous.*

A dramatic increase in your ambidexterity is "at hand." By practicing these simple exercises with your non-dominant hand/side, you'll soon be surprised by your improved balance, coordination and creativity. It's never too late to start enjoying a more synchronized and integrated body-mind-spirit.

Balance the body, balance the brain.
The future lies with the ambidextrous human!
Professor Raymond Dart, Australian anatomist and anthropologist

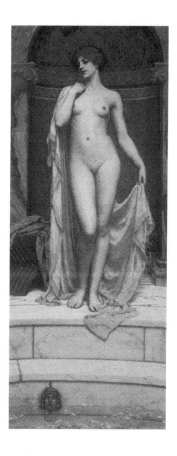

The timeless art of detoxification and

beautification, via hot bath and sauna.

Venus at the Bath by John William Godward.

7.

Detoxification

Elimination of undigested food and other bodily waste is just
as important as the proper digestion and assimilation of food.
Dr. Norman W. Walker, Nutrition & Health Pioneer

Detoxification is becoming more important every day, as we are constantly bombarded with increasing toxins from within and without. Luckily, our livers have the intelligence to detoxify metabolic waste products as well as environmental toxins and transform them into water-soluble substances that can be excreted in urine, bile, stool, sweat and breath. Water is the universal solvent that enables this process to occur. It's only when the degree of detoxification can't keep up with the amount of internally and externally generated toxins that problems arise. Our bodies have the ability to store toxins when we can't detoxify fast enough. However, at some point the storage capacity fills up and the toxins begin to inhibit efficient functioning of our metabolic machinery. Opportunistic microbes and parasites often arrive on the scene to feed on the sludge, which only complicates the situation. Then, varying degrees of unwellness begin to manifest: vague, low-grade symptoms like fatigue, headaches, insomnia, depression and subpar performance. Left unchecked, these low-grade symptoms can progress to actual pathologies like heart disease, asthma, cancer, diabetes, arthritis, Alzheimer's, Parkinson's or various immune system problems. However, by regaining Golden Ratio balance within each of the 9 main drivers of the Golden Ratio Lifestyle

Diet, we can rev-up our detoxification processes, eliminate the backlog of toxins and support the restoration of our health.

Breathing as Detoxification

The category of detoxification is woven through each of the top drivers in the Golden Ratio Lifestyle Diet. Each of the top categories has within it a detoxification phase, in order to maintain Golden Ratio balance of intake and output. In the case of driver #1, Air, breathing brings fresh oxygen into our bodies and also removes carbon dioxide/ CO_2. The exhalation phase of breathing not only gets rid of carbon dioxide, it also helps to regulate acid/alkaline balance. Without adequate respiration we would we be starved of oxygen and metabolic acids will accumulate, which then have many adverse downstream effects on our health. The rate of breathing is of course dependent on what our activity demands are at any given time. Our body continually monitors and tunes both our oxygen and CO_2 levels. Our bodies' Divine intelligence has the ability to dynamically shift in response to the demands of the moment, e.g., when exercising we naturally breathe faster; at rest we breathe slower.

Most of us get into trouble when we're at rest: we tend to hypoventilate or under-breathe. Over-breathing or *hyper*ventilation is a less common occurrence and is typically caused by anxiety. Under-breathing or *hypo*ventilation is usually exacerbated by poor posture, where rounded shoulders and a caved-in chest inhibit deep and adequate respirations. When we're not breathing deeply enough, acidity develops in the blood which then forces the kidneys to get rid of excess acids. Over time, this stress moves even deeper into our physiology, putting stress on our endocrine glands and even dips into mineral stores in our bones to buffer and keep our acid/alkaline balance in check. Our bodies are programmed with the homeostatic ability to maintain many different physiologic Golden Ratio set points. We're constantly striving to keep all of our set points in Golden Ratio balance, including oxygen/CO_2, acid/alkaline, blood sugar levels, hormones, blood pressure, temperature, hydration, etc. The first step in correcting hypoventilation—under-breathing— is to set up some constant reminder to scan your breathing and posture on a regular basis.

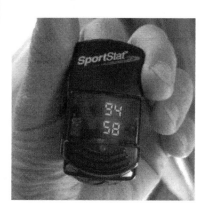

The pulse-oximeter monitors oxygen saturation and heart rate.

You might want to set up a cue; perhaps each hour stand up, stretch and do a few cycles of Golden Ratio Breathing. An easy way to actually measure hypoventilation is to get a pulse-oximeter. This is a simple home device that clips on your finger and measures oxygen saturation in your blood and your pulse rate after just a few seconds. It does this through your skin via a painless laser light. It can also be used when exercising. You will be amazed at how quickly your oxygen saturation will increase to healthier levels after just a few rounds of Golden Ratio Breathing.

Water, the Alkahest: Nature's Universal Solvent

Water, like Consciousness, is clear, tasteless and odorless, yet essential for life.
Robert Friedman, M.D.

Classical alchemists believed that there was a universal substance that had the ability to dissolve all other substances, gold included. They called this magical substance the "Alkahest," a word coined by Renaissance physician and alchemist Paracelsus. Alchemists were especially interested in its medicinal potential and projected onto this hypothetical substance the label of the much sought after philosopher's stone. Like the ancient alchemists, we too are interested in the medicinal potential of the Alkahest, except in our case the universal solvent is the ubiquitous compound of water. Water—commonly known as H_2O—has chemical properties that make it a true universal solvent. On a practical level, although water can't dissolve all substances as the Alkahest theoretically could, it has the ability to dissolve enough substances that our physiology has taken advantage of this property to assist with bodily detoxification. Toxic substances from both external sources like environmental pollutants and internal metabolic waste products are dissolved in water so that they can be excreted through urine, breath, sweat, bile and stool. It makes sense that we would want to give our system enough fresh water to keep up with detoxification demands. In this day and age, the importance of adequate water intake cannot be overemphasized. As Dr. Rashid Buttar, D.O., Vice-Chairman of the American Board of Clinical Metal Toxicology states,

I can now very comfortably and definitively state to you that, in my opinion, based on the evidence,

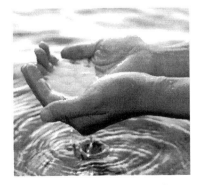

Water, Nature's universal solvent.

every single chronic insidious disease process is related to one word: toxicity. You cannot address the issues of aging unless you address detoxification.

Dr. Buttar's insights into toxicity are all the more relevant when we take an honest look at sources of toxicity that are less than apparent. The Associated Press reported in their 5 month investigation that over-the-counter and prescription drugs have been found in the drinking water supplies of 24 metropolitan areas across the United States. Drugs including antibiotics, antiepileptics, antidepressants, steroid hormones, acetaminophen and ibuprofen, among others, were found in trace amounts in all drinking water samples. The public at large is being continually poisoned with micro-doses of medications. It so happens that water is a bipolar molecule (although it's neither manic nor depressed) with a net negative charge near the oxygen end and a net positive charge at the polar hydrogen end. This is what accounts for its universal solvent properties. Luckily, water's bipolar structure assists our detoxification mechanisms in getting rid of these and other unwanted pollutants. The Center for Disease Control's (CDC) landmark study in 2003 identified 116 chemicals in blood and urine samples from hundreds of Americans. The toxicology screens identified significant levels of heavy metals, secondhand smoke residues, plastic residues, pesticides and herbicides in *all* subjects. This sobering study highlights the pervasive degree of environmental toxicity in virtually the entire U.S. population. It also can redirect our focus to learn about detoxification protocols and remind us of the importance of the universal solvent, water—the Alkahest—in regularly flushing these toxins from our bodies.

7

Water's near-miraculous ability to dissolve so many substances allows our lungs, liver, kidneys, intestines and sweat glands to eliminate these toxins. All we have to do is make sure that we are drinking enough pure water throughout our day to satisfy this demand. Water intake varies according to age, size, activity level, ambient temperature and health status. Everyone has an ideal amount of fluid intake. We can think of this ideal amount as each person's Golden Ratio quantity where not too much and not too little water intake will facilitate optimum functioning. This ideal amount changes from day to day and hour to hour, depending on the circumstances. As we learned in chapter 2/Water, simply following your thirst impulse isn't accurate enough to monitor your body's water requirements since there is a lag time between dehydration and the awareness of thirst. So, you have to anticipate dehydration and always be rehydrating even when you're not actually thirsty. In addition, as we age the thirst mechanism may become blunted, making our awareness of thirst even slower and duller. Try and ask yourself throughout the day if your hydration level is at the Golden Ratio point:

not too dry and not too wet. For a review of optimal hydration techniques, see chapter 2/Water.

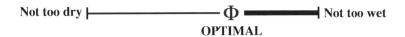

Not too dry ├─────────────── ⬤ ━━━━━┤ Not too wet

OPTIMAL

Der Goldene "Schnitt": The Golden Bowel Movement

Der Goldene "Schnitt" is German for the Golden Cut or Golden Ratio and also just happens to rhyme with the English word *Sh–t*. Nevertheless, the concept of the Golden Ratio can be applied to the subject of intestinal detoxification in order to give us some valuable insights. When considering the Golden Ratio there is always *quality* and *quantity* to consider. Let's consider quantity of bowel movements first. A study of over 20,000 people in *Public Health Nutrition*, 2003, by Miguel Sanjoaquin, et.al., revealed that vegan (a vegetarian who eats no animal or dairy products) males had an average of 11.6 bowel movements per week. That averages 1.6 bowel movements per day (11.6 ÷ 7 = 1.6), or what we call the Golden "Schnitt" (recall that 1.6 is the Golden Ratio). The size of a bowel movement depends on how much fiber is eaten in a given meal. The average American only gets about 15 grams of fiber per day in their diet, whereas a vegetarian can get upwards of 50 grams of fiber per day. Meat eaters fell significantly short of the Golden "Schnitt" at around 9 bowel movements per week, with a ratio of only 1.28 bowel movements per day. When bowel movement quantity is out of Golden Ratio, one is subject to a backup of toxic waste with various maladies manifesting that can affect our entire physiology. Regarding the out-of-ratio bowel movements of modern Americans, the renowned naturopath Dr. Richard Schulze remarked,

They will have an average of 2-4 bowel movements a week coming up 70,000 bowel movements short in their lifetime, definitely having diverticulosis and digestive and elimination problems.

Quality of bowel movements is influenced not only by *how much* fiber is in one's diet, but also by the type or *quality* of fiber. This is a critical distinction. The two classes of dietary fiber are known as soluble and insoluble, both indigestible. Soluble fiber is able to absorb water and is fermentable by intestinal bacteria. These fermentable by-products are known as SCFA (short-chain fatty acids) and are impressive in their ability to regulate blood glucose, lipids and cholesterol. They also favorably change the milieu of the intestinal environment, including the pH, reducing the risk of polyps and colon cancer. Insoluble fiber doesn't absorb water, but is mainly responsible for speeding the transit of toxins from the colon. Increasing both soluble and insoluble fiber in one's diet can either resolve or have a favorable impact on many conditions, including:

acne	diabetes	hemorrhoids
anxiety	diarrhea	IBS (irritable bowel syndrome)
arthritis	diverticulosis	immune dysfunction
bloating	eczema	indigestion
brain fog	fatigue	insomnia
constipation	gas	obesity
depression	heart disease	

Simply increasing the amount of fiber in your diet to the point where your bowel movement frequency approaches or exceeds the Golden "Schnitt" range—at least 1.6 per day—can be a major contributing factor in its own right in restoring healthy immune function and healing disease. The ratios of soluble and insoluble fibers varies greatly among foods. All fruits and vegetables have a mix of soluble and insoluble fibers; there are no unprocessed/whole foods with just one type of fiber. A few fruits have soluble/insoluble ratios that approximate the Golden Ratio, while most vegetables have much more insoluble fiber than soluble. Both types of fiber have the ability to increase the speed of bowel movements, thereby getting rid of toxic waste products faster. So if you want to approach the Golden "Schnitt," averaging or exceeding 1.6 bowel movements per day, just increase both your soluble and insoluble fiber intake gradually until you reach that target. Due to individual variations, some people may average more than 1.6 bowel movements per day. Soluble fiber has the special property of being able to bind toxins and bile acids in order to sequester and remove them from your body. Remember that soluble fiber always needs water in order for the fiber to expand and get to work; again, the universal solvent working its magic.

7

Insoluble/Soluble Fiber Ratios

Ample quality and quantity of fiber is clearly a vital dietary and internal cleansing requirement. Many of the following foods have insoluble/soluble fiber ratios close to the Golden Ratio; in the case of the remarkable apple, the ratio is exact to three digits. Others have ratios seen earlier in the Fibonacci Sequence, such as the 1.5 ratio. These are contrasted to examples like brown rice and pinto beans, which have relatively higher ratios of insoluble/soluble fiber. Note that wheat bran has the most lopsided insoluble/soluble fiber ratio; this should come as no surprise, as wheat bran is in fact quite a processed/refined food, missing all the other vital nutritional components of the *whole* wheat grain. This is one reason wheat bran can be an overly harsh fiber to eat, causing unnecessary intestinal irritation. You might try eating more of the Golden Ratio fiber-balanced foods to see if your digestion improves and bowel movements move into the healthy 1.6+/day range.

Food	Insoluble/Soluble Fiber Ratios
Wheat bran	11.3:1 *(wheat bran is overly processed and thus at the extreme end of the spectrum)*
Brown rice	8.0:1
Beans (pinto)	3.36:1
Flax seeds	2.0:1
Apple	**1.61:1**
The Golden Ratio	**1.618:1** *Nature's Secret Nutrient (NSN)*
Pear	**1.63:1**
Strawberries	1.55:1
Beans (black)	1.55:1
Cauliflower	1.5:1
Celery	1.5:1
Sesame seeds	1.5:1
Sunflower seeds	1.5:1
Grapes	1.5:1
Sweet potato	1.44:1
Carrots	1.38:1 *(Golden Ratio harmonic)*
Broccoli	1.3:1
Oats	0.92:1
Grapefruit	0.61:1 *(inverse Golden Ratio)*
Orange	0.61:1 *(inverse Golden Ratio)*
Asparagus	0.64:1 *(inverse Golden Ratio)*

(left axis, upper: More Insoluble Fiber; left axis, lower: More Soluble Fiber)

In actuality, both soluble and insoluble fibers work together through both binding power and elimination speed to detoxify your system and fine-tune your intestinal environment. So, if you want to better detoxify yourself simply increase fruits and vegetables to get both more soluble and insoluble fiber. Some people get fiber benefits from grains, however a growing body of evidence points to the possible negative immune-modulating and allergenic effects of grains. If you feel that you're not getting enough fiber through your diet, a wide variety of fiber supplements are available to augment your fiber intake. Remember to always increase your water intake when you use fiber supplements, since these products are dehydrated.

In Search of the "Golden Schnitt"

Renowned herbalist Dr. Richard Schulze was curious as to exactly what a Golden "Schnitt" was, so he set off on a world-wide journey to answer that question, since he hadn't been able to find one in America. Schulze reported:

I have traveled the world in search of the perfect bowel movement. I have traveled to the jungles of Central America and to China, India, Africa, and Asia. I wanted to see primitive, rural people living simple, natural lives, and I wanted to find out what their bowel habits were like, because I wasn't going to find normal and natural anywhere in America. Simple and natural people, who gather wood, eat natural food, and have relaxed, unstressed lives have between two and three bowel movements a day. They eat, and within 15 to 30 minutes after their meals, they wander off to their spots, squat, and have bowel movements. These are usually light in color, soft, and unformed, and they come out easily, with no straining, grunting, pushing, or meditation.

Schulze discovered that these "primitive, rural people" were having up to twice as many bowel movements than the average American vegan. They were super-vegans, in that they were consuming enough fiber to account for their increased stool volume and frequency. A possible side effect of consuming too much fiber is that some of the nutrients might not be absorbed since they would be bound-up in the fiber and excreted too rapidly. This malabsorption effect is probably of no consequence with the amount of fiber consumed by most American vegans.

7

Radiation Protection and Detoxification 101

Doctors know there is no such thing as a safe dose of radiation.

Helen Caldicott, M.D., co-founder, Physicians for Social Responsibility; author, *If You Love This Planet*

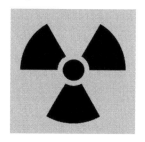

In light of the March 11, 2011 Japanese nuclear disaster at Fukushima, increased radiation levels will now be a factor affecting everyone on Earth for years to come. Besides being invisible, radiation is a cumulative toxin; fundamentally, there is no "safe" level of man-made radiation. While everyone's immune system is unique, there is always a threshold level of radiation in the body that once reached, automatically results in potentially life-threatening disease. Therefore, increased, targeted detoxification must now become a way of life for everyone as a matter of survival, let alone for optimal health and longevity. This will give your body the best shot at dealing with this latest increased radiation source, added to the "normal" toxic mix that is in our air, water, food and environment. Following are some concise tips on what you can do to help protect and detoxify yourself and your family from the growing menace of man-made radiation:

- Check radiation alerts frequently at: www.nuc.berkeley.edu/UCBAirSampling www.radiationnetwork.com, www.blackcatsystems.com/RadMap/map.html
- If airborne radiation levels are elevated, stay inside and avoid going out in the rain; exercise indoors and drive with windows closed
- Do sinus irrigation with salt water after being outside in questionable air
- Use an air filter for your house. Change the filter regularly and dispose of as per your local health department
- Use a water filter. Dispose of used filter as per your local health department
- Refrain from drinking or bathing in rain water
- Wash vegetables and fruits with biodegradable soap or baking soda
- Take frequent detoxing baths with Epsom salts, sea salt or baking soda
- Do an intestinal detox on a frequent basis
- Practice regular oral chelation, e.g., EDTA, garlic, chlorella, zeolite, vit-C
- Take antioxidants to prevent cellular and DNA damage, e.g., Vitamins B-C-E, Spirulina, R-lipoic acid
- Take iodine supplements if airborne radiation levels warrant it
- Foods may soon have Certified Radiation-Free labels in the grocery store; keep your eyes open for these, as avoidance is always the best medicine
- Reduce or eliminate all animal and milk products, as they are more concentrated radiation sources. Avoid seafood if from a radiation affected area
- Follow the Japanese custom of removing your shoes before entering your home. This simple practice prevents tracking radioactive particles into your house.
- Avoid exposure to ALL sources of man-made radiation, *unless absolutely necessary*, e.g., X-rays. Avoid airport radiation scanners and microwave ovens. Keep cellphones as far away from your body as possible; *always* use a headset. Remember: Radiation is a *cumulative* deadly toxin.
- Do whatever you can to end deadly nuclear power, before it ends us

7

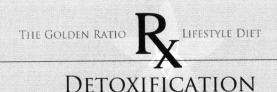

THE GOLDEN RATIO R_x LIFESTYLE DIET

DETOXIFICATION

Pick one or more of the following Rx's to add to your daily health regimen.

1. The A.M. BM (Morning Bowel Movement)

As we saw in chapter 3/Sleep, light is a most potent *Zeitgeber*, or time giver. It is a powerful cue that our brains rely on to reset our biorhythms on a daily basis. Regular bowel movements can also be used to reset and maintain our biorhythms, especially if they happen in the morning. We need some way of tuning our internal clocks to ensure bowel movements in the A.M. Morning bowel movements are essential to detoxify waste products collected from the previous day and night. Here are several helpful ways to assist a sluggish colon.

- Do 5-8 minutes of Golden Ratio Breathing upon arising: Inhale fully to the count of 3, exhale to the count of 5. Bonus: a sense of relaxation and inner peace follows naturally.

- Drink one or two glasses of pure warm water upon arising.

- Activate your colon by doing 30 seconds of stomach pumps: after a deep exhalation, roll your stomach muscles up and down 5-8 times. Rest and repeat 3-5 times. This motion will activate your colonic reflex.

- Increase the amount of fiber in your diet. This can be easily accomplished through the addition of one to two tablespoons of fresh ground flax seed to your meals, e.g., mixed into oatmeal, sprinkled over salads or mixed into most any dish. Eating more raw foods is also advised; experiment with increasing your intake. Go slow, as it can take weeks to months for your digestive system to adjust to an increase of raw foods.

- Colon cleansing may be advantageous. You may benefit from some gentle herbal colon cleansing formulas which also provide laxative assistance. Recommended products are Intestinal Formulas #1, #2 and #3, from Dr. Richard Schulze. These are excellent intestinal fiber/cleansing products and can be used in conjunction: www.HerbDoc.com

7

- Add fermented/cultured foods to your diet, such as yogurt, kefir, kombucha tea, sauerkraut, pickles, miso, kimchi or powdered or encapsulated probiotics.

- If your colon is particularly sluggish, you may want to get a series of colonic irrigations to help jump-start the detoxification process and reestablish regularity.

- Have a cup of coffee or tea. The resetting of your *Zeitgeber* is more important than the possible side effects of a small amount of caffeine, unless you have a particular sensitivity or medical condition that precludes morning/A.M. caffeine usage.

2. The Thermal Pump: Detoxification with Hot & Cold Water Therapy

Cold water stimulates and hot water relaxes! Together, they are like a hydrostatic pump that makes blood flow! Circulation produces cures! Herbs cannot cure, if the blood cannot circulate! Hot & Cold Water Therapy can bring about better circulation, because the hot water stimulates blood flow to the surface of the body, while the cold water stimulates blood flow to the core of the body, thus bringing fresh blood to the organs and glands and all parts of the body! In other words, OXYGEN & NUTRIENTS IN + TOXINS & PATHOGENS OUT!—Dr. Richard Schulze

This treatment is adapted from one of Dr. Richard Schulze's hydrotherapy exercises. It's a great way to harness water's unique abilities for healing—its amazing capacity to absorb and transfer heat through your body, as well as being the solvent for transporting nutrients to your cells and getting toxins out through perspiration. We have incorporated Fibonacci numbers and ratios into the exercise in order make it more fun and easy to remember, as well as to bring Nature's maximum efficiency principle into physiologic action.

1. At the end of your warm or hot shower, switch to full cold water for 13, 21 or 34 seconds. Start your cold water treatment on your extremities, then front, back and finally your head.

2. At the end of your 13, 21 or 34 second cold water treatment, switch back

to warm/hot water for the next higher Fibonacci number of seconds, e.g.,

13 cold to 21 warm; 21 cold to 34 warm; 34 cold to 55 warm

3. Do 3, 5 or 8 repetitions, remembering always to end with cold water.

4. For optimal detoxification, do the showers 1-2 times per day.

5. Drink a glass of pure water before and afterto facilitate your detox.

3. Triathlon Detox

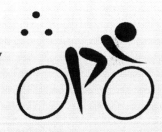

This potent detox isn't the familiar swim, bike and run—although that would also be a good one—it's the triad of sweating, water and exercise. Since many environmental toxins are stored in fat tissue, the only way to eliminate them is through exercising. Once the fats are mobilized by aerobic exercise, the toxins are released into general circulation. Only at that point will they be able to come out in sweat. So, if you were to walk, jog, swim or bike for 20–30 minutes before going into a sauna, you would be able to get rid of fat-soluble toxins that normally are hard to detox. Sweat glands and sebaceous glands are a great pathway for the exit of many fat-soluble toxins. Make sure to drink adequate water while exercising and sweating to replace fluid losses. You can add electrolytes such as Emergen-C to your water in order to maintain mineral balance as well as take advantage of Vitamin C's ability to bind toxins in the gut and kidneys. This can help prevent possible reabsorption of toxins from the blood and gut back into your body.

Here's a summary of the process:

• Aerobic exercise for 15+ minutes.

• Fluid replacement before, during and after exercise and sauna.
  Add electrolytes, such as a packet of Emergen-C (find at Whole Foods
  or Trader Joe's), to a large glass of water.

• Sauna or steam sweating. Use a dry skin brush to speed toxin release.
  Alternate going in and out of the sauna or steam room as tolerated. Take
  a cold shower during sauna breaks for 21, 34 or 55+ seconds for a great

thermal pump boost. Remember not to overdo it. Use Fibonacci Ratios for your sauna in-and-out and cold shower times, to avoid monotony.

Examples of possible sauna in/out and cold shower ratios:

5 minutes in, 3 minutes out;

21 second cold shower, then;

8 minutes in, 5 minutes out;

34 second cold shower, then;

13 minutes in, 5 or 8 minutes out;

55 second cold shower to finish.

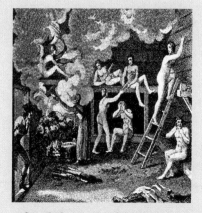

Swedish sauna, 19th century.

Note: If you have a medical condition or don't have sauna experience, check with your physician before trying this form of detox.

4. Soak Your Toxins Away

Another easy and enjoyable way to detox is taking a warm Epsom salt (magnesium sulfate) bath. Epsom salt has many beneficial properties, including relaxation and detoxification. The magnesium helps with muscle relaxation and the sulfate is important for detoxification. Skin becomes more permeable in warm water, so absorption of magnesium and sulfate can occur, as well as passage of toxins out of the body. Epsom salt soothes tired, overused muscles and induces a feeling of calm. It's also great for travelers and as a post-workout soak for athletes.

To prepare your soak: run a warm/hot bath and add 1 to 3 cups+ of Epsom salt, available at drug stores and many food stores. Soak 13-21 minutes; longer if desired. To enhance your soak, add a few drops of an essential oil into the running

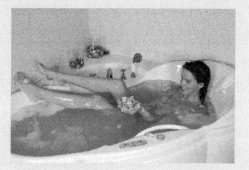

A relaxing Epsom salt detox soak.

water as your tub fills; eucalyptus oil is a common favorite. Before and after your bath, make sure you have a large glass of water to replenish fluid lost through sweating. If your bath is in the evening, notice the quality of your sleep and how you feel upon arising the next morning.

5. Liver Detox

Everything we eat or drink passes through our liver, to be metabolized, filtered and detoxified/prepared for removal from our body. Toxins are made water-soluble by the liver and secreted into bile and then into the stool. Water-soluble toxins may also be cleared through the kidneys. The liver is also our largest and heaviest internal organ (about 1/40 of body weight), weighing an average of 1.6 kilograms or 3.5 pounds (note that 1.6 is the Golden Ratio in two digits and 3-5 are early numbers in the Fibonacci Sequence). As the liver is our main organ of detoxification, it can become overworked, sluggish and occasionally clogged, leading to compromised immune function and numerous health challenges. One of the most effective and powerful ways to both maintain and restore healthy liver function is to do a liver detox. We recommend Dr. Richard Schulze's Liver DeTox system, available at: www.HerbDoc.com

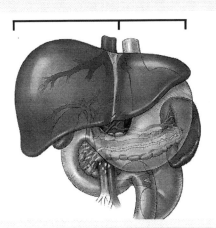

Note how the adult liver is bisected by the falciform ligament at the approximate Golden Ratio point of its length. A little known fact is the liver's remarkable connection to the Golden Ratio point of an infant: the fetus receives nutrients through the umbilical cord via the umbilical vein directly to the liver; within 2-5 days of birth, that vein is transformed into the falciform ligament.

6. Parasite Screening & Detox

Many chronic health conditions are related to undiagnosed intestinal parasites. Parasite testing became popular in the 1990's as a result of the best-selling book *Guess What Came to Dinner*, by Ann Louise Gittleman, Ph.D., CNS. Gittleman utilizes the Parasite Flexi-Test to screen for many types of bacteria, funguses, protozoa and worms. In the privacy of your home, 3 stool samples and 2 saliva samples are collected and sent to the lab. Results go directly to Dr. Gittleman's office; you then receive a personalized letter of recommendations to rid yourself of any discovered parasites: www.annlouise.com, www.unikeyhealth.com. Dr. Hulda Clark was another noted health specialist who formulated a targeted protocol for effective parasite eradication: www.HuldaClark.com

7. Smoke Free in 21 Days

The Golden Ratio principle exhibits equally powerful expansive and contractive potentials. As a unique method to go smoke-free, the following pattern of accelerated reduction follows the Fibonacci Sequence in reverse, down a 21-Day reduction spiral to zero 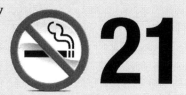 cigarettes. To start, pick the nearest Fibonacci number below the number of cigarettes you currently smoke per day. For example: If you currently smoke a pack a day (20 cigarettes), then 13 is your closest lower Fibonacci number. 13 is the number of cigarettes you would then smoke for the first eight days of your deceleration cycle. For the five days following those first eight days, you would then drop down to 8 cigarettes a day. Three days later, 5 cigarettes; two days later, 3 cigarettes; one day later, 2 cigarettes; one day later, 1 cigarette—and, on the last day, 0 cigarettes. The Fibonacci Sequence is used for determining both the number of cigarettes smoked, and the days on which you reduce that number. If you are smoking significantly more or less than in the above example, you will need to create a custom deceleration cycle, to allow for modifications of the standard 21-Day new habit cycle.

8. Nicotine Withdrawal a-la-Fibonacci

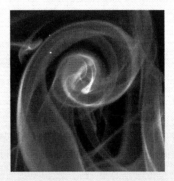

Smoke following the Path of Least Resistance by curling in Golden Spirals.

If you're using a nicotine patch to control withdrawal symptoms, you might experiment with decreasing dosages, sequenced to Fibonacci days. A friend of the authors chose to wear nicotine patches to help stop smoking. He changed the strength of his patches every five or eight days, which kept him aware that he was achieving his habit change in tune with Nature's Path of Least Resistance. Nicoderm® nicotine patches are the closest of the smoking reduction medicines offered in decreasing dosages: 21mg.–14mg.–7mg, approximating the Fibonacci Sequence of 21, 13, 8...

Nicotine is a unique drug in that it exhibits homeostatic or balancing properties. It acts as a mental, emotional and physical body balancer. So if you're tired, a cigarette will give you a lift; conversely, if you're nervous or anxious, it will calm you down. Yet since nicotine and smoking's negative health impacts are well known, so we need to find a healthful alternative— a new habit—to take its place. As we've learned, you can never fully extinguish a habit; you can only replace or "overwrite" it with a new, more deeply ingrained behavior.

We suggest replacing smoking with Golden Ratio Breathing, a natural, healthful way to regain balance in your autonomic nervous system. During the 21-Day smoking deceleration cycle, the carbon monoxide that has been blocking your body's oxygenation processes will be rapidly replaced with healthy oxygen. This process supports detoxification without throwing your body into physiologic withdrawal. Utilizing Golden Ratio Breathing during this time as well will support a smooth transition to a smoke-free life.

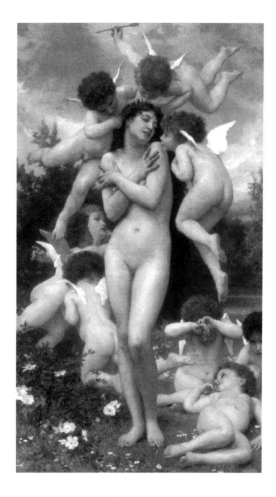

Blissful happiness in William-Adolphe Bouguereau's

Return of Spring.

8.

HAPPINESS & INNER PEACE

Genes that govern happiness must exist latently within everyone.
The genes are just waiting to be switched on.

Kazuo Murakami, Ph.D., Leading Geneticist
& Author, *The Divine Code of Life*

DNA and The Golden Ratio of Happiness

The Golden Ratio can be discovered in virtually every scientific discipline, including the field of human behavior. One of the more fascinating insights relating to the Golden Ratio is in the understanding of factors that determine happiness. In Sonja Lyubomirsky's intriguing book, *The How of Happiness*, she summarizes the general consensus of psychological research as to what are the most important determinants of happiness. Everyone has a happiness "set point," around which contentment hovers during their lives. The general consensus from many longitudinal twin studies reveals that approximately 50% of one's happiness is dependent on genetic factors (e.g., from our parents), 10% due to life circumstances and an astounding 40% is due to one's behavior and thoughts.

Surprisingly, life circumstances such as socioeconomic status, educational attainment, family income, marital status and religious commitment had minimal effect

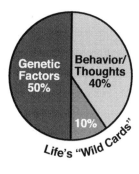
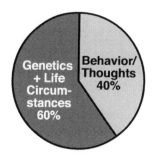
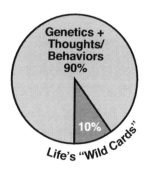

(*left*): Causal factors of happiness, general consensus.
(*center*): Causal factors of happiness, Golden Ratio distribution.
(*right*): Causal factors of happiness, quantum perspective: Up to 90% of our happiness may be genetically influenced through the combination of hard-wired genetic predisposition plus modifiable thoughts and behaviors. The remaining 10% of happiness is connected to our life outlook and how we handle the seemingly random "Wild Cards" life throws our way.

on one's overall well being. Even for people blessed with favorable circumstances—such as wealth or exceptional beauty—happiness is not guaranteed. A phenomenon called *hedonic adaptation* seems to effectively neutralize these fortunate life circumstances over time. We become accustomed to the same input over time, no matter how wonderful, and invariably gravitate back to our natural happiness set point. Conversely, Lyubomirsky says that a saving grace of hedonic adaptation is that in times of the reverse—such as illness or accident—adaptation also occurs, returning us to our genetic happiness set point. According to Lyubomirsky, by paying attention to and cultivating positive, life-affirming behaviors and thoughts, the malleable behaviors and thoughts can make up for potential poor predispositions in our genetic happiness set point. For people who are naturally blessed with a rosy disposition, cultivating positive behaviors and thoughts can lead to especially fulfilling lives. For those less fortunate, cultivating such behaviors can be nothing short of transformational. If we look at this distribution a little closer, we see that the ratio is along the lines of the Golden Ratio. The breakdown can be regrouped as follows:

Genetics 50% + Life Circumstances 10% = 60%; Behavior and Thoughts = 40%

This gives a 60/40 ratio—within 2% of the more exact Golden Ratio distribution 62/38. In other words, one's tendency towards happiness falls under the influence of the Golden Ratio. This is not surprising, since even our genetics are based on the precise, Divinely-Coded shape of our DNA: the primary structure of DNA's double helix has a length/width ratio of 34/21 angstroms. This 34/21 Fibonacci Ratio approximates the Golden Ratio of 1.618.

8

Our DNA is Modifiable

One of the world's top geneticists, Kazuo Murakami, Ph.D., has proven that our DNA is not just a static data bank. On the contrary, it has the dynamic potential to have desirable latent regions activated—or active, undesirable regions silenced—*by psychological input alone.* For example, Dr. Murakami proved that diabetics could lower their blood sugar simply by watching comedy movies. The molecular mechanism had to do with the activation via laughter/good emotions of 23 genes that have roles in controlling blood sugar. This calls to mind journalist and world peace activist Norman Cousins' successful treatment of his heart disease and other illnesses through comedy movie laughter therapy (and mega-doses of Vitamin C). Cousins explored the biochemistry of emotions in his best-selling book *Anatomy Of An Illness.* The modification of gene expression by conscious psychological input has revolutionized traditional concepts of our DNA as being a static, unalterable destiny control system. In essence, this research shows that we are *not* held hostage by our family's genetic heritage. Dr. Murakami says that we can activate our beneficial genes through positive or "genetic thinking," as he states in his book *The Divine Code of Life:*

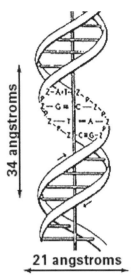

DNA molecule with Golden Ratio dimensions. Our Divinely-Coded DNA is modifiable through our thoughts and behavior.

> *My hypothesis is that an enthusiastic approach to life leads to success and activates the genes that make us experience happiness.*

Among the methods for activating the good or positive genes in our DNA, Dr. Murakami suggests:

> *Keep your intentions noble... Live with an attitude of thankfulness... Keep your thoughts positive* [which he believes is the most important]. *The trick is to take a broader perspective... we need to see the bigger picture and endeavor to see the positive in everything that happens to us in life... Let yourself be inspired. If nothing inspires you in the moment, think back to a time when you were deeply moved... I believe that when we are inspired, our genes never move in an adverse direction... [another method is*

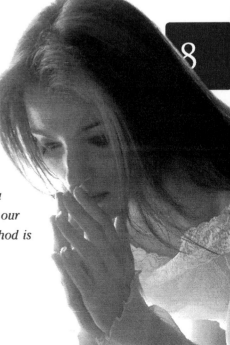

231

Our Hardwired 62/38 Golden Ratio Perspective

[Psychologist] B.A. Kelly proposed in 1955 that every person evaluates the world around him using the system of bipolar constructs. When judging others, for instance, one end of each pole represents a maximum positive trait and the other a maximum negative trait, such as honest/ dishonest, strong/weak, etc. Kelly had assumed that average responses in value-neutral situations would be 0.50. He was wrong. Experiments show a human bent toward favor or optimism that results in a response ratio in value-neutral situations of 0.62, which is phi. Numerous binary-choice experiments have reproduced this finding, regardless of the type of constructs or the age, nationality or background of the subjects...

When [psychologist] Vladimir Lefebvre... asks subjects to choose between two options about which they have no strong feelings and/ or little knowledge, answers tend to divide into the Golden Ratio proportion: 62% to 38%... When subjects are given scenarios that require a moral action and asked what percentage of people would take good actions vs. bad actions, their answers average 62% [towards the good actions]. 'When people say they feel 50/50 on a subject,' says Lefebvre, 'chances are it's more like 62/38.'

Essentially, this intriguing research means that our general, default ratio of positive opinions/perspective vs. negative reflects the Golden Ratio: 62% positive and 38% negative.

Source: *The Wave Principle of Human Social Behavior*,
by Robert Prechter, Jr.

8

to] shake up your habits regularly to become refreshed and invigorated—mentally and physically. A change in environment can also make you see new things and become the start of a new life... Our genes can even make possible those things we think are impossible... We are all born with the potential to become living miracles...

Dr. Murakami's inspiring work underscores the value of consciously, daily increasing the ratio of one's positive to negative thoughts. It calls to mind the importance of strengthening our ability to dwell at or above the 62% Golden Ratio point of positive, inspiring thoughts and feelings. This is especially true in light of the prevailing blizzard of negativity we are subjected to on a daily basis. Indeed, even the negative-to-positive ratio of emotion words silently conspires to pull us into the negative, as Chip and Dan Heath point out in their book *Switch: How to Change Things When Change is Hard:*

> *In an exhaustive study, a psychologist analyzed 558 emotion words—every one that he could find in the English language—and found that 62 percent of them were negative vs. 38 percent positive. That's a pretty shocking discrepancy. According to an old urban legend, Eskimos have 100 different words for snow. Well, it turns out that negative emotions are our snow* [note the 62/38 Golden Ratio at work].

In the above example, it is clearly imperative that we consciously focus on the "meaningful minority" 38% positive words in our daily language. Dr. Murakami says that we can dramatically improve the quality and perhaps even the quantity of our life through further activation of the Divine Code of Life within us all. This means we must choose to minimize or even avoid exposure to the way-out-of-ratio negativity of mainstream media. It can also cause us to healthfully reduce the amount of time we spend around negative people and situations. Regarding the unlimited wonder of genes and DNA, Dr. Murakami's work highlights the sublime role of what he calls "Something Great" plays in the evolution of humanity and the Universe.

Sleep Deprivation: A Surprising Major Cause of Unhappiness

When interviewer Charlie Rose asked author and former Harvard University president (1971-1991) Derek Bok what causes people the most unhappiness, Bok replied that there are three afflictions that seem to cause real unhappiness, as long as they persist: **1. Clinical Depression 2. Chronic Pain 3. Sleep Disorders** (deprivation or sleep apnea). The Golden Ratio Lifestyle Diet provides a solid framework for addressing all three of these conditions. Note: Derek Bok is the author of *The Politics of Happiness: What Government Can Learn from the New Research on Well-Being.* Excerpt from *The Charlie Rose Show*, PBS, 4/30/10.

8

The 90% Happiness Ratio

In Bruce Lipton, Ph.D.'s book, *The Biology of Belief*, he makes the case that cell membranes are the gatekeepers that control the environmental and psychological inputs into the cell. Environmental inputs could be anything from hormones, nutrients or toxins. Psychological inputs are what Candice Pert, Ph.D., calls *Molecules of Emotion*, which is also the title of her landmark book on the subject. Pert, one the featured speakers in the film *What the Bleep Do We Know!?* states that molecules of emotion are peptides that circulate in our blood in response to mental-emotional activity. In other words, our beliefs and emotions can generate molecules that can interact with our cell membranes causing an intracellular cascade effect that can turn various DNA switches on—or off. Bruce Lipton makes the convincing case that our DNA only *indirectly* controls what happens in our systems. He proposes that external inputs, environmental and/or psychological, which interact with the cell membrane are the *real* determinants of our health and happiness.

Now that we know that happiness is modifiable through positive behaviors and thoughts, let's reconsider the percentages of factors that determine our happiness. If 40% of the determinants of our happiness are due to our daily, cumulative behaviors and thoughts, which are actually having their effects through the mechanism of genetic modification, that means that our genes have the potential to activate *up to 90% of our happiness*: 50% inherited + 40% modifiable!

The Happiness and Beauty Connection

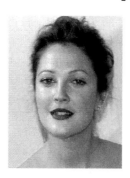 Enchanting actress Drew Barrymore topped *People* Magazine's list of the world's 100 most beautiful people in 2007. Barrymore attributes her beauty to her happy frame of mind and fun-loving approach to life: *Cheerfulness helps you look and feel pretty. People with a joyful nature always look beautiful.* It's no surprise that Barrymore's face also features the Golden Ratio in abundance. Glamorous Oscar-winning actress (and ping-pong enthusiast) Susan Sarandon echoes Drew's happiness and beauty perspective: *At the heart of looking good is, more than anything, having fun and greeting each day saying 'yes.'*

8

> *Happiness depends upon ourselves.*
> **Aristotle**

There is in actuality a push-pull relationship going on between our genes on the one hand and environmental factors and psychological inputs on the other. This scenario is in accordance with Dr. Murakami's "genetic thinking" concept, and reminds us that we have more power than we realize in altering our life perspective, thereby resetting our happiness set point to an upward, expanding Golden Spiral. Since the structure of our genes (DNA) is designed with Golden Ratio parameters, we can surmise that DNA may functionally operate by Golden Ratio principles as well.

The more alignment that we have with the Golden Ratio, the more positive resonance will be possible with our DNA. That is why by incorporating the easy-to-apply recommendations from the Golden Ratio Lifestyle Diet, it is possible to access more of Nature's Secret Nutrient (NSN) and turn *on* genes that are connected to our happiness, health and longevity.

Inner Peace and the Mona Lisa's Smile

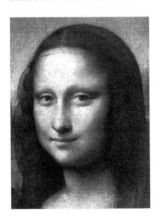

Taking the essence of happiness to a more refined level brings us to the quality of Inner Peace. The peaceful state denotes a subtle contentment that transcends the more buoyant nature of happiness. Leonardo Da Vinci captured this peaceful and contented quality in his masterpiece, the *Mona Lisa*. Mona Lisa's smile has fascinated people across the globe for centuries. If you look at her alluring smile carefully, you will notice that it isn't exactly halfway between a full-blown grin and a sorrowful frown, but has a slightly upward hint.

8

In her smile, Da Vinci skillfully captured the asymmetric point of Golden Ratio balance. Just by having Mona Lisa gaze upon you with her peaceful countenance, you might notice that you feel a little better than before. This Da Vincian blessing can be used as a quick inner attunement anytime you need to transcend your present circumstances and feel a lift.

Happy For No Reason

Author Marci Shimoff shows how happiness manifests along a spectrum in *Happy For No Reason*. This happiness continuum is shown in the following graph adapted from her book:

Unhappy	Happy for Bad Reason	Happy for Good Reason	Happy for No Reason
☹ ←————————————————————→ ☺			
Depressed	High from unhealthy addictions	Satisfaction from healthy experiences	Inner state of peace and well-being, not dependant on external factors
	External Source		**Internal Source**

The ultimate goal is Happy for No Reason or the state of Inner Peace. The distinction between happiness for any reason and Inner Peace is highlighted by the insightful quote that Marci found from the Upanishads:

Happiness for any reason is just another form of misery.

By aligning yourself with the Golden Ratio you will increasingly radiate and attract greater happiness, contentment and Inner Peace. Perhaps as more people become aware of the unifying principles of the Golden Ratio and begin to implement them in their lives, their personal state of Inner Peace will increase and spread throughout the world. This is exactly what seems to be happening with many artists, as they incorporate various aspects of the Golden Ratio into their creations.

8

> *Nothing in the future that happens to you is dependent on anything that's happened in the past.*
>
> **Robert Friedman, M.D.'s human evolution**
> **interpretation of Markov's Chain Theory**

The Golden Ratio of Peace

Imagine all the people, living life in peace...
You may say I'm a dreamer, but I'm not the
only one...

John Lennon, *Imagine*

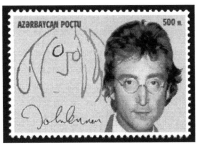

John Lennon, from a 1995
Azerbaijan postage stamp.

In October 2005, the New Jerusalem Foundation in Israel unveiled a Golden Ratio-based 50 ton sculpture called *Ratio* in Jerusalem. Thirty-two 1.5 ton limestone square stones modeled after certain stones in the Western Wailing Wall were arranged in a formation reflecting the Golden Ratio. The vertical arrangement of the blocks in the sculpture mirrors the beginning numbers in the Fibonacci Sequence, edges beautifully gilded with gold to catch the rays of the rising and setting sun. Sculptor Andrew Rogers of Australia had this to say about his unique work of gold-fringed stone:

I came at the invitation of the New Jerusalem Foundation. This is a very special city for me. I came here to create a stone sculpture called "Ratio"... "Ratio" demonstrates a mathematical formula, which helps us understand the compositions of plants and how they grow, the proportions of plants and the human body. In everyday terms it helps explain the curve of a snail shell or seashell, the sections on a pineapple,

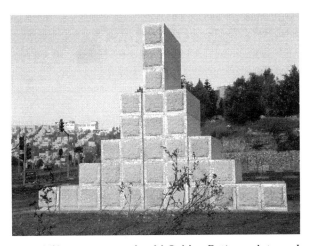

Andrew Rogers' 50 ton stone and gold Golden Ratio sculpture, Jerusalem.
The number of stones in each column are stacked vertically according to a rising
and falling Fibonacci Sequence: 1-1-2-3-5-8-5-3-2-1-1. This sculptural Fibonacci
sequence mirrors the FIT exercise patterns, as seen in chapter 6/Exercise Rx's.

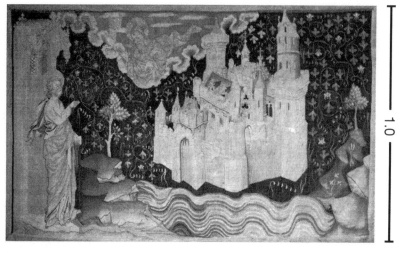

John of Patmos watches the descent of the New Jerusalem from God in a 14th century tapestry. The dimensions of the tapestry conform almost exactly to the Golden Ratio (1.618).

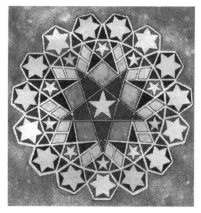

John Michell's *New Jerusalem* pentagonal, Golden Ratio diagram.

the proportions of our body, and it helps explain in my case a lot of sculptures that I'm creating around the world.

I started a project in contemporary art initially in the Arava desert, and to explain this project, we set out the mathematical formula in stone… I thought that because this is such a universal city and the Golden Ratio is such a universal explanation that there was a synthesis and symbolism of having it here… after all, it's one of the cradles of civilization and this is one of the universal theories…

Jerusalem is a city where three major world religions and cultures intersect. In our current era, this intersection has been one of ongoing war, separation and chaos. The principle of the Golden Ratio—of parts coming together in such a way as to form a harmonious, greater whole—can be seen as a key principle of the New Jerusalem concept. Prophecies in the Bible describe New Jerusalem as a place of peace and harmony that will descend from the heavens.

English author John Michell speaks eloquently about the New Jerusalem in his book *The Dimensions of Paradise: The Proportions and Symbolic Numbers of Ancient Cosmology*. This emerging new consciousness, grounded in the applied science of sacred geometry inclusive of the integrative Golden Ratio, would serve to unite the discordant fragments of world culture and religion, reorganizing them into a peaceful, inclusive whole. Perhaps as a timeless symbol of unity, the sculpture *Ratio* may act as a catalyst for the New Jerusalem to come of age in our time. For those of us not actually living in Jerusalem, the concept of the New Jerusalem can be thought of as being synonymous with awakening to a personal sense and enjoyment of the sacred, Divine Proportion. Identical Golden Ratio sculptures are being established by Andrew Rogers in twelve countries around the world, in conjunction with UNESCO's World Heritage project. Other countries that will have their own Golden Ratio sculptures include Chile, Peru, Great Britain, the United States, Australia, Sri-Lanka and Iceland.

Hopefully, as more people become aware of their divine nature and interconnectedness with all life, the positive effects will become evident throughout the world. Visionary artisans like John Michell and Andrew Rogers are among the modern-day Golden Ratio pioneers, helping people reawaken to their personal sense and stewardship of the New Jerusalem, within and without. Interestingly, the peace symbol has connotations similar to Lyubomirsky's Golden Ratio pie graph of happiness. The peace symbol, in addition to implying peace, reflects Golden Ratio balance in that it is also a pie graph that divides a circle into Golden Ratio.

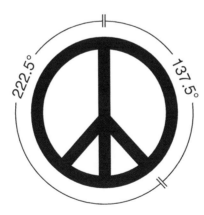

The Peace Symbol exhibits angles that directly reflect Golden Ratio angles: a circle can be divided into Golden Ratio with angles of 137.5° and 222.5° (222.5÷137.5=1.618). The resurgent popularity of this iconic 1960's symbol heralds not only the obvious increasing hunger for peace in our time, it also signals the more subtle re-emergence of Divine Code consciousness.

De-stress for More Happiness with *The 4-Hour Workweek*

There is no lack of time, only a lack of priorities.

Tim Ferriss

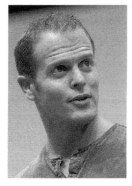

Lifestyle Design pioneer Timothy Ferriss, author of the bestselling book *The 4-Hour Workweek.*

For many, the word Work is similar to the word Diet in its negative connotations. While most people spend an extreme ratio of their waking hours at, travelling to or thinking about work, far too few would describe their work as a source of happiness, fulfillment and inner peace. Clearly there is room for improvement in both the quality and quantity of work time for many. Taking work quantity to an intriguing opposite extreme, visionary anti-workaholic author and optimal lifestyle designer Timothy Ferriss has developed paradigm-shifting ways of whittling down one's working time to an amazing 4 hours per week. How is this possible? In his bestselling book, *The 4-Hour Workweek*, Ferriss explores the time we routinely waste in our work and life and shows how to ruthlessly reclaim it. His innovative time reclamation techniques can rapidly revolutionize your work-to-personal-time ratio. To begin reclaiming wasted time, we have applied the Golden Ratio in a work-reduction graph to assist you in moving towards Ferriss' 4-hour workweek. While you may not want to go all the way down to 4 hours a week (or feel initially capable of doing it), you can use the Golden Ratio work reduction graph to gauge your own appropriate decremental progress towards a healthier work/personal time ratio. As many people are working in excess of 45 hours a week, this means that they are still working outside of the first Golden Ratio reduction, with insufficient personal/recreational/recharge time. Invariably, we end up

8

Golden Ratio work reduction graph, applying Golden Ratio reductions to Tim Ferriss' 4-Hour Workweek concept. Each reduction is multiplied by .62 to arrive at the next lower level.

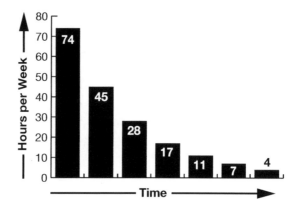

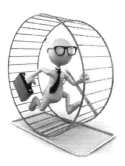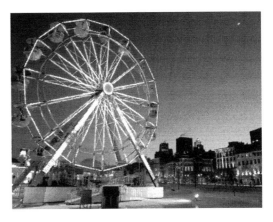

(*left*) While running on a hamster wheel might be fun for hamsters, humans generally prefer more stimulating and enjoyable pursuits. If you've ever felt like this in your work-life, know that there *is* another way. (*right*) By applying Tim Ferriss' 4-Hour Workweek principles, you can begin to step off the traditional work hamster-wheel and onto the more fulfilling and fun Tim Ferriss-wheel.

"robbing Peter to pay Paul," compromising or rushing our sleep, grooming, eating and our personal time. If this applies to you, it is well worth taking a closer look at how you could dial back your working time towards healthier, lower Golden Ratios of work to personal time. Start by incorporating more "white space" into your life and daily schedule—rest, relaxation, regeneration and personal/family time. While it's possible to burn the candle at both ends for years—working 50, 60, 70+ hours a week at work you may not enjoy—the long-term effects on your health, happiness and longevity can be far more serious than you allow yourself to think. If this describes you, perhaps it's time to take a cue from Apple and *Think Different*.

> *Get satisfied with doing less of what matters least,*
> *and more of what matters most.*
> **Frank Sabato**

8

Enhancing Healthy Work/Life Ratios

Like an athlete who over trains without sufficient rest and recovery (leading to poor performance, burnout or injury), poor work/life ratios invariably lead to under performance and unhappiness, not to mention potentially deadly health challenges. One study of 7,095 British civil servants revealed that long/overtime working hours increases the risk of coronary heart disease by a whopping 67%. Mika Kivimaki, professor of epidemiology and public health at University College London and lead author of the study published in the *Annals of Internal Medicine* put it this way:

We knew there was an association between working long hours and coronary heart disease, but we were really surprised that it was such a strong predictor.

Clearly, maintaining a healthy work/life ratio is an imperative for health, happiness and longevity. While everyone's work/life ratio needs are unique, many are both overworked and insufficiently fulfilled, with inadequate personal/recharging time. Whether you're interested in the 40+ or 4 hour (or less) workweek, the following strategies can offer support towards achieving your ideally fulfilling work/life ratio.

Kaizen: Small Steps for Greater Happiness

A journey of a 1000 miles begins with the first step.

Lao Tzu

Hoshin and The First 15%, inspired by Dr. Deming, are also at the root of Kaizen (Japanese for Continuous Improvement), consisting of taking small steps of improvement towards a goal. In his Deming/Kaizen-inspired book *One Small Step Can Change Your Life*, Dr. Robert Maurer illustrates how taking small steps can lead to big progress, as large steps often cause a fear-of-change, shut-down reaction in the brain. Kaizen's small steps are also at the heart of this book's 21-Day Quick-Start Checklist System. By taking small daily steps in support of the 9 health and longevity drivers, the butterfly effect of increasing returns is engaged. Like the ripples in the surface of a lake after a pebble is tossed, the waves start small and then grow exponentially. Energy and momentum builds in a cross-reinforcing chain reaction.

Kaizen's power is that the steps need not be big ones; again, the most effective steps are paradoxically often the smallest. For example, if your work is unfulfilling you are more likely to take the small step of spending 2 minutes a day visualizing the key details of more fulfilling work or polishing up your resume vs. taking the bigger step of quitting your current job. Such small steps invariably set the stage for the big change desired; they prime the pump and get you in the game. The key to Kaizen's success is to take *meaningful* small steps. How to start doing this leads into the next strategy for better work/life happiness, a key element in Tim Ferriss' 4-Hour Workweek.

8

242

The 80/20 Principle: Working Smarter (and Happier) vs. Harder

Anyone can be more effective with less effort by learning how to identify and leverage the 80/20 principle— the well-known, unpublicized secret that 80 percent of all our results [and happiness] in business and life stem from a mere 20 percent of our efforts.

Richard Koch, *The 80/20 Principle*

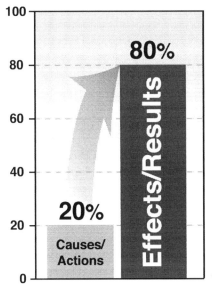

The 80/20 Principle: 80% of the results come from 20% of the actions.

First observed in 1906 by Italian economist Vilfredo Pareto and championed by quality genius Dr. Joseph Juran, the 80/20 Rule (aka the Pareto Principle) can transform your work and life. Pareto initially observed that 80% of the land in Italy was owned by 20% of the people, closer to home noting that 80% of the peas in his garden came from 20% of the pods. Ten words summarize this principle: *80% of the results come from 20% of the actions.* This dynamic of uneven distribution is at play everywhere in the Universe. Whether 80/20, 60/40, etc., the Universe seems to operate according to a seesaw of small-to-large ratios of causes to effects, actions to results, e.g.,

- 20% of activities/work delivers 80% of happiness
- 20% of customers generate 80% of business
- 20% of people known generate 80% of general relationships fulfillment

Identifying and enhancing the 20% "vital few" minority causes/actions which lead to the majority of desired outcomes is magic for greater happiness. Increased focus on the 20% of activities which deliver 80% of the desired results multiplies your productivity and results. 80/20 authority Richard Koch calls applying this principle to life and work *80/20 Thinking*, which leads to the popular *working smarter vs. harder* maxim becoming real. Combining kaizen's small steps with 80/20 focus on the *best* steps allows us to step into the Golden Ratio synergy zone: a greater whole which exceeds the sum of its parts.

8

Order From Chaos: A Human-Scaled System for Enhanced Productivity

Picture		Vase
	Monitor	
Hot File	Keyboard	Phone
Work Space	Chair	Work Space

The Order From Chaos system upgrades working space to enhance productivity. Positioning key desk items using a Golden Ratio grid can provide an added boost.

In *Order from Chaos: Six Steps To Personal & Professional Organization*, organizational expert Liz Davenport presents a proven system which greatly increases the ratios of creativity and productivity to chaos. Not surprisingly, some of Davenport's research echoes the Golden Ratio. For example, she notes that mistakes increase about 40% when most people try to do multiple things at once, aka multitasking. Another example is a U.S. survey showing that about 60% of people are habitually disorganized. While chaos is not always a bad thing—a certain proportion often fosters creativity—the challenge comes when the *ratio* of creative chaos to productivity and fulfillment falls out of proportion. When this happens, frustration and stress levels rise and inner peace and happiness inevitably suffers.

Davenport's approach better integrates you into your working environment, enhancing calm and confidence. One's desk and working space is tuned to basic human proportions, e.g., everything used daily is placed within hand's reach; weekly, arm's reach; monthly, in the room (out of hand's or arm's reach). This supports the 80/20 Principle at work: 80% of the time we work with just 20% of our papers/files. Davenport's system also includes optimizing one's to-do list and scheduling/calendar systems. Integrating Golden Ratio dynamics boosts the system even further, e.g., the small step of positioning key objects on your desk (monitor, phone, pen cup, picture, etc.) according to approximate Golden Ratio grid points. Greater productivity and happiness—Nature's Path of Least Resistance and Maximum Performance—are more predictable, pleasant results of this easy-to-implement system.

8

Adding Time To Our Life and Life To Our Time

We all get the same gift of 168 hours per week: 7 days x 24 hours/day. If you figure the Golden Sleep Ratio of about 9 hours of sleep/rest for every 24 hours (63 hours/week), 3 hours/day for meals prep/eating (21 hours/week), and 1.5 hours daily for bathing/bathroom/grooming (10.5 hours/week), it adds up to 94.5 hours/week—

for just the basics. This leaves 73.5 hours/week of waking time for work, commuting, exercise and all personal activities. It's logical that in order to improve the quality of your life, you'd want to increase your personal time ratio in order to arrive at your individual ideal ratio of work to personal time. Of course, everyone's idea of the ideal ratio will vary, depending on the rewards obtained from work vs. personal activities.

Hours worked per day and week through the centuries (US and Europe).			Average hours worked per week in different countries (2008/pre-recession data).	
Time Period	Work hours per day	Work days per week	Country	Work hours per week
Middle Ages	8	6	USA	35
1800	14	N/A	Poland, Czech Republic	38
1840	10	N/A	Greece	41
1919	8-9	N/A	South Korea	44
1936	8	5	Spain, Denmark, Ireland	31
2010	5-8	4-5	France, Belgium	30
Ferriss 4HWW	<1	.5	Netherlands, Norway	27
			Ferriss 4HWW	4

Life is precious and our days are numbered. We have a total of about 29,000 days to live when we're born, assuming an 80 year life span. If you're 40 years old, this means you have around 14,500 days to go—14,500 sunrises and sunsets. It goes pretty fast, especially if we fail to appreciate the quality of the moment. And to top it off, none of us knows for sure when the screen of our life will read: *Game Over.* But hold on—here's the great news: if you learn and apply the Golden Ratio Lifestyle Diet, you can vastly increase the quality of your life along with your odds of living 100+ *healthy* years. This translates into enjoying 36,250 days of life from birth or about a 20% increase over the "norm" of 29,000 days. Since most people spend the majority of their waking time working, doing work that's fulfilling and meaningful ought to be high on everyone's list, whether it's for 4 or 40+ hours a week.

Along with upgrading the quality of your work to be more enjoyable, de-stressing via upgrading your work-to-personal time ratio is clearly a major modifiable happiness/longevity behavior you can control. Greater happiness, health, inner peace and longevity are among the inevitable results.

> *Happiness is the meaning and the purpose of life,*
> *the whole aim and end of human existence.*
>
> **Aristotle**

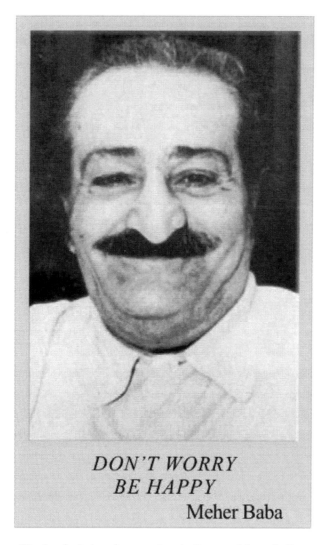

DON'T WORRY
BE HAPPY
Meher Baba

Words of wisdom from an inspiration card from Indian
mystic Meher Baba (1894–1969), which inspired Bobby
McFerrin's 1988 hit *Don't Worry, Be Happy.*

THE GOLDEN RATIO **Rx** LIFESTYLE DIET

HAPPINESS & INNER PEACE

Pick one or more of the following Rx's to add to your daily health regimen.

1. DNA Reactivation Mandala Meditation

The use of mandalas is an ancient and powerful method of focusing to de-stress, ground and center yourself. Simply by gazing at this image of a DNA cross-section immediately gets you away from your thinking mind and into a more right-brained state of relaxation.

Gaze at the DNA image on the next page in a relaxed frame of mind, as you breathe slowly and deeply for 3-5 minutes. Then, close your eyes and continue to see this beautiful latticework pattern of life in your mind's eye until it fades. When you're ready, slowly open your eyes. You will now feel more deeply relaxed and in sync with your innate Golden Ratio biorhythms. May your day now unfold in greater and more effortless harmony.

Next page: Cross section of DNA; note multi-petalled decagonal Golden Ratio geometry. Since a decagon is essentially two 5 pointed stars overlaid, we could say that we are all superstars, right down to our DNA design level.

8

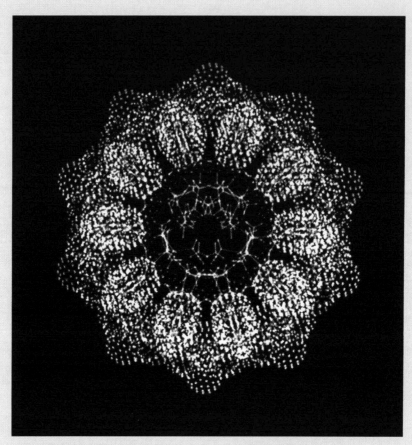

DNA cross section, with decagonal Golden Ratio symmetry.

2. Upgrade Your Working/Personal Time Ratio

Consider the amount of time you work in relation to your personal time. Is the proportion healthy and fulfilling? The easiest way to get a sense of this is to simply record the actual hours you spend on work and work-related activities in any given week in your daily planner (work-related activities would include things like lunch and travel time to and from work). Then, simply divide your total time spent working vs. your total non-working/personal time. If you feel that your working time is out of ratio and is stressing you out, try these small steps to restore a healthier balance:

Kaizen's Small Steps for Continuous Improvement

Select and review for a few moments ONE of your current top challenges. Next, surface ONE small meaningful yet manageable step that would move you forward regarding your challenge or aim. Next, take the step! Then, ID another small step. Schedule your next small step to set it in place as necessary. Read Dr. Robert Maurer's book *One Small Step Can Change Your Life: The Kaizen Way*.

The 80/20 Pareto Principle

Start thinking 80/20 by taking targeted small steps to enhance the 20% causes/actions which lead to the 80% desired outcomes/results. For example:

- 20% of activities/work delivers 80% of happiness:
  ACTION: ID and expand the key 20% to increase happiness/fulfillment.
- 20% of customers generates 80% of business:
  ACTION: ID and focus more on the 20% to grow your business.
- 20% of people known generate 80% of fulfillment.
  ACTION: Clarify the 20% group & increase meaningful time spent with them.

Combining 80/20 focus with small steps sets the stage for breakthrough results. Read Richard Koch's book *The 80/20 Principle* and Tim Ferriss' *The 4-Hour Workweek*.

Order From Chaos

Take the following small step to begin upgrading your workspace to the Cockpit Office, point #1 from Liz Davenport's Order From Chaos system:

1. Clear your desk of all items currently within both hands and arms reach.
2. Place all items/papers/files you access daily to be within easy Hands Reach.
3. Place all items/papers/files you access several times a week within Arms Reach (beyond the Hands Reach zone).

Read *Order from Chaos* or visit Liz's site to take the next simple step: www.OrderFromChaos.com

3. Fibonacci's Reverse Psychology for Happiness and Inner Peace

This exercise is a great way to reestablish your natural state of happiness and inner peace and takes a just few minutes. By using Nature's Path of Least Resistance, i.e., the Fibonacci Sequence, to balance your emotional state before going to bed or upon awakening, subtle stresses on your nervous system can be released. Many of us have people who, at one time or another, caused us a bit of grief. It may be just one person or there may be many with whom we are at odds. The perceived injustice to us may be real or there may be some projection involved. In either case, the subtle effect on our nervous system is insidious and detrimental to our health and peace of mind. However, there's a unique and easy way to short-circuit this unhealthy, negative reaction. By reversing Fibonacci's Sequence and using it to discharge your projections and feelings, you can clear your nervous system of needless psychological stress.

Here's the process:

Imagine that your feelings towards a particular person with whom you are at odds are at their most intense—we'll call this "level 21." With a deep in-breath, feel that intensity for about five seconds and then as you exhale feel the intensity drop all the way down to a 13. Whew! That feels *much* better. Take another deep breath and as you exhale, feel the intensity drop down to an 8. Now that the intensity is lessening, you can feel a deep relief and relaxation emerging in your nervous system. With another deep inhalation and exhalation, feel the intensity drop down to level 5. The negative emotional pattern is really weakening now, especially as you take another breath, in and out and move down to 3. Those invisible knots in your nervous system are almost totally unraveled, as you continue breathing and drop to level 2.

Now it's just one more gentle in and out breath and you can let go down to 1…and breathing through 1 another time… and one last deep breath in and out, and the intensity is all the way down to 0. Now, just breathe gently 3 more times while you let those good feelings of release and inner peace resonate through your body.

Fibonacci's Reverse Psychological Stress Reduction Sequence

21——————————13————8——5—3—2-1-1-0

| Enemy–Negative Charge–Problem | Friend–Neutral Charge–Resolution |
| *Disharmony* | *Peace* |

You have just harnessed Fibonacci's Reverse Psychology to dissolve a negative emotional charge, which was potentially damaging to your health and transmuted it to a state of enhanced inner peace. Now you can act without reacting the next time you interact with your friend. Repeat the process as often as desired if you feel any residual charge or recurrence.

4. The Power of the Mona Lisa Smile

Look at *Mona Lisa's* smile. For a few moments you might try to mirror her smile—approximately 60% happy. See if you can find that subtle balance point that defines the Golden Ratio. Try it first without a mirror and then with one. This is a playful way to raise and balance your emotions throughout your day. How does it feel when you smile like *Mona Lisa*? You may want to get a small picture of *Mona Lisa* to keep on your desk so you can fine-tune your inner state of mind whenever you like. Of course, if you feel the need to expand your range or balance a smile-less day, you can always take *Mona Lisa Smile* star Julia Robert's cue and unleash your best megawatt superstar smile :))

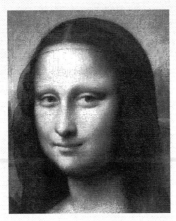 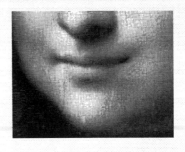

Mona Lisa's Divinely-Coded smile.

5. The Vitruvian Wo/Man Happiness & Inner Peace Exercise

Take a look at Da Vinci's *Vitruvian Man* and Hedden's *Divine Code Vitruvian Woman*. Then, mirror either image by standing with your feet slightly wider than shoulder-width apart and your arms extended from your sides, so that your silhouette forms a five-pointed star—a timeless, classic symbol of the Golden Ratio. Close your eyes for a moment and breathe deeply. Feel your idealized five-fold symmetry and know that your entire being is reflecting the Golden Ratio. Know that this Code links you with everything in creation, from the tiniest atoms to the great spiraling galaxies in the heavens. Allow a feeling of love, gratitude, happiness and inner peace to spiral out from your heart, spreading into a vibrant connection with all that is, giving thanks for the precious gift of your life and all the people and magic within it.

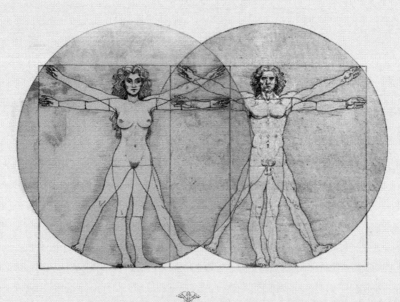

6. Candle Gazing Exercise

This is a simple and relaxing method for strengthening your sense of inner peace. The exercise is adapted from mindfulness master Dr. Phil Nuernberger's *Strong and Fearless* and describes how to both calm and focus your mind:

1. Practice in a dark, quiet room. Your candle should be an even-burning dinner candle placed at about arms length in front of you. The flame should be level with your eyes, so you can hold your head steady and gaze straight ahead. If you're lucky and the wick of your candle is the right length, your candle flame will divide itself into Golden Ratio by natural color and temperature gradients. This allows you to subtly tune into your sense of Divine Proportion.

2. Sit quietly with tall, relaxed posture. For a few moments, close your eyes and breathe slowly and deeply. Mindfully focus on your Breath Awareness: note the gentle coolness of the air as it flows over your upper lip and nostrils upon inhalation, followed by the gentle warmth of the air on your upper lip upon exhalation. This clears your mind and steadies your concentration.

3. Open your eyes and gaze without blinking at the flame. If you blink within a few seconds after beginning, ignore it and continue to gaze. Focus on the flame and ignore all other thoughts, sensations and feelings. Keep your gaze steady and unblinking.

4. When you blink or your eyes begin to water, stop the external gaze. Close your eyes and visualize the flame in your mind's eye as long as you comfortably can. The smaller, clearer and more defined the image of the flame, the better the training for meditation. Don't worry if at first the image of the flame is undefined or vague. With practice, the image of the flame will become clearer and more defined. By internalizing the image of the flame, you change the exercise from one of *concentration* (external orientation) to one of *meditation* (internal orientation). Begin by gazing at the flame for 5 minutes with eyes open and then visualize for 3 minutes with eyes closed. Gradually increase the length of your external concentration/internal meditation segments according to Fibonacci Ratios, i.e., 5/3...8/5... and finally as your concentration/meditation skills improve, work up to 13 minutes eyes open and 8 minutes eyes closed, 21 minutes in total.

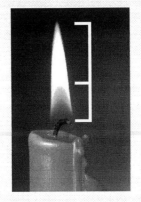

The exercise should be performed in a totally effortless and relaxed manner—avoid any straining during the exercise. To achieve maximum benefits, try to practice twice a week or more. Your new powers of concentration and relaxation will noticeably transfer to improvements in concentration and creativity in your work and life in general.

Note: Do the candle gazing exercise in a room that has some ventilation, but not so much that your flame wavers. To avoid excess smoke and perfume smell, use clean burning fragrance-free candles, made of natural substances like beeswax. Also, make sure that your candle is in a stable candle holder and that there is nothing near or above the candle that could catch fire.

7. The Sacred Sites Inner Peace Exercise

What do the Great Pyramid, Stonehenge, Mexico's Pyramid of the Sun, the Parthenon and New Mexico's Chaco Canyon all have in common? In addition to being places of profound peace and majesty, all of these ancient sacred sites integrate the Golden Ratio in their design and/or layout (see *The Divine Code of Da Vinci, Fibonacci, Einstein & YOU* for a more in-depth analysis). Sacred sites are visited by many as a means of connecting with their visible and energetic link to the highly advanced wisdom encoded in their geometry along with their mysterious beauty. Such sites hint at the vast canon of the timeless, mysterious wisdom of the ancients.

Select the site that appeals to you on the next three pages and contemplate it for a few moments. Then, close your eyes and see it in your minds eye. Allow your mind to gently explore the site, being aware of any sensations or meaning that surfaces for you. Let your own inner peace and presence be strengthened by your mind's journey to your chosen sacred site. Two highly recommend picture books are *Sacred Earth: Places of Peace and Power* by Martin Gray and *The Sacred Earth* by Courtney Milne. Both feature large, beautiful color pictures of the world's sacred sites, offering an enjoyable opportunity to connect with their silent wisdom and peace. Next time you're planning a vacation, you might try to include a sacred site in your itinerary.

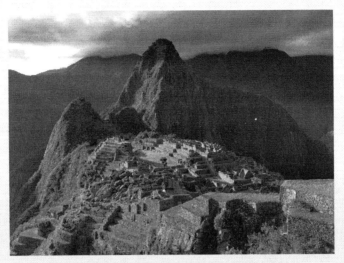

Machu Picchu, lost city of the Incas in Peru.

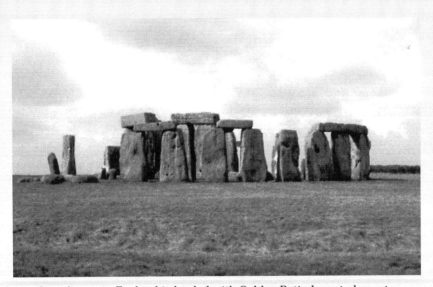

Stonehenge in England is loaded with Golden Ratio layout elements.

8

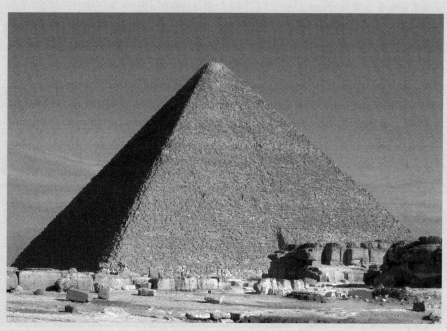

The Great Pyramid, Egypt. To this day no one knows for sure who built it, or why.

8

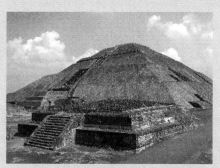

Pyramid of the Sun, Mexico. Its footprint
exceeds that of Egypt's Great Pyramid.

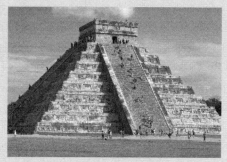

Pyramid at Chichen Itza,
Yucatan, Mexico.

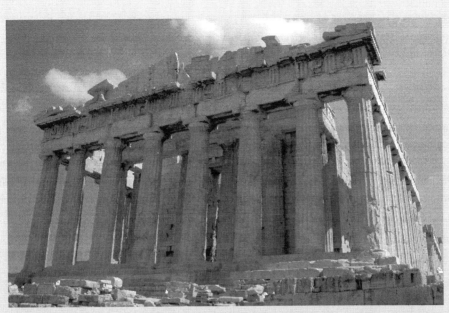
The Parthenon in Greece, whose front façade fits neatly within a Golden Rectangle.

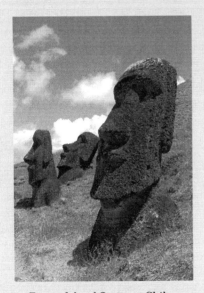

Easter Island Statues, Chile.

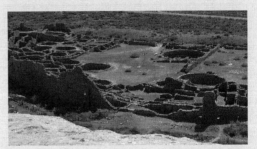

Pueblo Bonito ruins, Chaco Canyon, NM USA.

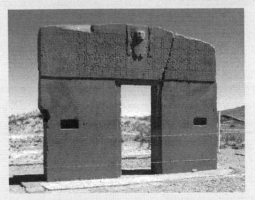

Gate of the Sun, Bolivia.

8

8. The Golden Doors of Your Day

When you awake each morning, you are presented with the priceless gift of another day. Then, at the end of your day when you lay down to sleep, you are preparing to relax deeply and recharge for the next day. How can you set the stage to make the most of these twin "Golden Door" opportunities? Try this simple daily practice for 21 days and see the difference for yourself.

• For at least 3 minutes after waking up (in bed with eyes closed, just after using the bathroom if needed): Imagine the day ahead. See yourself accomplishing all you wish with ease, grace and great enjoyment. See any possible barriers or challenges that may arise melt away, as if by magic. Allow yourself to fantasize about incredibly wonderful things happening in the day ahead that would make it a most fantastic day. Spend a few moments feeling deep gratitude for your life, the day ahead, the people close to you and all known and unknown opportunities. When you're ready, take a few long deep breaths and slowly open your eyes...

• For at least 3 minutes before falling asleep: What are you most grateful for in your life? Let the images, sounds, feelings wash over you. Then, see yourself enjoying great health, wealth and happiness, in whatever forms and experiences are most meaningful and inspiring for you. Remember, the subconscious mind cannot tell the difference between what is "real" and what is passionately imagined. For these precious minutes before you fall asleep, give yourself permission to let go and imagine, in multi-sensory detail, all that you most desire to be, do and have in your ideal life...

9. Focus: Happiness, Gratitude, Appreciation

As 1964 Olympic 10K Champion Billy Mills points out, *the subconscious mind cannot tell the difference between reality or imagination.* Said another way: *Whatever you APPRECIATE (regularly focus your heart and mind on, value) APPRECIATES (grows, like assets in a bank).* Mills rehearsed his victory in his mind daily for four years, leading to his achieving one of the greatest upsets in Olympic history. There is enormous hidden power in using our imagination to focus on what we most want to create and grow in our lives. Focused appreciation, gratitude and expectancy are like super magnets which attract their counterparts. When you clarify and focus on what you want and are most grateful for in life, you attract more of it. Focusing on happiness attracts more of the same. Try this easy exercise from co-author Matthew Cross' Personal Hoshin workshop: write down 1-2 items each on the following Appreciation Focus List. Then, appreciate—*focus with feeling*—on as many as you wish with eyes closed for a few moments. Remember to sit tall and breathe deeply. Let your mind flow over your Appreciation Points. Feel them as if they are real, *now*. Then, open your eyes and release those good feelings into your day and future. Next day, or whenever you need a boost, repeat. As Oprah Winfrey said:

> *The more you praise and celebrate your life,*
> *the more there is in life to celebrate.*

My Appreciation Focus List

My Best Memories (*any*):

_____

_____

_____

My Greatest Strengths:

_____

_____

_____

Inspiring Activities (*things I love to do*):

_____

_____

_____

Inspiring People (*past or present*):

_____

_____

_____

Inspiring Places (*places where I feel great*):

_____

_____

_____

I am most Grateful for:

_____

_____

_____

I am Happiest when I:

_____

_____

_____

My Wild Dreams (*any, e.g., circle the world, climb Everest, write a book*):

_____

_____

_____

My Unique or Hidden Talents:

_____

_____

_____

8

My Greatest Triumphs (*any*):

_____

_____

_____

10. 5-Point Inner Peace Meditation

Meditation is one of the oldest methods known to regain and maintain inner peace and support enlightenment. Its benefits are profound and scientifically proven to also enhance total health and performance. There are many meditation practices to choose from, e.g., Benson Relaxation Response, Transcendental/TM, Vipassana, Zazen, etc. Try this easy Golden Ratio 5-point version for 13 to 21 or more minutes a day to reap the rewards of meditation.

- Choose a place and time where you won't be disturbed.

- Relax… Sit tall, with comfortable, buoyant posture. Ideally, sit cross-legged on a carpeted floor, using a cushion if desired.

- With eyes closed, begin to deepen and slow your breath. Experiment with Golden Ratio Breathing: breath in deeply into your belly to the count of 5; breath out fully to the count of 8. Do this for a few breaths until your body gets used to the ratio of a shorter inbreath and longer outbreath. Let the count go whenever you like.

- Gently focus on your breath. When any thoughts come into your mind, simply return to focusing on your breath and let them pass. Variations can include focusing on one word, image, sound or feeling, along with your breath. Experiment and find what works for you.

- When the time feels right to finish, raise your hands together and bring them up a few inches in front of your eyes, palms facing your face. Slowly open your eyes and allow them to acclimate first to your palms; after 5 or so seconds, gently lower your hands.

- Allow yourself a few minutes to return to your activities, refreshed and calm. Jot down any insights you may have received while they're still fresh.

8

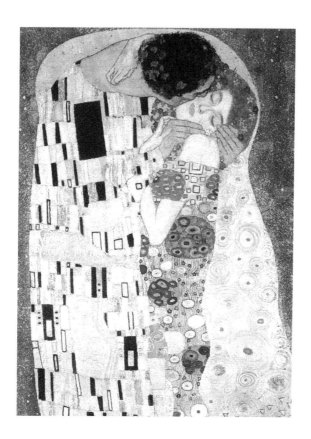

The Kiss, Gustav Klimt's masterpiece.

9.

NATURAL BEAUTY & ATTRACTION

...it can be said that wherever there is an intensification of function or a particular beauty and harmony of form, there the Golden Mean will be found.
Robert Lawlor, author, *Sacred Geometry: Philosophy and Practice*

The Golden Prime Zone: Ages 19–31

From ages 19 to 31, Nature ingeniously fine-tunes our hormonal physiology and sexual attractiveness to maximally reflect the Golden Ratio. Nature's elegant Golden Ratio engineering has designed the attraction of the opposite sexes to be a force that is too strong to resist, thus ensuring the passage of one's DNA to the next generation.

The numbers 19 and 31 generally define the boundaries of our prime physical 13 year lifecycle phase and are also known as "prime" numbers. Prime numbers are numbers that are only divisible by themselves and the number 1. However, 19 and 31 are special prime numbers: when 31 is divided by 19, the result is 1.63: within 1% of the Golden Ratio. In essence, our most robust years—the period between ages 19 and 31—is our "Golden Prime Zone." This double entendre highlights the fact that the physical robustness and sexual vitality that virtually everyone experiences in their Golden Prime Zone (between ages 19-31) is the ideal state to which all health, exercise, diet and lifestyle programs aspire—the Golden Ratio Lifestyle Diet included. Natural beauty and attraction are but two of the many outcomes that result from aligning with the

9

Golden Ratio. One's inherent genetic potential is optimized once the primary drivers of the Golden Ratio Lifestyle Diet are aligned and activated. Yet the external beauty associated with the Golden Ratio doesn't stop with one's appearance and physiology. It can powerfully manifest in one's behavior, creativity and character as well. The Golden Ratio attributes of "beautiful people" are only an external hint of the excellence that anyone can display in any of the multitude of human endeavors. As a reminder of how beautiful the reflections of the Golden Ratio can be in the human form, let's look at some well-known examples and some of the reasons underlying their natural beauty and power of attraction.

Marilyn Monroe and Sean Connery: Divinely Proportioned Sex Symbols

Marilyn Monroe and Sean Connery are two of the 20th century's most well-known sex symbols. They both strongly epitomize Divine Proportions in their archetypal physical attractiveness and magnetism. Monroe's Golden Ratio attributes are very apparent in the accompanying photo from the 1957 movie, *The Prince and the Showgirl*. One's attention is immediately drawn to her shapely waist and bustline. Her waist accentuates the Golden Ratio dividing point between her shoulders and knees, while the width of her shoulders to waist displays Golden Ratio proportions as well. Monroe's ability to arouse the opposite sex was no doubt based on a subconscious Golden Ratio recognition by her fans. In spite of her short career, she won the 1960 Golden Globe Award for Best Actress for *Some Like It Hot*. Her image is forever etched into America's collective unconscious as the archetypal beautiful blonde female of her generation.

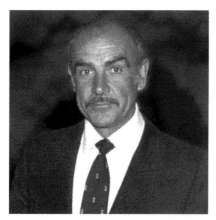

The ever-suave and debonair
Sean Connery.

Sean Connery developed his rugged masculinity early in his career by sculpting his body with serious weight training. He also learned to master and express graceful movements, which set him apart from other actors. All of these techniques complemented his innate animal magnetism to produce one of the era's most iconic sex symbols. As *GQ* magazine describes Connery:

All the actors who've inhabited the role of James Bond have enjoyed the trapping of style—killing bad guys in Savile Row bespoke—but only one of them can truly be said to have style... Sean Connery

9

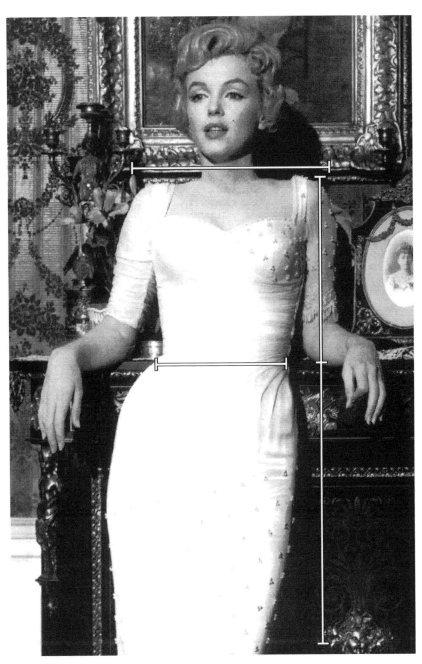

Marilyn Monroe's displays her shapely Golden Ratio attributes in *The Prince and the Showgirl*, 1957. Shoulder width/waist width = the Golden Ratio, and her waist is also the Golden Cut point between shoulders and knees.

9

is still the yardstick by which all other Bonds are measured—the arched eyebrow, the dry wolfish smile. But we at GQ think it mostly has to do with the way he moved. It only looked effortless: Before he was cast in Dr. No, Connery was an ardent student of the Swedish movement teacher Yat Malmgren, whose book on body technique became Connery's bible. That's how the former bricklayer from a hardscrabble section of Edinburgh learned to walk with (in one observer's memorable phrase) the threatening grace of a panther on the prowl.' Read it as a gloss on his penchant for violence or his sexual prowess: It works both ways.

Connery used his Divinely Proportioned attributes to great advantage, from his suave and debonair James Bond role to many other movies, including his 1987 Academy Award-winning performance as Best Supporting Actor in *The Untouchables*. Many critics and fans alike have said that the quality of Connery's acting has only improved with time. Certainly his personal appeal has. In 1989, at almost 60 years of age, he was voted *People* Magazine's Sexiest Man Alive; in 1999, at the age of 69, he was voted Sexiest Man of the Century. He has also received a Crystal Globe for outstanding artistic contribution to world cinema. On a fun side note, Sean Connery stands 6'2" tall—62 being the numbers used to represent the Golden Ratio when referring to percentages, e.g., 62% to 38%.

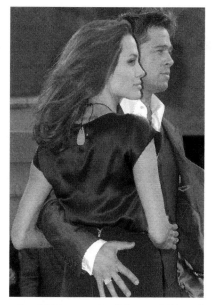

Brad Pitt scored a 9.3 out of 10 and Angelina Jolie scored a 7.7 on Oprah Winfrey's *Laws of Attraction* special.

The Golden Ratio Facial Scores of Brad Pitt and Angelina Jolie

America's most famous television host and media mogul, Oprah Winfrey, has discovered the science of the Golden Ratio. In March, 2009, she presented a series of shows on the *Laws of Attraction*, on which she hosted biostatistics professor Dr. Kendra Schmid. By using 29 precise facial measurements, including several Golden Ratio parameters, Dr. Schmid is able to assess anyone's level of attractiveness. For example, to get a higher score, the length of the face compared to the width should be 1.6, the Golden Ratio. She then takes other key measurements of proportion and symmetry to come up with a composite score on a scale of 1–10, with 10 being the ideal.

9

Two of the highest scoring celebrities, Brad Pitt and Angelina Jolie, scored 9.3 and 7.7 respectively. Brad Pitt's 9.3 is the highest score received by any celebrity so far. Dr. Schmid noted that Angelina's famous "full lips," [although voluptuous], were what lowered her score. Dr. Schmid said that *the width of a mouth should be twice the height of the lips.* Other notables were Halle Berry at 7.4 and Hugh Jackman at 6.5.

Anastasia Soare: Hollywood's Golden Ratio Natural Beauty Expert

My goal is to make the eyebrows beautifully symmetrical and proportionate to a person's own natural symmetry and bone structure, because even when features are asymmetrical—as they often are—well-shaped brows will bring a harmony, proportion and balance to the face.

Anastasia Soare

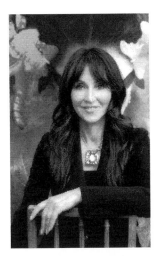

Anastasia Soare, Golden Ratio beauty expert to celebrities worldwide. Her work has transformed the art and science of natural beauty enhancement.

A Divine Code Genius is someone who has been inspired by and applied the Golden Ratio in a unique and original way. In our first book, *The Divine Code of Da Vinci, Fibonacci, Einstein and YOU*, we featured some of the more prominent Divine Code Geniuses in history, including Da Vinci, Fibonacci and Einstein. We are always pleasantly surprised when a new and innovative Divine Code Genius arrives on the scene. Anastasia Soare, Hollywood's Golden Ratio natural beauty expert, has joined the ranks of history's Divine Code Geniuses with her Golden Ratio-inspired innovations in the fields of beauty, aesthetics and cosmetology.

Anastasia and her family emigrated from Romania to America in 1989. Despite not yet speaking English, she soon found work in a Los Angeles salon as a cosmetologist. By 1997 she had opened her own salon, with an emphasis on eyebrow sculpting. As a result of her innovative approach, she quickly became the rave of Beverly Hills, in high demand by the world's top celebrities. Some of her notable clients include Oprah Winfrey (whose eyebrows Anastasia sculpted live on Oprah's show), Madonna, Jennifer Lopez, Jennifer Aniston, Naomi Campbell, Kim Kardashian, Reese Witherspoon and Ryan Seacrest.

9

What was it that compelled Hollywood's most beautiful and influential people to have Anastasia sculpt their brows and upgrade their look and appearance? While it's true that Anastasia has an eastern European flair to her personality and work, what really distinguishes her peerless approach is her underlying mastery of the Golden Ratio. In Romania, Anastasia studied architecture, engineering, drawing and mathematics, including an emphasis on the works of the two Leonardo's: Da Vinci and Fibonacci. These were the seminal imprints that would later inspire her breakthrough insights as an aesthetician and cosmetologist. While studying proportions of the human face, she had the intuitive flash to apply Golden Ratio proportions to eyebrow sculpting. This Golden Ratio upgrade enhances the intrinsic beauty inherent in anyone's natural facial proportions and bone structure, and became the underlying concept that has revolutionized the field of aesthetics and cosmetology. Anastasia discovered that anyone's eyebrows could be sculpted to Golden Ratio proportions by determining three key landmarks:

❶ An imaginary line running vertically through the middle of the nostril determines the medial eyebrow border.

❷ The high point on the eyebrow arch can be found on a line connecting the tip of the nostril to the center of the iris. The high point divides the eyebrow into Golden Ratio proportions.

❸ The point that lies on a line running through the edge of the corresponding nostril through the outer edge of the eye determines the lateral eyebrow border.

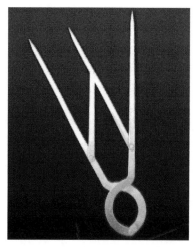 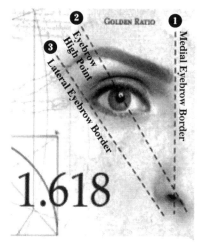

Golden Ratio calipers (left); detail from Anastasia's educational materials (right), illustrating her patented formula for Golden Ratio eyebrow sculpting. Note how Anastasia's dotted facial lines mirror the Golden Ratio calipers' design.

> *Beauty is not Perfection. Real beauty is Proportion.*
> **Anastasia Soare**

Although most people's facial proportions deviate to varying degrees from the Golden Ratio, Anastasia's eyebrow sculpting technique can reorient anyone's facial features towards Divine Proportion. This reveals their own natural beauty and attractiveness, cross-reinforcing an upward spiral of enhanced inner and outer self-esteem. Regarding the universal applicability of her discovery Anastasia said,

Studying technical design and art in Romania gave me the ability to see things in 3-D. Back then, we didn't have computers—we figured things with pencils. Once I became an aesthetician, I took that knowledge and studied the bone structure of every ethnic group. It helped me to find the perfect shape for anyone's bone structure... I became really obsessed with the eyebrow, because nobody thought that it was important... Taking all the knowledge I learned from Leonardo Da Vinci and Leonardo Fibonacci, I was able to get at the perfect Golden Proportion on anybody's face.

Anastasia's genius was to superimpose Golden Ratio caliper geometry over the nose, eyes and brow in order to find the precise Golden Ratio divisions of the brow. Golden Ratio calipers have two prongs that are parallel and one prong at a variable angle. When you look at Anastasia's facial lines graphic you will see that, just as with Golden Ratio calipers, two lines are parallel and one line is at an angle. In addition, the three lines running from the nose to the eyebrow do not originate from a single point, just as the three prongs of Golden Ratio calipers don't originate from a single point. This unique linear array makes it possible to integrate and enhance nasal, eye and eyebrow features within the context of Golden Ratio proportions.

When you make contact with someone, your attention first goes naturally to their eyes. If their eyes are framed by the eyebrows above and the nose below—all in Golden Ratio proportion—the beholder receives the message that the Golden Ratio always conveys, that of beauty, harmony and unity. Anastasia's profound epiphany was to fuse the Golden Ratio with the insight that the eyebrow is the single most impactful feature to upgrade facial symmetry towards Divine Proportion. Essentially, Anastasia created a universal, noninvasive, high impact method for restoring and accentuating anyone's natural beauty and attractiveness, male or female.

9

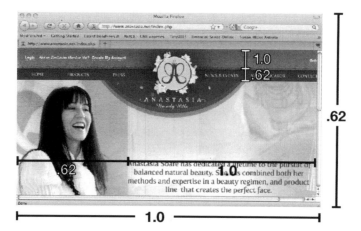

www.Anastasia.net "browser" window in Golden Ratio (1:62 width-to-height ratio) illustrates two elements: 1. The ease of sizing your web browser to the Golden Ratio, which anyone can do in moments. 2. Embedded Golden Ratios, which are clearly present in Anastasia's web site design.

In the process, she revealed a profound new beauty truism (and created the remarkable method to bring it to life):

*Beauty is in the eye of the beholder **and** in the eyebrows of the beheld.*

Not only has Anastasia's day-to-day salon practice benefited from her breakthrough insights into the Golden Ratio, she's also reaping the financial rewards that inevitably follow aligning one's work and passion with it. Her growing line of products are featured in over 400 locations in the United States, including Nordstroms, Sephora and Ulta, as well as globally. While her beauty empire grows in a graceful upward Golden Spiral, Anastasia also keeps giving and receiving in Golden Ratio: she is associated with many charitable foundations, including *Oprah's Angel Network* and *The Blue Heron Foundation* (benefiting Romanian orphans).

> *The mathematics of the Universe are visible to all in the form of Beauty.*
> **John Michell, Golden Ratio Genius; Author, *How the World Is Made: The Story of Creation According to Sacred Geometry***

9

The Golden Beauty Ratio

New Jersey-based Orthodontist Dr. Yosh Jefferson is a Golden Ratio medical pioneer focusing on orthodontics. He developed a standardized system for the ideal position of the jaw and facial bones and a temporomandibular joint (TMJ) realignment therapy based on the Golden Ratio. Such realignment has been shown to alleviate a host of conditions such as chronic headaches, mouth breathing, myofascial pain, TMJ dysfunction, scoliosis, skin disorders and chronic fatigue syndrome. It can also improve respiration, memory, mental and hearing acuity, as well as lessen depression. His theories are described in the *Journal of General Orthodontics* (June 1996), for which he wrote the cover article, *Skeletal Types: Key to unraveling the mystery of facial beauty and its biologic significance.* In that article, Dr. Jefferson speaks on the Golden Ratio beauty connection:

All living creatures, including man, are intimately connected by a biologic phenomenon known as Divine Proportion [Golden Ratio]. We are all genetically encoded to develop into this ideal shape and form for many reasons.

Dr. Jefferson further states that individuals who conform to the Divine Proportion/ Golden Ratio are biologically and physiologically arranged to be profoundly efficient and healthy. In his view, most physical variations from Divine Proportion, especially extreme ones, are environmentally induced. Restoration therefore should closely approximate the biological standard that is both aesthetically pleasing and physiologically healthy. He observes that all living things, including humans, are genetically encoded to develop into an ideal and defined proportion. This proportion

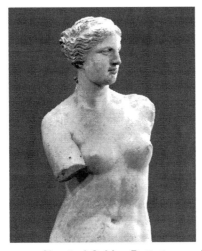
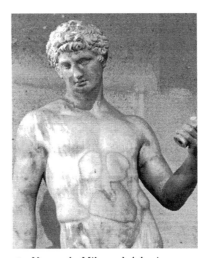

Classical Golden Ratio icons of beauty *Venus de Milo* and *Adonis*.

is universal, applying to all individuals regardless of race, age, sex, and geographic or cultural variabilities. Yet because of various environmental factors, most living creatures deviate somewhat from the ideal. As an example, Dr. Jefferson notes:

Infants suckling on a latex bottle nipple develop unnatural swallowing patterns and possible [tongue] thrust, which can cause abnormal facial and dental growth and development.

Bottle-fed babies also tend to be mouth breathers, which can lead to various types of facial and dental abnormalities. Artificial influences during the First 15% of early childhood such as the above can obviously cause development away from the Golden Ratio. In a perfect world, free of extreme environmental conditions such as high stress, abnormal biomechanical habits, pollution, toxins, radiation, allergens, and latex bottle nipples, etc., most people would naturally develop closer to the Golden Ratio. Dr. Jefferson also notes that many studies have proven the universality of beauty:

A number of recent cross-cultural researchers have shown that the basis for judging facial attractiveness was consistent across cultural lines. Furthermore... babies as young as three months can distinguish between attractive and unattractive faces. Because babies at this age are deemed too young to be substantially exposed to cultural standards of beauty, these studies indicate an innate ability of all human individuals to appreciate facial form and balance that have universal appeal.

> *It is impossible to join two things in a beautiful manner without a third being present, for a bond must exist to unite them, and this bond is best achieved by a proportion.*
>
> **Plato**

Dr. Jefferson believes this carries enormous social implications: We are instinctively inclined to search for mates whose features conform more closely to the Golden Ratio. By looking for partners that are Divinely Proportioned, we are at the same time unknowingly looking for partners who are vibrantly healthy, thereby ensuring the health and survival of our offspring. We are all apparently predisposed to the lifelong appreciation of and search for beauty. The social implications of being perceived as beautiful are staggering, as Diane Ackerman describes in *A Natural History of the Senses*:

Attractive people do better: in school, where they receive more help, better grades and less punishment; at work, where they are rewarded with higher pay, more prestigious

Monica Dean's Golden Ratio Facial Proportions

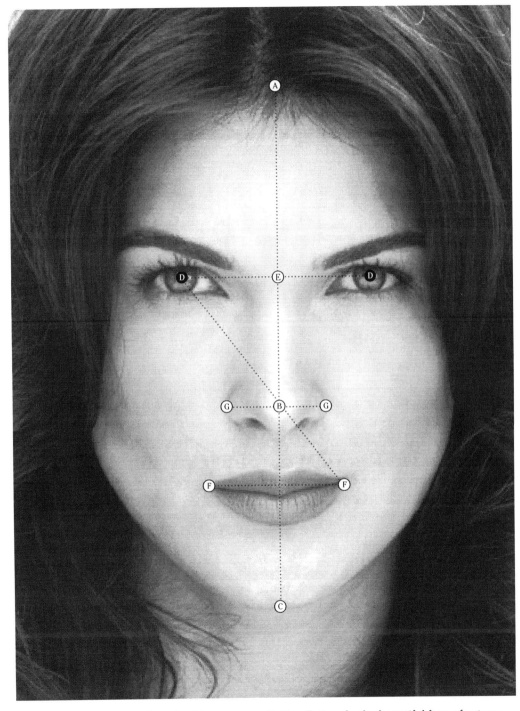

The human face is endowed with numerous Golden Ratios. In the beautiful face of actress Monica Dean, we highlight four. Line segments shown are in Golden Ratio to one another.

1. ⒶⒷ:ⒷⒸ=1.618 **2.** ⒺⒸ:**DD**=1.618 **3.** **D**Ⓑ:ⒷⒻ=1.618 (*diagonal*) **4.** ⒻⒻ:ⒼⒼ=1.618

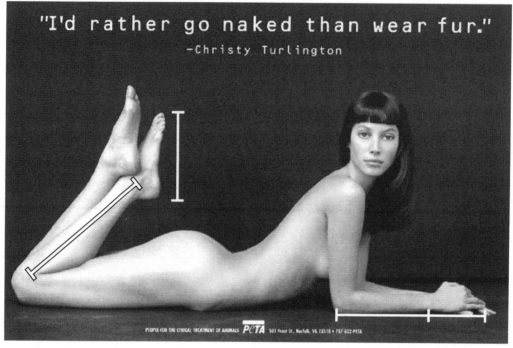

Christy Turlington, supermodel and author (*Living Yoga*) exhibiting some of her furless
Golden Ratio proportions for PETA (People for the Ethical Treatment of Animals).
Golden Ratios added by the authors.

*jobs and faster promotion; in finding mates, where they tend to be in control of the
relationship and make most of the decisions; and among strangers, who assume them
to be more interesting, honest, virtuous and successful.*

A brain imaging study led by Dr. Hans Breiter which was published in the November,
2001 issue of *Neuron*, revealed that when men were shown pictures of various faces,
only female faces deemed beautiful triggered activity in brain centers previously
associated with food, drugs and money. With one group of men, studied via a
brain imaging procedure known as functional magnetic resonance imaging (fMRI),
researchers found that only attractive female faces set off the brain's reward circuitry.
Dr. Nancy Etcoff, a coauthor of this study, noted that the research echoes previous
work suggesting that the human perception of beauty may be inborn. Dr. Etcoff added:

*While we know that experience, learning and personal idiosyncrasies all have an
impact on attraction between particular individuals; these results show that this basic
reward response is deeply seated in human nature.*

274

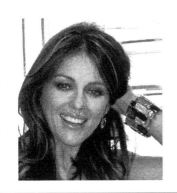

Elizabeth Hurley's Golden Ratio Face

Actor and author John Cleese (of *Monty Python* and *A Fish Called Wanda* fame) wrote and presented a fascinating program for the BBC called *The Human Face*, which showcases the secrets of the Golden Ratio and beauty. It features model and actress Elizabeth Hurley as a classic example.

Clearly, our responses to beauty and Divine Proportion are more instinctive than conscious. We have been programmed to recognize, love and delight in that which reflects our universal, divinely inspired Golden Ratio design. California-based Dr. Stephen Marquardt has taken practical advantage of our natural instinct for beauty. In his work as a leading maxillofacial plastic surgeon, Dr. Marquardt developed male and female "beauty mask" facial overlays utilizing the Golden Decagon (a ten-sided Golden Ratio-based geometrical shape) and its application to facial beauty. Faces that conform to the mask will be universally perceived as beautiful, regardless of race, age or nationality. His beauty mask can be utilized to guide the application of makeup, to aid in the evaluation of a face for orthodontic or dental treatment or facial surgery, or simply to see how closely a face conforms to the Golden Ratio. Dr. Marquardt's beauty mask and work has attracted international attention, validating yet again the universality of the Golden Ratio as a touchstone of beauty.

Drs. Oz and Roizen on Beauty, the Immune System and the Golden Ratio

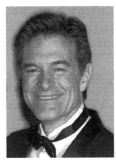

Bestselling author and television show host Dr. Mehmet Oz shares here some of his insights on the Golden Ratio's connection to beauty, healthy immune function and genetics. Dr. Oz is co-author with Michael Roizen, M.D., of the popular *YOU: The Owner's Manual* health book series and is one of *Time* magazine's *100 Most Influential People* (2008) and *Esquire* magazine's *75 Most Influential People of the 21st Century*. From *YOU: Being Beautiful*:

Dr. Mehmet Oz.

9

The theory is that the more symmetrical a face is, the healthier it is… the formula for beauty is that precise Golden Ratio (go ahead and pull a ruler and a calculator on your next date). The same ratio holds for the width of the cheekbones to the width of the mouth… [similarly] the width of the mouth should be roughly 1.6 times the width of the bottom of the nose… Scientists also believe that symmetry is equated with a strong immune system—indicating that more robust genes make a person more attractive. Of course, that's the element of beauty that you typically can't control. You have what you were born with. But that doesn't mean that you can't make changes—changes to enhance your beauty and, along with it, the way you feel about yourself.

Michael Roizen, M.D., author of the award-winning *RealAge* books and Dr. Oz's co-author in the *YOU* health book series, shared these insights on the Golden Ratio's beauty connection in the audiobook *YOU: Being Beautiful,*

The omnipresence of phi [the Golden Ratio] throughout our world creates a sense of balance, harmony and beauty in the designs we see naturally and artificially. Phi is also a driving force in human attraction—men and women around the globe prefer a mate whose face is symmetrical and follows this ratio (more than 2,000 years ago, Pythagoras developed a formula for the perfect female face, which included such stats as this one: The ratio of the width of the mouth to the width of the nose should be— tada!—1.618 to 1).

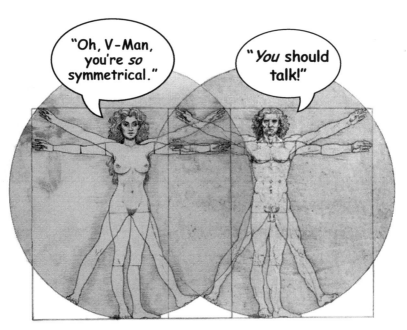

Vitruvian Woman and Man comparing notes.

The Fashion Code

The Fashion Code is based on the timeless secret for beauty [the Divine Proportion] that has inspired everyone from Da Vinci to today's top fashion icons. Once women know what this secret is and how to use it, they will have the power to create the perfect outfit everyday.

Sara and Ruth Levy, Developers of The Fashion Code

In our previous book, *The Divine Code of Da Vinci, Fibonacci, Einstein and YOU*, we described the two complementary aspects of the Golden Ratio known as The Golden Twins. Dual aspects of the Ratio allow it to be seen alternately as 1.618:1 and other times as 0.618:1, depending on the context. The Golden Twins are like two sides of a coin, their complementary natures forming a unified whole. Likewise, in the world of haute couture, twins Ruth and Sara Levy, both beautiful brunette fashion designers, have taken a hint from Da Vinci's *Vitruvian Man* and created a

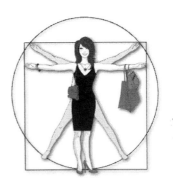

The Fashion Code logo.

breakthrough in the art and science of fashion. Ruth and Sara discovered that 10 Golden Ratio division points—superimposed over a client's body—reveal the most flattering clothing lengths and proportions, from necklines to hemlines.

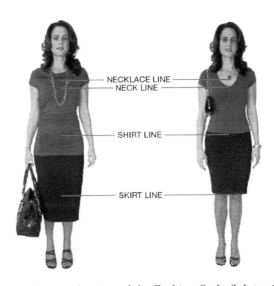

Before and after application of the Fashion Code (left to right).

> *It's a real jaw-dropper [the Divine Proportion-based Fashion Code]... I'm a believer!...*
>
> **Rachel Ray, commenting on the live presentation on her popular talk show of Sara and Ruth Levy's Fashion Code.**

As these Golden Ratio Fashion Stylistas say,

These days, there's an instruction manual for everything—except how to dress... Sure, there are tips and tricks for looking good, but nowhere is there an actual foolproof formula for dressing beautifully... until now.

On their debut on the *Rachel Ray Show* on April 15, 2010, the twins said that with the Fashion Code any woman can instantly

...look 10 pounds thinner, 10 years younger and 10 times more stylish.

Several models, including the twins, showed how Golden Ratio Fashion makeovers accent anyone's hidden Divine Proportions. A visibly impressed Rachael Ray noted that the Fashion Code is *where the Da Vinci Code meets fashion*. This is a truism, since the simple mathematics of the Golden Ratio work on virtually everyone. Not to worry, because the twins have taken care of the math. To take advantage of the twin's timeless Golden Ratio knowledge applied to dress and fashion, all you need to do is enter your height on their website—www.TheFashionCode.com—and they'll supply you with an elegant, customized chart of the magical necklines and hemlines for all of your outfits and accessories.

Julia Roberts and the Mona Lisa Smile

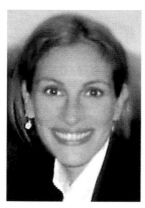

Julia Roberts.

At the front end of the 21st century, Julia Roberts is one of the highest paid actors in the world, commanding twenty-five million dollars for her starring role in 2003's *Mona Lisa Smile*. In our time, Julia Roberts' trademark smile easily rivals Da Vinci's *Mona Lisa* smile in recognition, however different they may be. What Julia and the *Mona Lisa* have in common is their ability to encompass and express many quantifiable as well as unquantifiable aspects of the Golden Ratio. In the *Mona Lisa*, Da Vinci masterfully embedded the Golden Ratio in many levels of the painting's geometrical composition. First coming to global prominence in the hit 1990 movie

Pretty Woman, Roberts revealed a rarely seen charm that only enhanced her broad, dazzling smile. Actor Tom Hanks commented on her remarkable stage presence, as reported by HollywoodReporter.com:

> *When you share the screen [with her], you might as well be a waffle iron in a tree… No one is ever looking at you… Everybody loves Julia Roberts, absolutely everybody.*

Winner of the 2001 Academy Award for Best Actress for *Erin Brokovich*, Roberts has been voted to *People* magazine's list of the world's "Fifty Most Beautiful People" eleven times. Julia Roberts reminds us that the Golden Ratio shows up not only in quantifiable physical appearance, but also in many immeasurable and intangible personal qualities. George Clooney had this to say in 2010 about Robert's secret to staying lovely:

> *It has nothing to do with the way she looks. It has everything to do with who she is.*

What I study is photographic, two-dimensional attractiveness, photos with no dimension or sense of time or personality… In the real world, beauty has to do with elegance, sense of humor, how a person carries herself. It's something completely different.

Mounir Bashour, M.D., Ph.D., Plastic Surgeon and Author of *Is an Objective Measuring System for Facial Attractiveness Possible?*

George Clooney: The Ideal Male Face

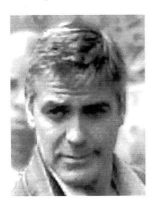

George Clooney.

In 2003, the American Academy of Facial Plastic and Reconstructive Surgery polled its membership to find out which stars embody present-day appeal and everlasting allure. Twenty-five percent of the facial plastic surgeons selected actor George Clooney as the male "modern-day ideal face of beauty" (Brad Pitt and Mel Gibson were tied for second place, at twenty percent each). Plastic surgeon and AAFPRS President Dean M. Toriumi, M.D. was quoted on www.aafprs.org:

George Clooney was selected because he possesses a strong jaw, deep brown eyes, an "ever-perfect" olive complexion, and a strong and straight masculine nose… Clooney is known for his sense of humor, often seen in interviews making wry comments, jokes, and pulling pranks, thus, his appeal seems partially to stem from a persona, which is a blend of warmth and humor.

9

Like his friend and co-star Julia Roberts, Clooney's appeal is a mix of physical attractiveness, wit and charm. His Golden Ratio-chiseled good looks also got him honored not only as *People* magazine's Sexiest Man Alive (twice), but also as one of *People's* Most Beautiful People (2007). In 2005, Clooney won an Academy Award for Best Supporting Actor for *Syriana*. George Clooney's career showcases, in elegant proportion, his multifaceted talents which include acting, directing, screenwriting and producing.

The Golden Dental Ratio

In order to optimize the appearance, structure and function of their patients, more leading-edge doctors are incorporating Golden Ratio principles in their treatments. Dr. David Frey is a top Beverly Hills-based Golden Ratio dentist who utilizes the Golden Ratio to restore healthy proportion to his patient's teeth. This results in increased bite efficiency, more relaxed jaw, face and head muscles and enhanced beauty and appearance. In his book *Revitalizing Your Mouth*, Dr. Frey notes,

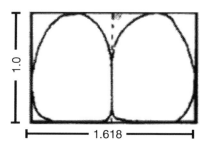

Front teeth in height-to-width Golden Ratio.

Combining the Golden Proportion with modern-day full mouth restoration techniques enables you to find the smile that is in proportion to your face. For example, the Golden Proportion can be applied to your two front teeth by measuring their width and mathematically determining the proper length. If the teeth have worn down, porcelain veneers can add the necessary length to restore them to Golden Proportion. It has been discovered that when your mouth is positioned in the physiologically correct

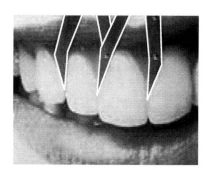

Our teeth have multiple Golden Ratio relationships.

bite, your top and bottom teeth can generally be placed in Golden Proportion— or Golden Vertical Dental Index—when the teeth are closed together.

9

Beauty is the splendor of truth.
                                        Plato

Xylitol and the Teeth and Longevity Connection

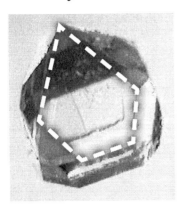

Xylitol crystal magnified, showing pentagonal structure.

The importance of maintaining healthy teeth in a healthy mouth environment for longevity cannot be overstated. Not only is the mouth the First 15% of healthy digestion, due to proper mastication (chewing), it turns out that the same bacteria which causes tooth decay and gum disease can migrate to the heart, leading to inflammation and heart disease: the #1 cause of death in America.

Dr. Mark Briener, a Connecticut-based dentist and author of *Whole-Body Dentistry*, points out that the health of our teeth and mouth are directly connected to the health of our whole body. Essentially, tooth health is a key fractal and predictor of total health. Dr. Briener's visionary and life-changing work has received extensive media coverage and is endorsed by many leading health authorities, including Nicholas Perricone, M.D., Bernie Siegel, M.D., Stephen Sinatra, M.D. and Gary Null, Ph.D. Reducing/eliminating white sugar and refined/processed foods along with practicing healthy oral care (including daily flossing is of course vital. It turns out that including xylitol, a naturally occurring sugar substitute, in our oral health regimen adds clinically proven support to tooth and total health. Xylitol, a unique 5-sided crystal originally discovered in 1896, is available in toothpaste, gum, mints and as a sugar substitute. What makes xylitol so remarkable is that it tastes as sweet as sugar *and* actually kills the bacteria which cause tooth decay and gum disease (unlike regular refined sugars, which accelerate tooth decay). Xylitol also does not cause blood sugar levels to spike, so it's safe for diabetics and hypoglycemics. To learn more about xylitol's proven dental and health benefits, read Dr. Briener's book *Whole-Body Dentistry*; also visit www.WholeBodyMed.com and www.EpicDental.com

9

Divine Symmetry and Movement

We are clearly predisposed to the appreciation of and the search for beauty, and the Golden Ratio is beauty's foremost blueprint. Those whose appearance and movements more closely mirror the Golden Ratio/Spiral inevitably attract more attention and interest from the world at large, and the opposite sex in particular. The following excerpt from Jeanie Davis' *WebMD* article *Men Who Dance Well May Be More Desirable As Mates* (December, 2005) describes the research of William M. Brown, Ph.D. This study highlights the importance of bodily symmetry in dance as it relates to mate selection:

> *Dancing is believed to be important in the courtship of a variety of species, including humans, writes researcher William M. Brown, Ph.D., an anthropologist with Rutgers University. Mating studies revealed that women seek out males with bodily symmetry, he explains. If the potential mate has a great degree of asymmetry, he or she is judged to be less than optimal. In numerous species, asymmetry is linked to greater rates of disease and early death, and lesser success in fertility—all-important to their selection as mates. A guy's or girl's symmetry (or lack of it) affects their attractiveness in other ways, too—like odor, voice, and facial appearance... Why is symmetry so important? 'We do not know,' writes Brown: 'Perhaps it indicates good coordination or good health, including freedom from parasites. Attractive dances may be more difficult to perform, more rhythmic, more energetic, more energy efficient, or any combination of these factors.'*

An Archives of Sexual Behavior study reveals that woman are most attracted to muscular men whose shoulders measure 1.6 times [the Golden Ratio] the size of their waist.

John Barban, *The Perfect Body Formula;* Men's Health Magazine, July/August 2008

The Golden Ratio of Attraction

Jackie Summers is the founder of Jack from Brooklyn (purveyors of Sorel® and other fine spirits) who also writes poetically and frankly on love and life. His blog post about the Golden Ratio of character and charisma in healthy relationships caught our eye:

> *Charisma makes us swoon but might lead us to disaster. Character is steadfast and honorable but often wooden, and dull. How do we resolve this? With Phi Φ. An irrational number (along with it's more famous cousin, π pi) if you think you're unfamiliar with the concept of phi, you're mistaken. The equation which represents perfect symmetry is everywhere you look, if you're looking. Ratios can be defined as the proportion of one thing to another; it's knowing how much Jack Daniels to add to a*

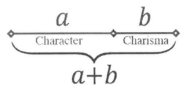

Coke to have just the right balance of sweetness and potency. Phi, the aptly named Divine Proportion, is simply the best ratio to combine any parts. So, why not apply the concept of ideal proportions to a lover? When set upon a predominant base of character, charisma provides the stage to perform its seduction over and over. The ability to identify these qualities and their relative proportion to each other is key, not just in seduction but in securing healthy, stable, sustainable relationships. The capacity for character and charisma exists in each of us, as does their right ratio to one another. Instead of simply searching for an ideal mate, begin by adjusting the sliding scale in yourself to ideal proportions. Souls of a like nature seek each other out, so if you truly want to find The One, start by becoming The One.

The Golden Ratio of Character and Charisma.

Jackie's message is clear: we must work on The One—ourselves—first. If we do this with desire and dedication, we cannot help but attract (or keep) the other One. Most people focus on the movie, the projection, instead of the projector (ourselves). This invariably leads to chasing shadows. Try making a short list of those qualities you most desire in another and then do everything you can to cultivate, refine and strengthen those exact qualities in yourself. Like attracts like or, as the ancients said: as above, so below.

Golden Ratio Relationships

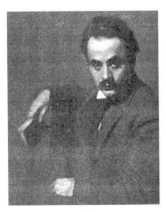

Khalil Gibran (1883-1931) hints at Golden Ratio relationships in *The Prophet*.

Khalil Gibran wrote in his timeless classic *The Prophet*:

Let there be spaces in your togetherness, and let the winds of the heavens dance between you... Love one another but make not a bond of love: Let it rather be a moving sea between your shores... Sing and dance together and be joyous, but let each one of you be alone, even as the strings of a lute are alone though they quiver with the same music... And stand together, yet not too near together: For the pillars of the temple stand apart, and the oak tree and the cypress grow not in each other's shadow.

9

As Gibran beautifully illustrates, a dynamic balance, a ratio, must exist in space, energy and time in order for relationships to become fulfilling and ultimately unifying states. Interpreting his wisdom through the lens of the Golden Ratio, we can see that harmonious relationships require a dynamic symmetry—a ratio or proportion—and it's not a static 50:50 ratio. For example: Consider the possibility that a healthy relationship might benefit with 62% of total time being spent with a partner, and 38% spent apart. This could set the stage so that you could better enjoy the "spaces in your togetherness" and thus better appreciate one another, especially over time. The ratio could of course be flipped or modified in those relationships where people want to spend either more time together or more time apart.

One must also consider the balance or ratio of power in relationships of every kind. For example, our world is now struggling to reestablish a dynamic divine balance by moving away from near-total male dominance in the areas of leadership and decision making. Yet this can only occur when the feminine perspective is restored to its proper proportion. The key word here is dynamic. Like the play of the tides, the various ratios of interactions within healthy relationships manifests and moves through endless expressions of the Golden Ratio. These include time together vs. time apart, giving vs. receiving, action vs. rest, etc. These cycles flow between the Golden Ratio's "low tide" side (38%) to its "high tide" side (62%). In reality, all relationships reflect this continuous dance, and all relationships can benefit from greater conscious sensitivity to these natural ebb and flow cycles.

Golden Intimacy: The Feel-Good Health & Longevity Supernutrient

An orgasm a day keeps the doctor away.
Mae West, legendary early Hollywood actress

It should come as no surprise that lovemaking reduces stress, boosts immune function, promotes sounder sleep, increases optimism and releases hormones beneficial for health, happiness and longevity. Study after study confirms that lovemaking offers so many health benefits it could literally qualify as a supernutrient. Regular doses of this feel-good nutrient may even save your life: in 2002, the *Journal of Epidemiology and Community Health* reported that 914 men in the U.K. were monitored for 20 years. At the end of the study, the ones who had enjoyed lovemaking at least 2 times a week had a 50% less chance of having a fatal heart attack, compared to those whose lovemaking frequency was once a month. Golden Ratio aficionado Dr. Michael Roizen, author of *RealAge: Are You as Young as You Can Be?*, states that *having sex at least twice a week can make your RealAge 1.6 years younger than if you had sex only once a week.* Dr. Roizen defines 'real age' as *an estimation of your age in biologic terms, not chronological years.*

Other studies reveal sexual dissatisfaction as a predictor of the onset of cardiovascular disease. For example, a study published in the November-December 1976 journal Psychosomatic Medicine compared 100 women with heart disease with a control group. The result? Sexual dissatisfaction was found in 65% of the coronary patients, yet in only 24% of the control group.

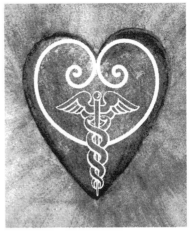

Every heart is composed of two Golden Spirals.

In a long-term study of 3,500 people ages 30 to 101, published in his book *Secrets of the Superyoung*, Scotland's Dr. David Weeks revealed the age-reversing power of intimacy. In his study, he discovered that those who were enjoying satisfying intimacy with the same partner about 4 times a week on average were perceived by others to be 4 to 7 years younger than their actual age. This was arrived at through impartial ratings of the study subject's pictures. This is interesting data, as the Golden Ratio point falls at approximately 4.3 times per week (7 days ÷ 4.3 = 1.62, the Golden Ratio). Dr. Weeks, a clinical neuropsychologist at the Royal Edinburgh Hospital, attributed the perceived age reversal to significant stress reduction, greater contentment and sounder sleep, stating that:

> *The key ingredients for looking younger are staying active… and maintaining a good sex life.*

Since everyone's libido is unique and tends to rise and fall over time, no one can say for sure what a "perfect" regular lovemaking frequency is. Everyone must find their own Golden/Divine Ratio in this personal life area based on desire, condition and partner. However, the above data highlights the important role intimacy can play in a healthy lifestyle diet. In light of this, you might consider adding intimacy as a tracking category to your 21-Day Quick-Start Checklist.

9

The Golden Ratio Orgasm

The lover is drawn by the thing loved, as the sense is by that which it perceives...
Leonardo Da Vinci

The ultimate purpose of sexual intimacy, as Dr. Wilhelm Reich, 20th century sexual psychology and life energy pioneer proposed in *The Function of the Orgasm*, is a loving communion. The divine sharing of intimacy is meant to result in both partners experiencing a full and ecstatic energetic release, renewal and union with one another. Reich, a one-time protégé of Sigmund Freud, theorized that a lack of healthy sexual intimacy is a root cause behind much of humanity's dysfunction, repression and dis-ease. Orgasm can be likened to a strong outgoing wave or tide of energy, followed by a natural resolution or afterglow stage when the tide comes back in. The post-orgasmic afterglow time allows us to integrate the vital regenerative energies of which Dr. Reich spoke. Early scientific research by Masters & Johnson and others into the physiology of the human sexual response identified five primary stages of lovemaking:

1. Foreplay > 2. Excitement > 3. Plateau > 4. Orgasm > 5. Afterglow

When the Golden Ratio is superimposed over these 5 stages of lovemaking, we find that the onset of orgasm occurs at a point approximately 62% of the way through lovemaking. This means that in order for enjoyable lovemaking and mutually fulfilling orgasms to occur, both partners must honor the early stages of lovemaking, especially foreplay. Chaos theory pioneer Professor Edward Lorenz could easily have been referring to the importance of foreplay when he said,

When a butterfly flutters its wings in one part of the world [if the initial conditions are right] it can eventually cause a hurricane in another.

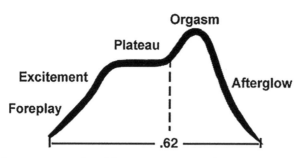

Five-stage sexual response graph, with orgasm onset at the approximate Golden Ratio point. Note: this graph only a stylized version of how an orgasm could be represented graphically.

286

9

As if to reinforce the importance of a healthy ratio between foreplay and orgasm, *Esquire* Magazine conducted a survey of 2000 women in 2003. Given a choice between cuddling and making love, 62% preferred to cuddle while 38% preferred to more immediately make love. This study reinforces what many women have been saying to their partners for years. Healthy foreplay is the foundation that supports a loving and mutually fulfilling union.

The Leonardo Da Vinci of Contraception

The challenge was daunting. How to design and manufacture a means of dependable contraception and STD protection that would be both regularly used *and* actually enjoyed by both partners. As it turned out, the innovative answer would end up being based on the Golden Spiral. Named Inspiral,® it became the best-selling condom in America for many years running. It features an unusual Nautilus shell/helix design, which resulted in it being hailed by most reviewers as the best condom ever made. The Inspiral® was created by Dr. Alla Venkata Krishna Reddy, M.D., whom the *New York Times* named "The Leonardo Da Vinci of Condoms." The Inspiral's® unique twisting design has received much international praise, including:

- The History Channel's *Modern Marvels* program stated that the Inspiral® was *designed to improve, rather than get in the way of sex.*
- Rated #1 in *Men's Health, GQ, Maxim* and *Cosmopolitan* magazines; rated best choice in a University of Virginia survey.
- A Marie Stopes International study stated that Inspiral's® shape helped women achieve easier and quicker orgasms.

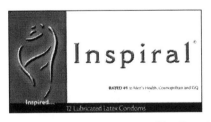

It is indeed a stunning work… a Nautilus shell.
The New York Times, on the Inspiral® Condom.

9

Golden Ratio Aphrodisiac and Life Extender: Chocolate

Chocolate turns out to have profoundly important healing powers.
John Robbins, author of the ground-breaking *Diet For A New America*

In Dr. Peter D'Adamo's bestseller *Eat Right For Your Type*, we find that 62% of chocolate's fat is saturated and the remaining 38% is polyunsaturated and monounsaturated. This 62% to 38% distribution falls exactly into Golden Ratio proportions. One of chocolate's main psychoactive chemicals is theobromine, literally "Food of the Gods"; with an antioxidant profile higher than red wine or green tea, it certainly qualifies for such a lofty title. Chocolate also contains small amounts of the marijuana-like chemical (cannabinoid) anandamide. Phenethylamine, otherwise known as the "love chemical" is also present in small amounts in chocolate. The combination of these elements, along with tryptophan and trace amounts of caffeine, give chocolate its characteristic addicting flavor and powerful mood elevating and aphrodisiac qualities. Some have questioned chocolate's purported aphrodisiac effects. Yet the popularity of movies such as *Like Water for Chocolate* and *Chocolat*, starring Juliette Binoche and Johnny Depp—to say nothing of Chocolate's undeniable connection to Valentine's Day—suggest that the amorous effects of chocolate are undeniable. With its mix of Divinely-Proportioned components, it's no wonder that so many people become chocoholics—which may actually be a healthy addiction, in moderation. A growing number of studies are revealing that minimally processed, dark chocolate (cocoa with a higher ratio of polyphenols) is beneficial for the prevention of heart disease, high blood pressure and stroke—and may in fact enhance longevity.

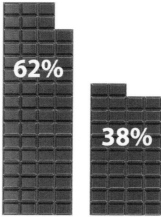

Chocolate is truly a Food of the Gods, with a Golden Ratio of 62% saturated
to 38% unsaturated fat composition (monounsaturated 35%, polyunsaturated 3%)
and more health and longevity enhancing antioxidants than red wine or green tea.

THE GOLDEN RATIO **Rx** LIFESTYLE DIET

NATURAL BEAUTY & ATTRACTION

Pick one or more of the following Rx's to add to your daily health regimen.

1. Golden Ratio Facial Beauty Enhancement

Our face is the primary point of focus and interaction with others. While everyone is gifted with their own unique facial features, most faces can benefit from a little extra TLC. With this in mind, let's look at several things you can do to enhance your natural Golden Ratio attributes. These simple techniques can make a meaningful difference in how you feel about yourself and how others perceive you. Remember, it's not the quantity of actions taken here, it's their quality and consistency. Here are a few good examples to consider; try adding one to your regimen for 21 days and see how it makes you look and feel, inside and out.

- **Facial Hydration:** Proper, daily facial hydration is a must in any health and beauty regimen. In addition to keeping your face glowing and youthful, facial hydration strengthens your skin's role as a resilient barrier against environmental toxins. Select a high quality facial moisturizer without toxic ingredients such as mineral oil, as creams and lotions can be absorbed through your skin directly into your bloodstream. Ideally, your moisturizer should be pure enough to eat,— if not, it really doesn't belong on your face. Many toxic ingredients are easily identified by being multi-syllabic, hard-to-pronounce and/or have CAPITALS or numbers in their names, e.g., PEG-13. Visit the Skin Deep website at: www.cosmeticsdatabase.com to evaluate most cosmetic or personal care products or ingredients to check their safety.

- **Anastasia's Eyebrow Sculpting Kits:** Anastasia Soare's easy-to-use Golden Ratio eyebrow sculpting kits make it fun and simple to sculpt your eyebrows to enhance the natural beauty of your face. Available at Nordstroms and Sephora, or at: www.Anastasia.net.

9

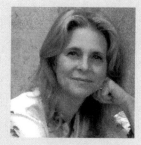

Lindsay Wagner.

- **The Accupressure Facelift:** *Lindsay Wagner's New Beauty: The Acupressure Facelift* is an excellent instructional book by the beautiful actress Lindsay Wagner (*The Bionic Woman*). This is an easy-to-learn method for facial rejuvenation, through gentle massage of facial acupressure points.

- **Sleep!** Honoring Golden Ratio Lifestyle Diet driver #3: Sleep, Rest & Recovery, is one of the huge hidden factors in maintaining a healthy, vibrant face. Many people continually compromise this high-priority health, longevity and beauty driver. Don't be one of them.

- **Eat Anti-Oxidant-Rich Foods (High ORAC):** ORAC is an anagram for Oxygen Radical Absorbance Capacity—a measure of the antioxidant potential of foods. Eating super-charged ORAC foods such as cloves, cinnamon, turmeric, curry, red beans, cranberries, blueberries, acai berries, goji berries, etc., can result in dramatic improvements in the health of your skin. See chapter 4/Nutrition, Rx section, for a more complete list of ORAC foods.

- **Exercise your facial muscles:** A fun and easy way to do this: make as many different faces as you can in front of a mirror for 1 minute. Try this daily for a week and see and feel the increase in the tone and flexibility of your face.

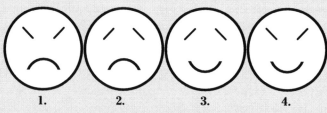

1.　　　2.　　　3.　　　4.

As a starting point, here are four simple smiley-like *emoticons* that you can imitate to take your facial muscles through the range of archetypal human emotional temperaments: **1.** Choleric (angry, irritated), **2.** Melancholic (gentle sadness, thoughtful), **3.** Phlegmatic (not easily disturbed), and **4.** Sanguine (happy, cheerful). Note: you might want to spend just 38% of your time exercising the left two examples (1-2) and 62% on the right two (3-4).

9

2. Activate Your Natural Beauty and Attractiveness

How can we best support and maximize our own innate Golden Ratio symmetry and magnetism? Simply by following the cornerstones of the Golden Ratio Lifestyle Diet, the presence and power of the Ratio will begin to flow naturally. Natural Beauty and Attractiveness is available to everyone at anytime by moving towards Golden Ratio balance in each of the Diet's 9 key drivers. Remember to always be mindful of your breathing, posture and movement. A few easy methods that support these three factors include:

• Golden Ratio breathing: inhale fully to the count of 3, exhale to the count of 5. A sense of relaxation and inner balance will naturally follow after 8 breathing cycles.

• Stand with your feet firmly grounded and allow your spine to rise to its full, natural length. You'll find that your neck and head are in a relaxed position and that your chest and heart are more open. This will tend to support and enhance the natural Divine Proportions in your body. As an added bonus, when you work on improving your static posture, it will automatically enhance your dynamic, moving posture.

• Move with grace and efficiency. When dancing for example, allow your movements to be in "flow-motion." Gentle circular or spiraling movements are one good way to allow your body to move with more fluid, attractive grace.

3. The 38/62 Golden Communication Ratio

Based on the pioneering work of UCLA Professor Emeritus Albert Mehrabian, the strength and impact of our primary channels of communication directly reflects the Golden Ratio: 55% of our communication power is in our body language, e.g., eye contact, facial expression, posture; 38% is in our voice tone, and only the remaining 7% is in the actual words we use.

This is an exact Golden Ratio distribution, as:

$$55 + 7 = 62 + 38 = 100$$

9

Since the top two categories equal the vast majority (93%!) of our communication power, this ought to inspire us to prioritize our communication enhancement efforts towards improving our non-verbal, body language and voice tone skills.

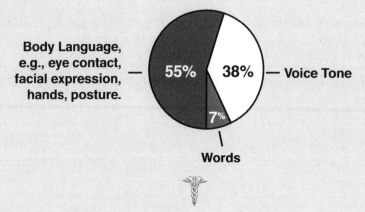

4. The 60/40 Power of Sight, Sound and Feeling

In *How To Make People Like You in 90 Seconds or Less*, author Nicholas Boothman explores how to optimize our ability to more rapidly and meaningfully connect with people. As it turns out, the three primary modalities we use to connect and communicate fall into approximate Golden Ratio. They are: Visual (pictures), Auditory (sounds) and Kinesthetic (feelings). These three modalities or frequencies are 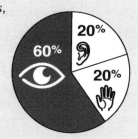 how we communicate with ourselves internally—and with others externally. However, each individual prefers to communicate predominantly via one of the three. It turns out that approximately 60% of people are visually dominant, with the remaining 40% being nearly evenly split between auditory and kinesthetic dominance: 60/40, approximating the Golden Ratio. This is yet another example of how human (and universal) structure and function align with the Golden Ratio, as we've explored throughout this book. In order to know yourself better and communicate with greater grace and effectiveness, become more aware of your communication preference and strength. How do you prefer communicating (sending and receiving) with others? How do those close to you prefer to receive communication? How can you best create strong bridges of understanding and value with others? The answers to these questions are golden keys which unlock life success skill #1: building meaningful communication and relationships with others.

5. The Divine Rose Spiral

Look at the multiple Golden Spirals in this picture of a rose. Notice how the petals gracefully trace the spiral leading into and coming out of the heart of the rose. Close your eyes for a moment. Take a deep, full breath. On your exhale, send this Golden Spiraling love energy to the heart of your beloved. Repeat 3 times.

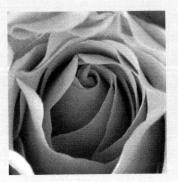 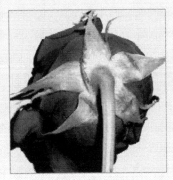

The rose sends a double imprint of the Golden Ratio: petals unfolding in Golden Spirals on the face and a five-pointed Golden Star on the back.

6. Golden Ratio Time-Sharing

• Become more aware of how much time you and your mate are spending together and apart, on a daily, weekly and monthly basis. Where do your time ratios fall with respect to the 38/62 or 62/38 Golden Ratio? If it feels right, continue what you're doing; otherwise, experiment by shifting the time ratio one way or the other to reflect Divine Proportion in your relationship.

9

- Experiment with other ratios in your relationship, such as decision making ratios, giving vs. receiving, action vs. rest, etc. If any of these ratios are not fulfilling/out of proportion, experiment with shifting the balance one way or the other toward the Divine Proportion (38/62 or 62/38).

7. Fibonacci's Foreplay

What would it be like to enjoy *infinite* foreplay? Impossible you say? Leonardo Fibonacci might have explained it as follows:

You are 10 inches away from your mate and you want to kiss him or her. In order to meet the lips of your love, you will need to progressively reduce the distance between you. However, by continually moving towards him or her in approximate Golden Ratio reductions, you would get infinitely closer... without actually touching. How is this so? You'd first move from 10 inches to 6.2 inches...then to 3.8 inches... 2.3 inches... 1.5 inches... infinitum frustratum... continually approaching each other, yet in theory never actually touching.

The inspiration for this playful exercise in extended foreplay is courtesy of Zeno and his famous paradox (Greece, 5th century, B.C.) This exercise also echoes the infinite nature of the Golden Ratio, which forever approaches, yet never actually arrives at the infinite number 1.6180339...

The illusory Fibonacci Foreplay or Zeno's Kiss. Look closely: what else do you see besides three shrinking candle holders?

9

9. NATURAL BEAUTY & ATTRACTION

8. Golden Afterglow

The resolution or afterglow phase of lovemaking should ideally be enjoyed and even prolonged, to allow your energies to replenish and rebalance. See if you can feel together when the afterglow has reached the Golden Ratio point of balancing the more active phases of lovemaking (see graph in the Golden Ratio Orgasm section).

9. Golden Ratio Foot Reflexology

Buddhist artisans obviously had knowledge of the Golden Ratio when they placed the Dharmachakra (Golden Flower design) and the Three Jewels design at the precise locations on the Buddha's footprint that correspond to Golden Ratio points. Armed with this knowledge, you can now treat your partner, friend or even yourself to a Golden Ratio foot massage. Be especially mindful to massage the charged points indicated on the Buddha's footprint. It's said that a good way to reach (and lift) a person's soul is through their soles.

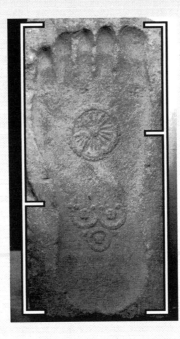

Footprint of the Buddha. Dharmachakra and Three Jewels are at Golden Ratio points of the foot. From the Gandhara, ZenYouMitsu Temple, Tokyo; 1st century.

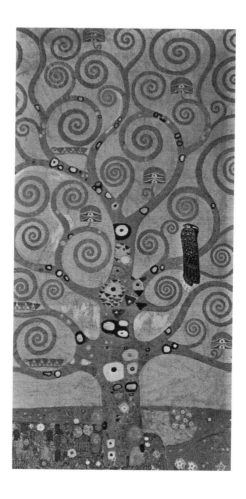

The Tree of Life, by Gustav Klimt, a legendary

tree planted by God in the Garden of Eden whose

fruit bestows everlasting health and longevity.

10.

Vibrant Health & Longevity

The water you touch in a river is the last of that which has passed and the first of which is coming. Thus it is with time present. Life, if well lived, is long.

Leonardo Da Vinci

The Golden Ratio Fountain of Youth

The Golden Ratio Lifestyle Diet has the ability to lift you to a level of extraordinary health, happiness and wellness heretofore unobtainable by any other means. By discovering Nature's Secret Nutrient (NSN) and how to apply it within the true context of Diet, boundless free energy becomes available. Free energy is usually thought of in the context of quantum physics; here we are focused on optimizing the function of our physiology and augmenting our energy—and thus our life force. As you practice and activate the optimum health driver sequence amplified with the Golden Ratio, you gain access to your own literal Fountain of Youth. The elusive Fountain of Youth is reputed to have restorative powers that confer eternal youth on anyone who drinks of its waters. In our case, the Golden Ratio Lifestyle Diet confers its profound health-giving and life-extending waters on all who learn and apply its principles.

How is it possible to increase our vital life force—our *élan vital*—to optimize our daily functioning and extend our longevity? The simple answer is to mimic Nature, whose efficiency is unparalleled. Nature is designed both structurally and functionally

10

with the Golden Ratio, at every scale. Thus, a unified field appears throughout Nature where the resulting whole is greater than the sum of the parts. This is where the free energy or élan vital appears. When two complementary elements of any system are brought into Golden Ratio balance, a unified relationship emerges which opens the door to a new realm of energetic efficiency, robust health and maximum longevity.

In the subsections of the Golden Ratio Lifestyle Diet, there are always opposing, yet complementary polarities that can be adjusted to Golden Ratio balance for optimal results. As we have seen, by tuning our sleep/wake cycle closer to the Golden Ratio—about 9 hours of sleep/rest and around 15 hours of wakefulness— we maximize our restorative and regenerative powers. We get more energy out of our days—and nights—than we would have otherwise. The increased energy obtained simply by optimizing the sleep/wake ratio can then combine and amplify with other Golden Ratio-adjusted drivers to support the ultimate in lifestyle synergy/energy. This lifestyle synergy/energy is really at the core of what is known as longevity. If you look at the longest-lived societies in the world, such as the Hunza in northern Pakistan, the Okinawans in Japan, the Vilcabambans in Ecuador or the Abkhazians in the Caucasus mountains, you will see that their lifestyle naturally includes all critical aspects—in healthy ratios—of the Golden Ratio Lifestyle Diet. Looking at our top drivers, fresh air is as abundant in their isolated, more pristine environments as is clean pure water. In many of the isolated mountainous valleys which are longevity hotspots, electricity is limited or unavailable, so the residents aren't disposed to late night hours or light in their sleeping environments. They are therefore more likely to maintain healthier Golden Ratio sleep/wake cycles. Due to often lean conditions, abundant food may not be available year round; thus, the people are subjected to unavoidable periodic caloric reduction—one of the scientifically proven top methods of life extension.

The mineral-rich water in the remote mountainous valleys of some of the longevity hotspots is known as "glacial milk," and has been found by researcher Dr. Patrick Flanagan to have an extremely low surface tension. This low surface tension allows for easier absorption and may improve cellular hydration. As we have seen in chapter 2/Water regarding body composition, a decreasing percentage of body water accompanies aging, obesity and many disease states. Mineral-rich glacial water prevents chronic dehydration from occurring. In addition, due to the low surface tension of the water, bodily toxins are more easily dissolved and excreted, thereby enhancing detoxification. Detoxification is one of the pillars of the Golden Ratio Lifestyle Diet, to which these centenarians are naturally adhering. Another promising scientific discovery that supports our emphasis on detoxification is from Polish and

10

Danish studies that found the main detoxification enzyme in the body—glutathione reductase—to be higher in centenarians.

Aquaporins: Our Molecular Fountains of Youth

Aquaporins are microscopic openings in our cellular membranes where water molecules move in and out of cells. Dr. Peter Agre won the 2003 Nobel Prize in Chemistry for his discovery of the aquaporin. In an interview with *The New York Times* (by Claudia Dreifus, 1/26/09), Agre said that on the suggestion of his old hematology professor Dr. John Parker, he should consider that his unidentified protein fragment could possibly be "the long-sought water channel." The scientific search for this cellular water channel is reminiscent of the age-old search for the elusive Fountain of Youth. These searches are actually quite similar, although on different scales of magnitude. Dr. Agre is a modern day Ponce de Leon, who focused his vision down to cellular levels and actually discovered molecular-sized Fountains of Youth *within* the human body. When water molecules move through aquaporins in an unimpeded manner, much like the water coming out of a fountain, cellular processes have a greater chance of flourishing.

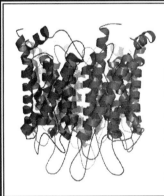

Aquaporins

Free-flowing aquaporins help maintain our intracellular-to-extracellular Golden Ratio water balance. About 63% of our total body water is intracellular, 37% is extracellular. If aquaporins aren't freely flowing, then this delicate Golden Ratio is upset and metabolic inefficiency results.

Over time, aquaporins are vulnerable to becoming damaged by free radicals or clogged with debris, such as heavy metals, environmental toxins or metabolic by-products. Just as a clogged fountain ceases to produce a strong and beautiful flow, the same can happen to aquaporins. When the aquaporins of millions of cells degenerate, we experience decreased performance, aging and ultimately death. Perhaps the secret to high-level wellness and longevity is to keep our molecular Fountains of Youth clean and freely flowing. All preventive measures are critical, such

10

as eating organic food and avoiding exposure to environmental toxins. Detoxification procedures are vital for eliminating cellular toxic debris and restoring aquaporins to full function. Cellular detoxification augments blood flow, lymphatic drainage, urination, defecation, breathing and sweating. More extensive detoxification therapies can include chelation, colonic irrigation, liver and kidney flushes, the use of digestive enzymes and avoidance of allergic foods.

Jeanne-Louise Calment (1875-1997): Supercentenarian Champion

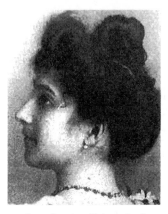

Jean-Louise Calment of France at 20. Calment lived to be 122, the world's oldest documented supercentenarian.

Although many societies like the Hunzans, Vilcabambans, Okinawans and Abkhazians claim supercentenarians (one who is over 110 years old), Jeanne-Louise Calment of France, who lived to 122 years of age, is the only supercentenarian whose age has been verified by official documents. In a *New York Times* article (8/5/97) Craig Whitney quotes French author and public health researcher Jean-Marie Robine regarding insights on Mrs. Calment's longevity:

The French, who celebrated her as the doyenne of humanity, had their own theories about why she lived so long, noting that she used to eat more than two pounds of chocolate a week, enjoyed a regular glass of port wine, poured olive oil on all her food as well as rubbing it onto her skin, rode a bicycle until she was 100, and only quit smoking five years ago... 'I think she was someone who, constitutionally and biologically speaking, was immune to stress,' he said in a telephone interview. She once said, 'If you can't do anything about it, don't worry about it.'

Clearly, one of Jean-Louise's most notable longevity factors was her "immunity to stress" and sense of inner peace. This attribute was likely a genetic behavioral predisposition. However, as explored in chapter 8/Happiness and Inner Peace, this quality of stress resistance can be cultivated through various methods. One's entire physiology can be modulated in a new, positive direction by reprogramming reactions to stress. Jeanne's orientation to humor was also very strong and though hard to measure or quantify, was probably a key factor enhancing her "immunity to stress." Here are a few of Jeanne's most memorable quotes which illustrate her positive, long-life attitude:

10

U.S. Longevity Champions Hall of Fame

Every culture has its own Longevity Champion's Hall of Fame. These are celebrated individuals who productively made it into their 89-144 Fibonacci Golden Years. Even without knowledge of the ratio, they excelled at one or more of the Golden Ratio Lifestyle Diet drivers. Perhaps, if they had practiced the integrated Diet, they would have lived as long or longer than long-life champion (age 122) Jeanne Calment of France. Here we present a few notable longevity examples from America:

Name	Career	Age lived to	Noted longevity support factor(s)
Dr. John Harvey Kellogg	Breakfast cereal pioneer, Loma Linda founder	91	Moderation in everything; had glass of water w/ lemon juice every morning; solar therapy, hydrotherapy
Dr. W. Edwards Deming	Quality leadership and management genius	93	Strong purpose, joy in work and learning
Dr. Linus Pauling	Chemist, peace activist, Vitamin. C proponent, double Nobel Prize winner	93	Vitamin C, great curiosity
Jack LaLanne	Father of the modern fitness revolution	96	Exercise, weightlifting in moderation, healthy living proponent, raw juicing
Kitty Carlisle	Singer, actress, *To Tell The Truth* panelist	96	Humor (stress reduction), dance /exercise
John D. Rockefeller	Oil magnet and philanthropist	97	Ample sleep; always eating to less than fullness; avoiding worry
Norman W. Walker	Raw food and juicing pioneer	99	Raw juicing, detoxification
Bob Hope	Comedian, philanthropist	100	Daily massage, humor (stress reduction)
W. Clement Stone	Businessman, philanthropist, self-help guru	100	Positive mental attitude
George Burns	Comedian, actor, writer	100	Humor (stress reduction)
Irving Berlin	Composer, lyricist	101	Music (stress reduction)
Dolores Hope	Philanthropist, wife of Bob Hope	102	Deep spiritual faith
Joseph M. Juran	Quality management genius and 80/20 proponent	103	Married 81 years; loved his work
Roy Neuberger	Financier, art patron	107	Business, art collecting, philanthropy
Bernando LaPallo	World's oldest blogger (age as of mid-2011):	109	Colon cleansing, raw diet/pescetarian
Leila Alice Denmark, M.D.	Pediatrician (age as of mid-2011):	113	Whole foods, low sugar diet; healthy hydration
Walter Breuning	Railroader	114	Healthy hydration habits, exercise

10

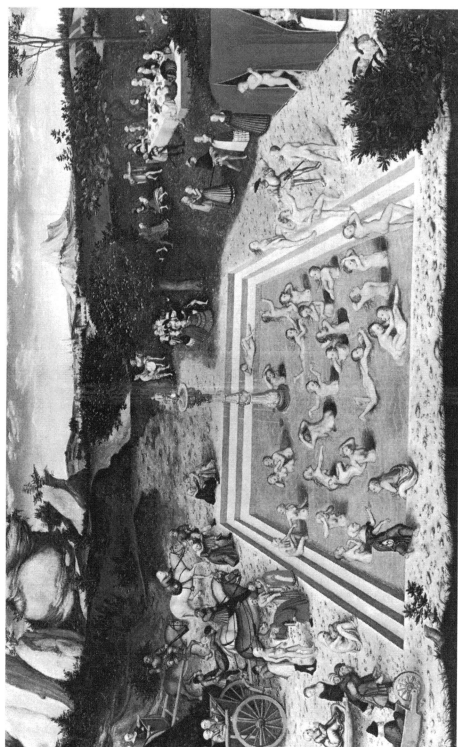

The Fountain of Youth, by German artist Lucas Cranach (1546). Note how the people enter the fountain pool as elders on the left and emerge on the right with their youth restored. Embarking on the Golden Ratio Lifestyle Diet is your lifetime VIP ticket to tapping your own virtual Fountain of Vibrant Health and Longevity.

10

- *I think I will die laughing.*

- *I never wear mascara; I laugh until I cry too often.*

- *I see badly, I hear badly and I feel bad, but everything's fine.*

- *Always keep your smile. That's how I explain my long life.*

- *I took pleasure when I could. I acted clearly and morally and without regret. I'm very lucky.*

- *I'm interested in everything but passionate about nothing.*

- *Not having children is one less worry.*

- *I'm not afraid of anything.*

- *I've only got one wrinkle—and I'm sitting on it.*

Longevity 3H

In keeping with the motif of the "3H" (Hips-Heart-Head) from chapter 5's Rx's, the 3H idea can also be conceptualized in the longevity essentials framework as:

Humor: Positive Attitude (Head correlation)

Happiness: Love, Community, Gratitude (Heart correlation)

Hot-Blooded: Passionate, Creative, Libido (Hips correlation)

Longevity Champion (and World's Oldest Blogger) Bernardo LaPallo

Bernando LaPallo of Mesa, Arizona is a retired master chef, podiatrist, herbalist, massage therapist, entrepreneur and, at 109, the world's oldest blogger. On his 109th birthday (August 17th, 2010) he commented on his blog:

I'm still traveling, still speaking in public, working on my second book and still drinking my SuperFood every morning. I have no plans to slow down, so stay tuned for what's next.

A selection of quotes from Bernardo offers a window into his health and longevity:

Health should be your first priority, and in order to do that, you eat properly and keep your colon clean.

You have to eat properly... not a bunch of stirred up, boiled-to-death food.

I was a protege of Dr. Schulze's mentor, Dr. Christopher. I and most of my family have been using Dr. Schulze's SuperFood since the 1980's.

10

Bernando wrote his book of lifestyle secrets, *Age Less, Live More*, at age 107: http://agelesslivemore.wordpress.com/   His longevity practices include:

• Eats mostly raw foods, fruits and vegetables and some soups
• He's a pescetarian (one who eats fish for protein) • Drinks cinnamon tea to keep his blood sugar controlled • Eats only two meals a day • Eats dinner around 4-5 pm
• Doesn't eat at night • Walks 1.5 miles a day • Rubs olive oil on his body and face to prevent wrinkles (just like longevity champion Jeanne Calment did)
• Takes Echinacea every morning • Eats Dr. Schulze's SuperFood daily.

Telomeres: Gateway to the Golden Ratio Years 89-144—and beyond

Telomeres are the DNA-protein caps at the ends of your chromosomes that protect them from deterioration as you age. With each cell division the telomeres continually shorten, until the DNA in the chromosome isn't protected anymore and begins to unravel, just like a frayed shoelace whose plastic tip—or *Aglet*—has deteriorated. At some critical point the cell approaches its Hayflick Limit: its maximal number of cell divisions (named after Leonard Hayflick, DNA research pioneer). As more and more cells lose their telomeres aging begins, with disease and ultimately death as the traditional final outcome. Scientists have come to the conclusion that the shorter the telomeres, the shorter one's life expectancy. Telomeres do have a repair process that is controlled by an enzyme called telomerase, yet this enzyme is usually not active in adult cells. Some cells do have active telomerase, like stem cells, reproductive cells and unfortunately, cancer cells. Telomerase is a double-edged sword: just enough can promote normal cell division and regeneration, but too much can enable cancerous cells to proliferate. Cancer cells have learned how to rebuild their telomeres by

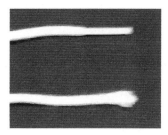 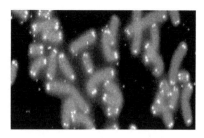

(*left*) Shoelace Aglets: normal (top) and frayed (bottom). (*right*) Chromosomes capped by telomeres. The telomeres are DNA-protein complexes that function like protective shoelace Aglets, preventing degeneration and aging. Professor Ramin Farzaneh-Far, M.D. of UCSF correlated higher levels of Omega-3 fatty acids with a slower rate of telomere shortening in patients with coronary heart disease. This finding may translate to a slowdown in overall cellular aging simply by increasing one's intake of Omega-3 oils.

10

activating their telomerase enzyme and have become essentially immortal. Scientists have perpetuated a particular line of aggressive, immortal cancer cells for medical research from a woman named Henrietta Lacks, who died of cancer in 1951. These so-named "HeLa" cells have become a standard cancer research cell line the world over. So prevalent in fact have the HeLa cells become that it's estimated that the entire mass of this immortalized cell line would weigh more than 100 Empire State Buildings. See the fascinating book *The Immortal Life of Henrietta Lacks* by Rebecca Skloot for more insight into telomeres, cancer and the ordeal Henrietta's family endures by having their mother's cells dispersed in laboratories worldwide.

Exploring Jeanne Calment's Longevity Factor

Among the many factors that have been attributed to Jeanne Calment's longevity, of particular note has been her immunity to stress. She once said,

If you can't do anything about it, don't worry about it.

Perhaps Jeanne's laid-back attitude had more to do with her becoming a super-centenarian than meets the eye. This life-enhancing psychological stance may actually be teachable to the average person as evidenced by the research of Herbert Benson, M.D. and Dean Ornish, M.D. They have discovered that stress reduction and positive lifestyle changes can modulate gene expression such that life-span can be significantly extended. Dr. Benson is the Godfather of Stress Reduction and Mind Body Medicine, inheriting the mantle from Dr. Hans Selye, author of the ground-breaking book *The Stress of Life.* Selye elucidated the physiological mechanisms of fight-or-flight responses and the General Adaptation Syndrome that occurs when flight-or-flight becomes chronic. Benson developed a practical and effective antidote to stress known as the Relaxation Response, which is a non-specific stress reduction technique based on meditation, deep breathing or prayer. However, Benson's research has now taken Hans Selye's fight-or-flight discoveries down to the genetic level. Stress reduction via the Relaxation Response has now been proven to favorably alter gene expression and possibly even affect apoptosis (programmed cell death). In his book, *Relaxation Revolution: Enhancing Your Personal Health Through the Science and Genetics of Mind*

> *The Ageless Body bears a quality of emotions that are light and joyous, willing to experience ecstasy and the richness of life at any moment.*
> **Chris Griscom, *The Ageless Body***

10

Body Healing, Benson shows that various genes responsible for high blood pressure, anxiety, depression, infertility, insomnia, hot flashes, back ache, headache and even phobias can be down-regulated (turned down) as a result of the Relaxation Response. Scientists have hypothesized that *increasing telomere length* may be the genetic mechanism through which stress reduction has its remarkable effects on longevity. In a related study, cardiologist Dean Ornish, M.D. showed that the telomerase enzyme could be increased by 29% in prostate cancer patients, simply by instituting a series of easy lifestyle upgrades including a diet low in refined sugars and fat and rich in whole foods, fruits and vegetables; aerobic exercise; breathing exercises and meditation. Ornish concluded that increasing telomerase through lifestyle modification may not be specific to only prostate cancer patients, it may in fact have similar powerful benefits for the population at large. Drs. Benson and Ornish have shown that stress reduction and lifestyle modification techniques can favorably influence gene expression and potentially preserve telomere length, thereby increasing life expectancy. The Golden Ratio Lifestyle Diet's approach of working with the optimal health driver sequence combined with Nature's Secret Nutrient builds on the work of these health and longevity pioneers. It gives us a head start into the future research of modulating gene expression, telomeres and life extension in simple and accessible ways. Being able to access the next Fibonacci Sequence level of life extension—the Golden Ratio Years from age 89 to 144 and even beyond—may now be close within our grasp. To ensure that you reach the next Fibonacci level of life span healthy and intact, make sure that you metaphorically tie your shoes—with your telomere's "Aglet" shoelace ends intact—by consciously reducing stress and increasing your inner peace and happiness.

Cross-Cultural Longevity Research
Supporting the Golden Ratio Lifestyle Diet

Scientific corroboration of many of the important factors in the Golden Ratio Lifestyle Diet are described by researcher and explorer Dan Buettner, who has lived among some of the longest-lived humans on Earth. Dan's cross-cultural research into the secrets of longevity led him to many of the centenarian hotspots or what he terms "Blue Zones" on the planet, including Sardinia, Okinawa, Costa Rica, Loma Linda, California, and Ikaria, Greece. In his compelling book *The Blue Zone: Lessons for Living Longer from the People Who've Lived the Longest* and in multiple issues of *National Geographic Adventure Magazine*, Buettner reveals some of his most consistent findings leading to longevity. After each of Buettner's key findings we list important Golden

10

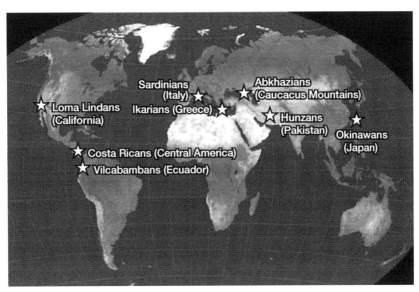

Centenarian Hotspot "Blue Zones," as reported
by longevity researcher and author Dan Buettner.

Ratio Lifestyle Diet factors, drivers or chapters that are supported by his research. While certainly not the last word on ultimate longevity, Buettner's research provides a compelling framework for writing—and living—our own optimal health and longevity lifescript. As Buettner suggests,

Set up your life, your home environment, your social environment, and your workplace so that you're constantly nudged into behaviors that favor longevity [which we'd suggest are all included in the Golden Ratio Lifestyle Diet].

Key Universal Longevity Factors [brackets = chapter/section correlation]

- People who make it to a hundred tend to be nice people; cultivate kindness, humor and altruism [8. Happiness & Inner Peace; 10. Longevity]

- Happier people live longer than unhappy people [10. Longevity/story of Jeanne Calment, world's oldest recorded super centenarian]

- The effect of unhappiness on your body can be as harmful as a smoking habit [7. Fibonacci's smoking reduction technique; 8. Happiness & Inner Peace]

- Longevity is much more a function of what you *don't* eat than what you *do* eat. This is a HUGE point. As Buettner reports, eating less in general (caloric reduction, as it's scientifically called) is the only proven way to slow down aging

10

THE GOLDEN RATIO LIFESTYLE DIET

> *How old would you be if you didn't know how old you are? Age is a*
> *question of mind over matter. If you don't mind, it doesn't matter.*
> **Satchel Paige, American Baseball Legend**

Dr. Ellen Langer: Mindfulness, Time Travel and Longevity

Mindfulness—the simple act of noticing new things—is crucial to our health in several ways. First, when we're mindless, we ignore all the ways we could exercise control over our health.

Ellen Langer, Ph.D.

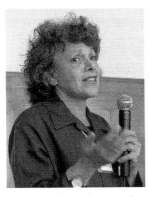

Harvard Professor of Psychology, Ellen Langer.

Harvard psychologist and professor Ellen Langer, Ph.D., author of *Counterclockwise: Mindful Health and the Power of Possibility*, performed a landmark study in 1979 that opened new frontiers into the science of longevity. Langer's fascinating work understandably also captured the imagination of Hollywood: actress Jennifer Aniston has signed on to produce and possibly star as Langer in the film *Counterclockwise*. In her experiment, Langer psychologically time-shifted a group of seventy and eighty year olds back in time 20 years—to the year 1959—by designing a totally realistic, isolated residential setting in rural New Hampshire that mimicked the visual, auditory and kinesthetic (seen/heard/felt) detail of that bygone era. The selection of all TV programs, magazines, radio and music, clothing—even the topics of their daily conversation—all reflected the ambiance of the late 1950's. Amazingly, after just *one* week of living in this time warp, the men showed the following significant improvements in key biomarkers of aging:

- Healthy weight
- Gait and posture improvement, with an increase in height
- Brain and sensory improvements in memory and hearing
- Less arthritic symptoms, with better dexterity and decreased inflammation
- Physiologic improvements, including decreased blood pressure
- A general sense of enhanced wellbeing
- A more youthful appearance at the end of the study, as determined by before-and-after photo comparison

10

Longevity Demographics and the Golden Ratio

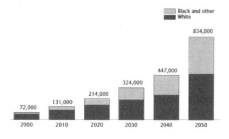

In the decades from:

- 2010-2020, the ratio of 214,000 to 131,000 is 1.63, virtually the Golden Ratio (1.62).

- 2030-2040, the ratio of 447,000 to 324,000 is equal to 1.38, a key Golden Ratio harmonic.

Number of projected centenarians in the United States by race, 2005 to 2050.
The exponential rise of centenarians conforms to the Golden Ratio.

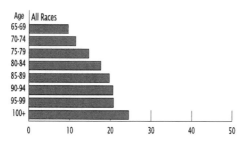

Percentage of people in the United States living below the poverty line, ages 65-100+ in 2000.

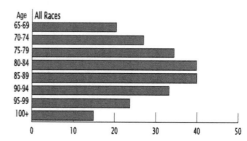

Percentage of people in the United States living alone, ages 65-100+ in 2000

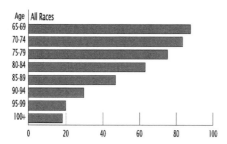

Percentage of people in the United States living with no disability limitations, ages 65-100+ in 2000.

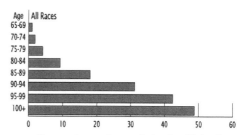

Percentage of people in the United States living in a nursing home, ages 65-100+ in 2000.

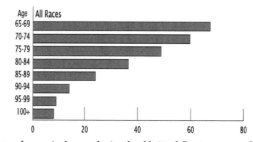

Percentage of married people in the United States, ages 65-100+ in 2000.

10

310

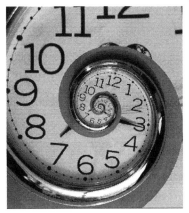

Langer's intriguing research invites us to reevaluate our concepts of the blurry division between mind and body, and the multi-directional flow of time. While many of us may not take the luxury of recreating actual physical stage sets of times past as Langer did for her study, we can nonetheless apply her work to our own lives. How? Through the powerful practice of mental/emotional time travel, to revisit times in our past when we were exceptionally happy, healthy and robust. By being mindful of and strategically revisiting memories that were especially invigorating to our psyches and hearts, we can support the re-release of those same enlivening neurotransmitters and hormones—

The benefits of mental/emotional time travel include tapping into your inner Fountain of Youth.

and thus experience their powerfully rejuvenating, healing effects *now*. An easy way to explore the intriguing genetic regeneration possibilities presented by Professor Langer's research is the Golden Prime Zone Meditation Rx 1 at the end of this chapter.

The Time Of Our Lives

As you can see from the following chart, human life expectancy has continually increased over the past 2000 years. Improvements in hygiene, nutrition and medical advances have been responsible for these increases and there is every reason to expect that future innovations in these and other areas will foster even longer life expectancies. The contrast is shocking between the 2009 U.S. life expectancy estimate of around 80 years for women, 75 years for men and the Swaziland estimate of just 32 years. The contrast between a supercentenarian—110 years old and over—and current U.S. life expectancy of approximately 80 years is food for thought.

Human Life Expectancy Over Time			
Year	Age	Year	Age
2000 BC	18	1900	50
500 AD	22	1946	67
1400	33	1991	76
1790	36	2009	80 Women; 75 Men (U.S.)
1850	41		32 (Swaziland)
			110+ (Supercentenenarian)

10

Fibonacci Sequence Lifestyle Stages

Kay Gardner (1941–2002) was a world-renowned musician, composer and author who had an insightful view into the stages of a woman's life, as seen through the lens of the Fibonacci Sequence. We have adapted Kay's original lifecycle chart to be applicable to both women and men. The Fibonacci numbers delineate the stages of life:

Childhood	8	Menopause/Andropause	55
Puberty	13	Elderhood	89
Awakening Sexuality	21		
Mother/Fatherhood	34		

The Golden (Ratio) Years: Expanding the Fibonacci Stages of Life

Human life expectancy has increased over the millennia and in order to accommodate this longevity, we can expand Kay Gardner's above Fibonacci life-cycle stages to the next higher numerical Fibonacci Sequence level. This becomes clear by following the Fibonacci Sequence to see what the next number would be, e.g., 0,0,1,1,2,3,5,8,13, 21,34,55,89,**144**... By looking at the spirals on a Nautilus shell and seeing that there's always another spiral that one can move to, we get a visual image of where our evolved lifecycle stage would be. Note that the first three stages stay the same, while the last three stages expand to the next level of the expanding life expectancy spiral:

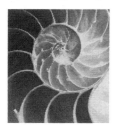

Childhood	8
Puberty	13
Awakening of Sexuality	21
Motherhood/Fatherhood	**34–89**
Menopause/Andropause	**55–89+**
Elderhood/Golden (Ratio) Years	**89–144**

Demographics of Longevity

By looking at the life expectancies of inhabitants of the longest-lived cultures in the world, e.g., Hunza, Vilcabamba, Abkhazia and Okinawa, we can see that the tendency to take a quantum Fibonacci jump in life expectancy is already happening. The number of centenarians in Okinawa is the highest in the world, at a rate of 50 per 100,000 population. The U.S. has a considerable number, yet lags behind, having a rate of around 18 per 100,000 population in the year 2000. However, the absolute number of centenarians will skyrocket to 834,000 by the year 2050, according to U.S. Census Bureau projections. Interestingly, the demographics of this exponential rise in the number of centenarians has some Golden Ratio aspects, as can be

10

seen in the accompanying diagrams. The demographics of longevity are alarming, as you can see in the centenarian graphs regarding disabilities, marital status, poverty and living situation. It may be hard to imagine yourself living to 100+, but if these U.S. Census Bureau data are accurate, many of us will become centenarians or supercentenarians and may have to confront living with disabilities, poverty, loneliness and compromised living quarters. Perhaps the Golden Ratio Lifestyle Diet can both help us become centenarians *and* overcome the challenges that longevity presents as we age. By applying the sequenced drivers in this book, you now have the ability to make a quantum evolutionary jump into *healthy* longevity. Can you imagine yourself transcending the accepted limit of an 80 year lifespan or becoming a parent in your 70's or 80's? The possibilities of what can be accomplished at any age expand preconceived lifecycle limits and need to be reevaluated and reimagined.

> *What you want to do is to regenerate and return to your*
> *true genetic blueprint, which has <u>no</u> age.*
> **Janet Krier, unlimited lifespan theorist**

Living into the 89–144–233 Fibonacci Sequence Range and Beyond

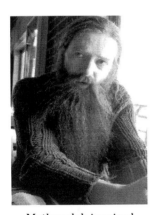

Methuselah-inspired maverick English longevity researcher, Aubrey de Grey.

Just as landing on the moon or running a sub four-minute mile were once "impossibilities," extending human lifespan well beyond current accepted limits is one of mankind's new frontiers. Considering that human life expectancy has been on an upward curve over time, especially in the last few centuries, it's not unreasonable to expect that we could see healthy triple-digit birthdays becoming the norm in the not-so-distant future. Maverick English researcher Aubrey de Grey is one of many pioneers pushing this longevity frontier forward. De Grey challenges us to expand our paradigm of possibility into the radical notion that *aging is optional*— and may instead be a culturally accepted disease. Called "The Prophet of Immortality" by *Popular Science* magazine, de Grey is a gerontology theoretician and co-author of *Ending Aging*. He works on the development of Strategies for Engineered Negligible Senescence (SENS), a tissue-repair strategy for human rejuvenation, prevention of age-related decline and extended lifespan. To this end, De Grey identified seven types of

10

molecular and cellular damage caused by metabolic processes. SENS is a therapeutic protocol to repair this damage. According to wikipedia.com, whose biography of de Grey includes an excerpt from LiveScience.com:

> de Grey argues that the fundamental knowledge needed to develop effective anti-ageing medicine mostly already exists, and that the science is ahead of the funding. He works to identify and promote specific technological approaches to the reversal of various aspects of ageing, or as de Grey puts it, 'the set of accumulated side effects from metabolism that eventually kills us,' and for the more proactive and urgent approaches to extending the healthy human lifespan.

Through regenerative medicine negating the deleterious effects of metabolism and a challenge to the "global pro-aging trance," de Grey champions research to reach "lifespan escape velocity." He submits there is a serious gap in understanding between scientists and biologists studying aging and those studying regenerative medicine. Through the application of leading-edge approaches like the Golden Ratio Lifestyle Diet, SENS and others, the celebration of triple-digit birthdays may well become as common as running a sub-four minute mile is today. By tapping the Golden Ratio's latent regenerative principle in our DNA, enduring robust health and more volitional longevity may be closer than we imagine.

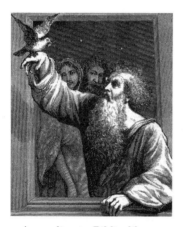

According to Biblical lore, Longevity Legend Noah lived to be 950 years of age. Noah was outlived however by his grandfather, Methuselah, who lived to a sprightly 969. Fantastic fiction or glimmers of ancient (and future) truth?

Biblical Longevity Legends: Myth or Reality?

Peppered throughout the Bible are dozens of examples of lifespan superheroes, pointing to the possibility of extreme longevity. They are grouped here into their respective "Generation Phi" categories by sequential Fibonacci Sequence number divisions. Methuselah is the Bible's archetypal elder... Enoch's son, Lamech's father and Noah's grandfather. Maybe longevity researcher Aubrey de Grey's supposition that *aging is optional* has some basis in the historical record (de Grey's longevity prize, with an award amount over $1 million dollars, is named the Methuselah Prize). Visionary *Star Trek* creator Gene Roddenberry referenced Methuselah in the *Star Trek* episode *Requiem for Methuselah*, which first aired in 1969. Most ironically, the last three digits of that year match Methuselah's

10

Generation Phi Φ age groups of Biblical Longevity Legends, as demarcated by adjacent Fibonacci Sequence numbers: 89–144, 144–233, 233–377, 377–610, 610–987.

610—987		233—377		89—144	
Name	*Age*	*Name*	*Age*	*Name*	*Age*
Methuselah	**969**	**Enoch**	**365**	Ishmael	137
Jared	962	Reu	239	Levi	137
Noah	**950**			Amram	137
Adam	930	**144—233**		Kohath	133
Seth	912	*Name*	*Age*	Laban	130
Kenan	910	Serug	230	Deborah	130
Enos	905	**Job**	**210**	Sarah	127
Mahalalel	895	Terah	205	Miriam	125
Lamech	**777**	Isaac	180	Aaron	123
		Abraham	**175**	Rebecca	120
377—610		Nahor	148	**Moses**	**120**
Name	*Age*	Jacob	147	Joseph	110
Shem	600	Esau	147	Joshua	110
Eber	464				
Arpachshad	438				
Salah	433				

reported life years reached: 969. The episode's main character, Flint, shared this thoughtful pearl of wisdom:

Death, when unnecessary, is a tragic thing.

Generation PHI Φ

We will see the emergence of a whole new generation of people with the ability to confidently access their higher Golden (Ratio) years—89 to 144 and even beyond—Generation PHI Φ. In addition to the immense personal implications of living longer, there will be profound social, political, environmental and global implications of extending your lifespan into the next higher Fibonacci Spiral of existence. The ideal way to age as proposed by life extension doctors is to live as healthy as possible, for as long as possible, with a compressed duration of morbidity. As Jeanne Calment, the world's longest lived person, might have said (paraphrasing Hunter S. Thompson):

Life should NOT be a journey to the grave with the intention of arriving safely in a pretty and well preserved body, but rather to skid in broadside—chocolate in one hand, a glass of wine in the other—body thoroughly used up, totally worn out, and screaming—WOW! What a Ride!

10

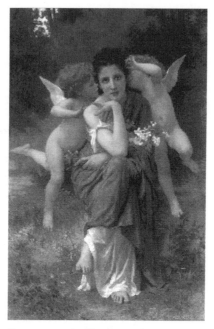

William-Adolphe Bouguereau's *Chansons de printemps* (*Songs of Spring*)
beautifully illustrates the feeling of communion with the idyllic realm of eternal youth,
while the quote below echoes the power of accessing this timeless state at will.

> *In my heart, I've never had room for envy nor for hatred, but only*
> *happiness that I could pick anywhere and anytime. I consider that what*
> *makes us live the most is the feeling of a permanent childhood in our life.*
>
> **Constantin Brancusi, internationally**
> **renowned Romanian sculptor**

10

THE GOLDEN RATIO ℞ LIFESTYLE DIET

VIBRANT HEALTH & LONGEVITY

Pick one or more of the following Rx's to add to your daily health regimen.

1. Golden Prime Zone Holodeck Meditation

In chapter 8/Happiness & Inner Peace, we identified the 13-year range from age 19 to 31 as the Golden Prime Zone. Recall that 19 and 31 are both prime numbers and 31 divided by 19 approaches the Golden Ratio of 1.618. This is the prime time range when our life force is especially strong and vibrant. All of our hormones are at their peak, including growth hormone and our sexual hormones. In the spirit of Dr. Ellen Langer's landmark 1979 Counterclockwise study, if we want to revisit a time of maximal health and potency, this 19 to 31 time frame is a great place to start. A simple and imaginative process for reactivating your Golden Prime Zone consists of creating and periodically visiting your own virtual Holodeck. A Holodeck is a virtual reality simulator that was popularized in the *Star Trek* movies and TV series, where a person can select and visit any chosen reality/timeframe and experience it as if it were real. Here's how to create your own personal Holodeck and reactivate your Golden Prime Zone:

1. **Set your TIME target coordinates**: On the TimeMap™ (next page), highlight your age 19 to 31 Golden Prime Zone years with a pen (if a little before 19 or after 31, that's ok). Then, select 3 to 5 of your favorite peak memories from within this timeframe and concisely note them on the graph in a few words, approximately when they occurred in your 19 to 31 year Golden Prime Zone. Your selected memories could be of particular people, places or events. Finally, select your ONE peak memory to work with in your Holodeck, write it at the top of a 3x5 index card (your Peak Memory Card) or large Post-It note, and proceed to step #2.

10

The TimeMap™ Graph: Blueprint for Activating
Your Inner Fountain Of Youth

Highlight your age 19 to 31 Golden Prime Zone years with a pen below. Then select 3 to 5 of your favorite, peak memories from within this time period. Concisely mark/note them on this graph in a few words, next to when they occurred in your personal Golden Prime Zone.

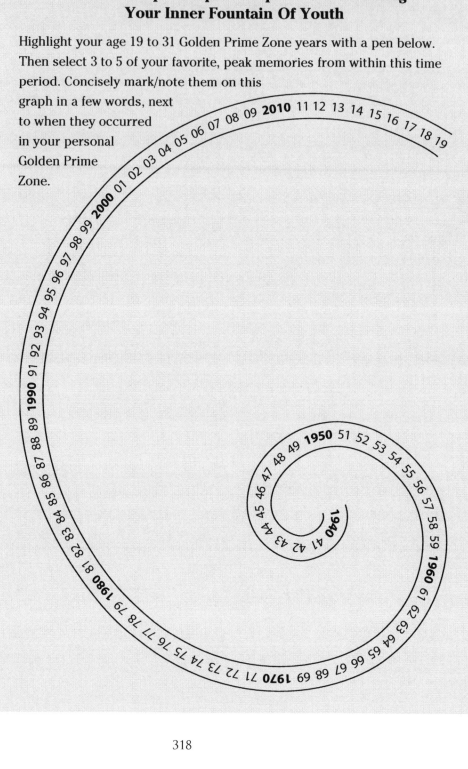

10

318

2. Next, **set your PLACE target coordinates**: Add the location of your ONE selected memory from step #1 to your 3x5 Peak Memory Card.

3. Now, **set your SENSORY target coordinates**:

Using your selected time and place memory coordinates, add a few sensory memory boosters from the following list to your 3x5 card:

 Visual: a favorite scene, person, picture, smile, painting; any evocative images.

 Auditory: a favorite song, a lover's voice, cheering crowds, laughter, sounds of nature—waves, wind, rain, crickets, etc.

 Kinesthetic: remember what you were wearing, the weather or how you were moving your body. Focus on how you felt in your body at the time. Pay special attention to how you *felt* in your selected memory. Bring those same feelings into this moment.

 Taste: a particularly wonderful meal or beverage and how it tasted: how delicious was it? sweet, spicy, cold, warm or hot?

 Smell: any scents or aromas associated with the scene—food, coffee, cocktail, flowers, perfume or cologne, smoke, freshly cut grass, the ocean, etc. Your sense of smell is intricately connected with emotional memories in the brain's limbic system. It plays a particularly powerful role in both encoding memories and in supporting their recall. Complete your 3x5 Peak Memory Card.

To begin your Holodeck time travel experience:

1. Set aside 8 to 21 minutes when you can be undisturbed and relaxed.

2. Sit with tall, buoyant posture and begin breathing deeply and slowly.

3. Review your 3x5 Peak Memory Card. When ready, gently close your eyes.

4. In your mind's eye, allow yourself to move fully into your chosen peak memory. Experience and enjoy it as if it was actually happening *now*.

5. As you surf the sensory waves of your memories, bask in any particularly intense and wonderful scenes when your physical, mental and emotional energies were at their PEAK. Know that you're fully protected and safe while in your Holodeck experiencing your targeted peak memory. Let the positive feelings that arise permeate your body, mind and soul. If you have areas of your body that aren't working up to par today, welcome

10

the wonderful feelings of robust times past into those areas. Feel the rejuvenating and regenerating qualities become a reality for you, NOW. Let your memory dwell on all of your senses: sights, sounds, touch, tastes and scents. This helps to amplify your feelings, which fuel and deepen your Holodeck journey and its impact.

When ready, prepare to return to the present. With eyes still closed, raise your hands and place them with the palms about 3 inches from your eyes. Slowly open your eyes so that all you see are the palms of your hands. Allow your eyes to adjust for a few moments before lowering your hands.

You may wish to jot down any insights on another 3x5 index card or Post-It to inspire you during your day and week ahead. Your Golden Prime Zone time travel meditations need only be a few minutes long—as little as 5 to 8 minutes—in order to reactivate your potent neurotransmitters and hormones. Practice your Golden Prime Zone Holodeck Meditation 1-3 times per week for maximal benefits. Over the coming weeks and months, you may be surprised at who's looking back at you in the mirror.

Note: If want to further amp-up your Holodeck experience, run through the prior 5-sense checklist *with your target peak memory timeframe in mind*:

- Find an associated picture, newspaper or magazine
- Select a favorite song from that timeframe
- Get a piece of clothing or something to hold or touch
- Obtain a specific taste item and/or an affiliated scent.

These would be the associated physical sensory items you'd review prior to commencing your Holodeck mediation, in addition to your Peak Memory Card. Once you've secured some or all of these items, you're ready to set up your own Integrated Holodeck Access Kit (iHAK). Keep these items together and handy in a special place or container. Your iHAK will amplify your fractal sensory activation keys and boost your mind's journey back into your selected peak Golden Prime Zone memories. This protocol effectively allows you to *hack* into your core Golden Ratio DNA operating system and upgrade your latent, infinite capacity for robust health, happiness and longevity.

10

2. Chocolate: Longevity Food of the Gods

Chocolate in various forms has enjoyed high esteem and popularity for thousands of years. Believed by the Maya to have been discovered by the Gods (its scientific name, *Theobroma*, means "Food of the Gods"), chocolate has been used as an endurance booster, aphrodisiac and even as a form of currency. Itzamna, legendary Mayan Sky God, founder of Mayan culture and early champion of chocolate, is said to have taught his people to grow maize and cacao, as well as writing, calendars and medicine.

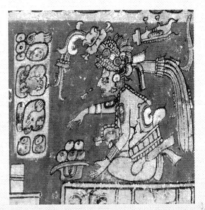

Mayan God Itzamna, early champion of chocolate.

The ancient Maya created a cacao concoction called *Kukuha*, which they flavored with chili and black pepper, spices and honey. It was consumed hot or cold by the Maya to boost their strength. Due to chocolate's potent mix of nutrients and divine flavor, it certainly fits the profile of a super health and longevity food of the gods—and humans. If we look deeper into the actual structure of cacao pods we find, to no surprise, that they exhibit Golden Ratio geometry in their design. There are 5 cacao beans in each pod, distributed in a Golden Ratio pentagonal array. Every cacao pod, and thus chocolate the world over, carries within it a distinct Golden Ratio imprint. To get the maximum benefits from chocolate, wikipedia.org recommends:

- *Buy cocoa in its raw form, instead of a highly processed/inferior form. Raw cocoa apparently contains roughly four times the number of antioxidants than [processed] cocoa powder and contains the largest antioxidant value of all natural foods worldwide.*

- *Raw cocoa has approximately double the number of antioxidants of red wine and about three times more than green tea.*

- *Chocolate's flavanols are also thought to help reduce blood platelet buildup and can balance levels of compounds called eicosanoids (special cellular signaling molecules), which may be beneficial to cardiovascular health.*

10

- *Cocoa beans are also high in magnesium...and sulphur. [magnesium is nature's valium, relaxing blood vessels and lowering blood pressure. Sulphur is a component of glutathione, our main detoxification enzyme.]*
- *Heat helps antioxidant release, so enjoy hot cocoa. Other benefits of drinking warm raw cocoa you may experience are having your mood enhanced—due to drinking the phenylethylamine in the cocoa—and feeling relaxed, as smelling chocolate/cocoa may increase theta brain waves, which can induce feelings of relaxation.*

Aim for the darkest, unprocessed organic cocoa powder you can find and consume it in a warm or hot drink, sweetened as desired with honey, agave or xylitol. When eaten in bar form, the darker-is-better rule applies—go for organic 62% or higher chocolate. Scharffen Berger actually makes a Golden Ratio percentage (62%) chocolate bar: www. scharffenberger.com. Enjoy a guilt-free daily portion of chocolate and savor the blessings of this Divine Food of the Gods.

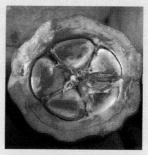

Cacao beans grow in a pentagonal Golden Ratio formation.

Itzamna's Golden Ratio Hot Cocoa Recipe: Aphrodisiac, Mood Booster and Super-Energizer, all rolled into one

3 cups milk (substitute almond, rice, oat, hazelnut or soy milk as desired)

8 tsp. organic darkest cocoa powder

3-5 tsp. agave nectar, honey, xylitol or organic sugar—sweeten to taste

1 vanilla bean (split), or a few drops of organic vanilla extract

1 or 2 cinnamon sticks (may substitute cinnamon powder, ¼ tsp.)

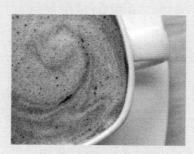

Hot Chocolate is a great way to bring people together (note the subtle Golden Spiral in the foam).

To invoke the power of the Mayan Gods, try adding ¼ tsp. cayenne pepper or chili powder.

10

In a saucepan on medium heat, add milk, cinnamon, vanilla (and cayenne pepper or chili powder as desired). Gently heat until warm, then reduce heat and add cocoa powder and sweetener, stirring ingredients until smooth. Pour into cups and garnish with a Golden Spiral of whipped cream. *Note the usage of Fibonacci Sequence numbers and attendant Golden Ratios in this recipe, to reactivate cocoa's special Golden Ratio imprint.*

3. The Master Golden Ratio Lifestyle Diet Prescription

Your master prescription for Vibrant Health and Longevity is simply the complete Golden Ratio Lifestyle Diet. By now you ought to have a good grasp on how to access Nature's Secret Nutrient (NSN) and prioritize and strengthen the 9 drivers of health and longevity. To review, they are presented here again in their relative order of top-down importance.

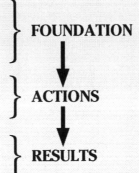

1. **Air & Breath**
2. **Water & Hydration**
3. **Sleep, Rest & Recovery**
4. **Nutrition**

FOUNDATION

5. **Posture**
6. **Exercise**
7. **Detoxification**

ACTIONS

8. **Happiness & Inner Peace**
9. **Natural Beauty & Attraction**
10. **Vibrant Health & Longevity**

RESULTS

All you need now is a practical, easy-to-use system that will help you implement the behavioral changes necessary to support the Diet. This system is the 21-Day Quick-Start Checklist in the next section. It has been extensively tested with Fortune 100 companies and lets you easily chart and support your progress. You will also get to see how your health and performance correlate and improve via application of key selected Diet Rx's. You will be amazed to see the growing improvement in your life by making the Rx's a part of your daily lifestyle. As you know, it takes 21 days to ingrain a new habit, so we have provided initial 21-Day charts for you to begin,

10

pre-loaded with a suggested top Rx addressing each of the nine health and longevity drivers. This 21-Day+ new habit pattern practice becomes in essence your master prescription for achieving and ensuring breakthrough health and longevity.

As the Golden Ratio-inspired ancient Pythagoreans would say,

HEALTH TO YOU

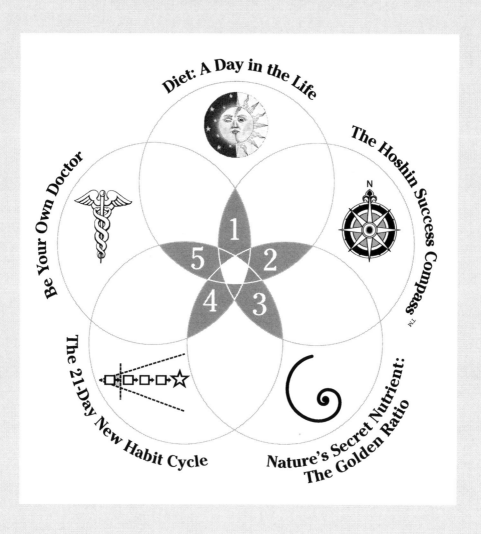

10

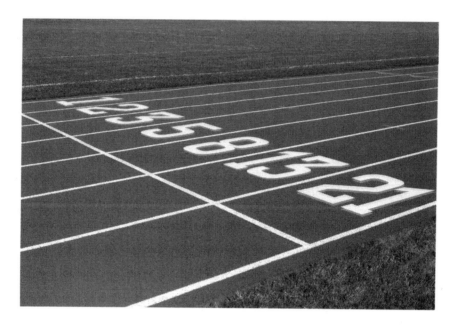

Ready, Set, Go!

The 21-Day Quick-Start Checklist system supports

new, healthy Golden Ratio Lifestyle Diet habits.

Nobody can go back and start a new beginning,

but anyone can start today and make a new ending.

Maria Robinson

11.

THE 21-DAY QUICK-START CHECKLIST SYSTEM

Most experts agree that it takes 21 days to set a desired new habit, in order for the new habit to enjoy the best chance of taking root. Yet the challenge for many is just getting to Day 21, e.g., most diets fail around Day 13. It seems that at about 60% (13 days) of the way to Day 21, old habits reassert themselves with a vengeance (another example of the Fibonacci Sequence and 60/40 Golden Ratio at work). Many of the Golden Ratio Lifestyle Diet action Rx's, while simple and even fun to do, are still new habits nonetheless. What is needed is an easy, visual system to help keep you on track and on target, so you can blast through day 13 and make it to that magical 21st day and beyond. This starts you on your way to adopting new habits that will support your successful upgrade into robust health and enhanced longevity.

The 21-Day Quick-Start Checklist system was originally designed by co-author Matthew Cross, to support peak performance habits for his corporate clients. In that arena, it's known as *The Hoshin Success Compass Peak Performance Passport.*™ Thousands worldwide continue to enjoy great benefit from this low-tech/high impact self-coaching system (a virtual version is imminent). It's an effective tool for upgrading your habits to support higher performance and life quality. Best of all, the system requires an investment of 3 minutes a day or less, which reflects the magic of Kaizen's small steps to success approach. The theory behind the system is simple: You must be able to *see* your progress in order to stay on track and on target. Further, when you start to see the correlation between acting on new habits and their impact on the quality of your life, it ignites a chain reaction of energy and inner commitment. It's simple: out of sight = out of mind—and therefore, out of action. On the flip side: IN sight (visible) = insight = action = follow through = results.

Here's how it works. Review the filled-in example on the opposite page for clarity.

1. First, **fill in the appropriate dates along the top of the graph.** Note that the graph is set to begin on a Monday.

2. You begin each daily recording session by Rating the Quality of Your Day (**Section 1**), in the top shaded row with the [1/low] to [10/high ranking]. At the end of each day, simply assign a "d●t" in the shaded 1-10 row across the top of the graph, correlating to the overall quality of that day. The aim: a simple, subjective rating of the day just passed; a quick visual indication of that day's "Emotional Altitude." As the days unfold, connect the d●ts, to form a simple run graph pattern. Patterns are powerful ways to learn and understand the impact of our actions, or lack of action. Visual patterns of your performance help you support your new actions to raise your game and predict better future results. *Patterns Predict.*

3. Track your Daily Rx progress (**Section 2**): Note the pre-filled in 10 suggested Golden Ratio Lifestyle Diet Rx actions. These are the "vital few" Rx's we've selected to get you going. These Rx's are drawn from each of the first 9 chapters. Feel free to modify this starter list or add additional items on lines 10-13 in the Checklist. You also have the option of selecting all of your own Rx's, on the blank daily Tracking System pages. Remember: *quality over quantity*. You don't need to fill in all 13 lines with action items; you might choose to start with just 3 or 5. In line with Kaizen, the secret is to choose small, managable yet meaningful steps.

4. After you assign your 1-10 day Quality Rating "d●t" in the top shaded area, you then simply check off each of your Rx Action Items, correlating to the date. For example, for most of the actions, you may choose to use a simple "check mark" to signify "I did it." For others you might fill in a number, e.g., number of hours of sleep/rest for that day (see example). If you missed doing an item for that day, leave that box blank (no "O's")—you need to see the patterns of the **blank** boxes as the days unfold. This offers valuable course-correcting data.

One important point: Do not judge yourself if you miss one or more items on one or more days. You're simply collecting data in order to upgrade and instill new habits.

11

Filled-in Example Pages

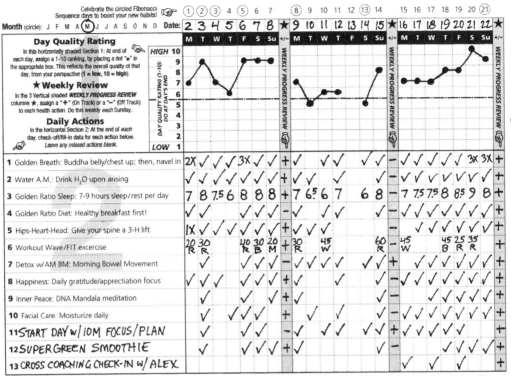

Celebrate the circled Fibonacci Sequence days to boost your new habits! ☞ ① ② ③ 4 ⑤ 6 7 ⑧ 9 10 11 12 ⑬ 14 15 16 17 18 19 20 ㉑

21-Day Quick Start Checklist

Daily Actions	M 2	T 3	W 4	T 5	F 6	S 7	Su 8	★ +/-	M 9	T 10	W 11	T 12	F 13	S 14	Su 15	★ +/-	M 16	T 17	W 18	T 19	F 20	S 21	Su 22	★ +/-
1 Golden Breath: Buddha belly/chest up; then, navel in	2X	✓	✓	✓	3X	✓	✓	+	✓		✓	✓				−	✓	✓	✓	✓	✓	3X	3X	+
2 Water A.M.: Drink H₂O upon arising	✓	✓	✓	✓	✓	✓	✓	+	✓	✓							✓	✓	✓	✓	✓	✓	✓	+
3 Golden Ratio Sleep: 7-9 hours sleep/rest per day	7	8	7.5	6	8	8	8	+	7	6.5	6	7			6	8		7	7.5	7.5	8	8.5	9	8	+
4 Golden Ratio Diet: Healthy breakfast first!	✓				✓	✓	✓	−		✓		✓	✓			−	✓	✓	✓	✓	✓	✓	✓	+
5 Hips-Heart-Head: Give your spine a 3-H lift	1X	✓	✓	✓		✓	✓	+	✓	✓	✓					−		✓	✓	✓	✓	✓	✓	+
6 Workout Wave/FIT excercise	20 R	30 R			40 R	30 B	20 M	+	30 R		45 W					60 R	−	45 W			45 B	25 R	35 R		+
7 Detox w/ AM BM: Morning Bowel Movement									✓	✓			✓		✓	+				✓			✓	+
8 Happiness: Daily gratitude/appreciation focus	✓	✓	✓			✓	✓	+	✓			✓					✓		✓	✓	✓		✓	+
9 Inner Peace: DNA Mandala meditation					✓		✓	+									✓			✓	✓		✓	+
10 Facial Care: Moisturize daily			✓		✓	✓	✓	+	✓								✓		✓	✓	✓	✓	✓	+
11 START DAY w/ 10M FOCUS/PLAN			✓		✓	✓		−	✓								✓	✓	✓	+	✓	✓	✓	✓
12 SUPER GREEN SMOOTHIE		✓			✓	✓	✓	+	✓										✓	✓	✓	✓	✓	+
13 CROSS COACHING CHECK-IN w/ ALEX																			✓		✓	✓	✓	+

Day Quality Rating
In this horizontally shaded Section 1: At end of each day, assign a 1-10 ranking, by placing a dot "•" in the appropriate box. This reflects the overall quality of that day, from your perspective (1 = low, 10 = high).

★ Weekly Review
In the 3 Vertical shaded WEEKLY PROGRESS REVIEW columns ★, assign a "+" (On Track) or a "−" (Off Track) to each health action. Do this weekly each Sunday.

Daily Actions
In the horizontal Section 2: At the end of each day, check-off/fill-in data for each action below. Leave any missed actions blank.

Month (circle): J F M A (M) J J A S O N D

DAY QUALITY RATING (1-10): HIGH 10 ... LOW 1

Progress Notes

Week 1	Week 2	Week 3	General Notes:
GOT OFF TO A GREAT START, THEN FELL BACK A BIT MID-WEEK DUE TO OVERNIGHT TRIP / LESS SLEEP... REACHING DAY 5 CELEBRATION WAS NICE - GLASS OF WINE ON THE WATER ☺	CRAZY WEEK! WAS ALL OVER THE MAP... ENOUGH SLEEP IS CLEARLY A MUST. FRIDAY WAS A 200, SO GAVE MYSELF THE OK TO LET THE TRACKING GO THAT DAY... GOOD NEWS IS I'M STILL IN THE GAME! WILL JUMP INTO NEXT WEEK w/ GUSTO + RENEWED COMMITMENT...	NOW WE'RE TALKING. FELT LIKE I WAS FIRING ON MOST CYLINDERS, ESP. SAT. - GREAT RACE! STILL ROOM FOR IMPROVEMENT, YET I'M FEELING LIKE I'M ON THE RIGHT TRACK	VERY ENLIGHTENING. BIG TAKE-AWAYS: • SLEEP: MUST MAKE IT A HIGHER PRIORITY! • SMOOTHIES ARE A HUGE FACTOR IN FEELING FOCUSED & ENERGIZED + A GREAT BREAKFAST ON THE RUN. • SHARING THIS DURING WEEK 3 w/ ALEX AND EXCHANGING INSIGHTS + COACHING KICKED EVERYTHING INTO A HIGHER GEAR. • PROGRESS FELT GREAT. GOING TO DO ANOTHER 21 DAYS TO TAKE IT EVEN HIGHER; LOOK OUT WORLD!

11

"Life Happens" and there may well be days when you're pulled off-track. On those days, you may miss doing one, many or even all of your new habits. Grant yourself amnesty, let it go, recommit and get back in the game—it's as simple as that. It's said that it's not how many times you get knocked down that counts—it's how many times you get back up on your feet. Keep your eyes on the Prize, no matter what.

5. Progress Notes (**Section 3**, optional). When done assigning your "d●t" in the top shaded graph and quickly filling in (or leaving blank) your appropriate Rx Action boxes, you may wish to jot down a few insights or notes regarding your progress, challenges and breakthroughs.

6. On Fibonacci Sequence Days 1, 2, 3, 5, 8, 13 and 21, take stock and do something special to affirm and celebrate your progress. On Day 21, do something especially memorable to commemorate your achievement. Thoughtfully review your progress over the past 21 days, looking for meaningful patterns and correlations. Commit to doing whatever it takes to close any "gaps" where you missed the mark. At the same time, keep doing what you've been doing where you consistently followed-through on a specific new habit/Rx Action.

When you're ready, feel free to begin another 21-Day tracking cycle, armed with fresh insights and higher commitment to upgrading your total lifestyle, health and longevity.

Optional: *Cut out the Checklist System page(s) from the book. Some prefer the ease of carrying just the single tracking page with them.*

> *We are what we repeatedly do.*
> *Excellence, then, is not an act, but a habit.*
> **Aristotle**

11

21-Day Quick-Start Checklist

Month (circle): J F M A M J J A S O N D **Date:** _____

Celebrate the circled Fibonacci ☞
Sequence days to boost your new habits!

WEEKLY PROGRESS REVIEW ☞ (×3)

Day numbers: ① 2 ③ 4 ⑤ 6 7 ⑧ 9 10 11 12 ⑬ 14 15 16 17 18 19 20 ㉑

Weekday columns: M T W T F S Su (repeated)

Day Quality Rating
In this horizontally shaded Section 1: At end of *each* day, assign a 1-10 ranking, by placing a dot "●" in the appropriate box. This reflects the overall quality of that day, from your perspective (1 = **low**, 10 = **high**).

HIGH 10
9
8
7
6
DAY QUALITY RATING (1-10): DO AT DAY'S END
5
4
3
2
LOW 1

★ Weekly Review
In the 3 Vertical shaded *WEEKLY PROGRESS REVIEW* columns , assign a "**+**" (On Track) or a "**–**" (Off Track) to each health action. Do this weekly *each* Sunday.

Daily Actions
In the horizontal Section 2: At the end of *each* day, check-off/fill-in data for each action below.
☞ *Leave any missed actions blank.*

1 Golden Breath: Buddha belly/chest up; then, navel in
2 Water A.M.: Drink H₂O upon arising
3 Golden Ratio Sleep: 7-9 hours sleep/rest per day
4 Golden Ratio Diet: Healthy breakfast first!
5 Hips-Heart-Head: Give your spine a 3-H lift
6 Workout Wave/FIT excercise
7 Detox w/AM BM: Morning Bowel Movement
8 Happiness: Daily gratitude/appreciation focus
9 Inner Peace: DNA Mandala meditation
10 Facial Care: Moisturize daily
11
12
13

11

Progress Notes

General Notes:

Week 3

Week 2

Week 1

11

21-Day Quick-Start Checklist

Month (circle): J F M A M J J A S O N D **Date:**

Celebrate the circled Fibonacci Sequence days to boost your new habits!

Circled day numbers: (1) (2) (3) 4 (5) 6 7 (8) 9 10 11 12 (13) 14 15 16 17 18 19 20 (21)

★ WEEKLY PROGRESS REVIEW ☞

Day Quality Rating

In this horizontally shaded Section 1: At end of *each* day, assign a 1-10 ranking, by placing a dot "●" in the appropriate box. This reflects the overall quality of that day, from your perspective (**1 = low, 10 = high**).

DAY QUALITY RATING (1-10):
DO AT DAY'S END

HIGH 10
9
8
7
6
5
4
3
2
LOW 1

★ Weekly Review

In the 3 Vertical shaded *WEEKLY PROGRESS REVIEW* columns ★, assign a "**+**" (On Track) or a "**–**" (Off Track) to each health action. Do this weekly *each* Sunday.

Daily Actions

In the horizontal Section 2: At the end of *each* day, check-off/fill-in data for each action below. *Leave any missed actions blank.*

Day columns: M T W T F S Su | M T W T F S Su | M T W T F S Su

1 Golden Breath: Buddha belly/chest up; then, navel in
2 Water A.M.: Drink H$_2$O upon arising
3 Golden Ratio Sleep: 7-9 hours sleep/rest per day
4 Golden Ratio Diet: Healthy breakfast first!
5 Hips-Heart-Head: Give your spine a 3-H lift
6 Workout Wave/FIT exercise
7 Detox w/AM BM: Morning Bowel Movement
8 Happiness: Daily gratitude/apprectiation focus
9 Inner Peace: DNA Mandala meditation
10 Facial Care: Moisturize daily
11
12
13

11

Progress Notes

General Notes:

Week 3

Week 2

Week 1

11

21-Day Quick-Start Checklist – Blank

Celebrate the circled Fibonacci Sequence days to boost your new habits!

Month (circle): J F M A M J J A S O N D   **Date:**

Day numbers: ①② ③ 4 ⑤ 6 7 ⑧ 9 10 11 12 ⑬ 14 15 16 17 18 19 20 ㉑

Days of week: M T W T F S Su (repeated for three weeks)

★ WEEKLY PROGRESS REVIEW ☞ +/−

DAY QUALITY RATING (1-10): DO AT DAY'S END

HIGH	10
	9
	8
	7
	6
	5
	4
	3
	2
LOW	1

Day Quality Rating
In this horizontally shaded Section 1: At end of *each* day, assign a 1-10 ranking, by placing a dot "●" in the appropriate box. This reflects the overall quality of that day, from your perspective (**1 = low, 10 = high**).

★ Weekly Review
In the 3 Vertical shaded *WEEKLY PROGRESS REVIEW* columns ★: assign a "**+**" (On Track) or a "**—**" (Off Track) to each health action. Do this weekly *each* Sunday.

Daily Actions
In the horizontal Section 2: At the end of *each* day, check-off/fill-in data for each action below.
Leave any missed actions blank.

Action rows: 1, 2, 3, 4, 5, 6, 7, 8, 9, 10, 11, 12, 13

11

Progress Notes

General Notes:

Week 3

Week 2

Week 1

21-Day Quick-Start Checklist – Blank

Month (circle): J F M A M J J A S O N D **Date:**

Celebrate the circled Fibonacci
Sequence days to boost your new habits!

① ② ③ 4 ⑤ 6 7 ⑧ 9 10 11 12 ⑬ 14 15 16 17 18 19 20 ㉑

★ WEEKLY PROGRESS REVIEW
M T W T F S Su   +/-

★ WEEKLY PROGRESS REVIEW
M T W T F S Su   +/-

★ WEEKLY PROGRESS REVIEW
M T W T F S Su   +/-

DAY QUALITY RATING (1-10):
DO AT DAY'S END
HIGH 10 / 9 / 8 / 7 / 6 / 5 / 4 / 3 / 2 / LOW 1

Day Quality Rating
In this horizontally shaded Section 1: At end of *each* day, assign a 1-10 ranking, by placing a dot ● in the appropriate box. This reflects the overall quality of that day, from your perspective (1 = **low**, 10 = **high**).

★ Weekly Review
In the 3 Vertical shaded *WEEKLY PROGRESS REVIEW* columns ★, assign a "**+**" (On Track) or a "**—**" (Off Track) to each health action. Do this weekly *each* Sunday.

Daily Actions
In the horizontal Section 2: At the end of *each* day, check-off/fill-in data for each action below.
Leave any missed actions blank.

1
2
3
4
5
6
7
8
9
10
11
12
13

Progress Notes

General Notes:

Week 3

Week 2

Week 1

11

GLOSSARY

21-Day New Habit Cycle: It takes about 3 weeks or 21 days—both Fibonacci numbers—to begin to successfully instill a new habit. Affirming the Fibonacci days within the 21-Day new habit-forming cycle—1, 2, 3, 5, 8, 13, 21—during new repatterning efforts consciously reinforces your desired new habit(s).

21-Day Quick-Start Checklist System: Innovative, kaizen-based small steps daily journaling system. Customized for this book to facilitate charting and implementation of simple Golden Ratio health and longevity drivers (see chapter 11, p.327). *Designed by co-author Matthew Cross.*

3-H (Longevity): Mnemonic for Humor/Happiness/Hot-blooded, longevity corollary to Head/Heart/Hips.

3-H (Posture): Mnemonic for Head/Heart/Hips, a simple alignment technique for postural awareness and correction.

40:30:30 (60:40) Zone/Golden Ratio Nutrition: 40:30:30 refers to the ratio of carbohydrates/protein/fat recommended by Dr. Barry Sears, bestselling author of the pioneering Zone nutrition book series. The 40:30:30 ratio can be reformatted as a 60:40 ratio that closely approximates the more precise 62/38 Golden Ratio.

5 Sense Nutrition: Our combined 5 primary sensory nutrient sources: visual, auditory, kinesthetic (touch), smell and taste.

80/20 or Pareto Principle: A predominant tendency of uneven distribution of causes/effects, actions/results throughout the Universe, commonly expressed as 80% of effects/results come from just 20% of causes/actions. First elucidated by Italian economist Vilfredo Pareto in 1906, the principle was later popularized by quality genius Dr. Joseph Juran. It was subsequently found to have valuable and ubiquitous application to all cause/effect, action/result relationships and allows for the identification and focusing on the "vital few" vs. "the trivial many." The principle is not locked to an 80/20 ratio, as it can express itself in any uneven ratio, e.g., from 51/49 to 99/1.

Aquaporins: Molecular water channels on cell membranes that act as microscopic fountains of youth.

Active Isolated Stretching (AIS): Aaron Mattes' stretching technique used by many professional and Olympic athletes. Mattes discovered that muscles can stretch 1.6 times (the Golden Ratio) their resting length before tearing.

AM BM: Morning Bowel Movement.

ANDI Scale: Acronym for *Aggregate Nutrient Density Index*, developed by Dr. Joel Furhman of Eat Right America; rates the relative healthy nutrient density of foods.

Calipers (Golden Ratio): A custom compass for measuring and designing according to the Golden Ratio.

Caloric Reduction This term is used in contrast to the more draconian phrase Caloric Restriction. In the more user-friendly yet effective practice of Caloric Reduction, overall caloric intake is reduced in varying degrees. Caloric Reduction results in significant activation of the "Skinny Gene" (SIRT-1), resulting in weight loss and normalization of many metabolic processes, including the aging process.

Chaos Theory: A theory for describing and understanding the often-invisible "higher order" that exists in seemingly random patterns or occurrences.

Chardonnay: Color standard used to measure urine water concentration. To make sure that your daily water intake is adequate and that metabolic wastes are being properly filtered, urine color should be similar to or lighter than the color of a pale Chardonnay wine.

Chiaroscuro: Painting technique contrasting light and darkness that is metaphorically adapted to the science of sleep and waking. It is used in the Golden Ratio Lifestyle Diet to assure that wake/sleep and light/dark cycles are adjusted to the Golden Ratio.

Dark Night: Optimal sleeping conditions of maximum darkness, necessary for optimal regeneration and rejuvenation.

Day and Night: Entablatures of the twin maidens Day and Night framing the four clocks which once adorned New York City's magnificent original Penn Station (1910-1963). Created by master sculptor Adolph Alexander Weinman, *Day and Night* beautifully represents the true holistic meaning of Diet: everything we do in our Day and Night.

Diet: Holistic, accurate concept of total daily living, represented by the classic sun/moon icon. The word Diet actually means *everything* we do in a day—breathing, hydration, sleeping, eating, exercise, relationships, working, etc. In the context of this book, Diet is short for the Golden Ratio Lifestyle Diet; *Lifestyle* is really the most accurate definition of the word *Diet*.

Divine: The word Divine is most commonly associated with its spiritual connotation, as in *Divine Guidance*. Lesser known is the word's equally powerful additional meaning: *To foretell through the art of divination; to know or presage by inspiration, intuition, or reflection*. Thus, *To Divine* means to foretell or predict future outcomes. In this context, the Golden Ratio/Divine Code Lifestyle Diet is a powerful way to *divine* optimal health and longevity, at any stage of life.

Divine Code: A term coined by the authors to describe the 5 combined primary, visual manifestations of the Golden Ratio: 1. The Golden Ratio 1.618:1, or more simply 1.62:1 or 62:38. 2. The Golden Rectangle, whose sides are in 1.62:1 ratio. 3. The Golden Spiral, which grows 1.62 larger each complete turn. 4. The Golden Star, whose every line bisects the other at their precise Golden Ratio points. 5. The Fibonacci Sequence 0, 1, 1, 2, 3, 5, 8, 13, 21... which showcases the Golden Ratio in the progressive ratios between its successive terms.

Divine Proportion: see Golden Ratio.

Driver(s): Sequenced priorities of lifestyle, health and longevity factors in the Golden Ratio Lifestyle Diet, as revealed through the Hoshin Success Compass™ process.

Elliott Wave Principle: Graphical wave representation of the cyclic growth/ retrenchment patterns in Nature, which are based on Fibonacci numbers, ratios and retracements. First described by R.N. Elliott in 1934 in relation to the stock market; championed in modern times by Robert Prechter, Jr., author and founder of Elliott Wave International, who advanced the principle further with his *Socionomics* concept. This principle can also be powerfully applied to health, lifestyle and diet.

FAB: Mnemonic for Foundation, Alignment, Buoyancy; for foot-to-head posture improvement towards healthier Divine Proportion. *Coined by co-author Matthew Cross.*

FAR Principle: The essence of the Hoshin Success Compass™ prioritization sequence is contained in the eponym FAR: Foundation>Actions>Results. The FAR sequence was used to determine the priorities of the core success drivers in the Golden Ratio Lifestyle Diet. *Coined by co-author Matthew Cross.*

Fatruvian Man/Homo Fatruvius: A play on words on Leonardo Da Vinci's famous drawing *The Vitruvian Man.* This concept juxtaposes an image of the prototypical modern obese person, *Fatruvian Man,* with the ideal body mass representation of mankind as seen in the *The Vitruvian Man.*

Fibonacci Sequence: The infinite Sequence of numbers created such that each successive number in the series is the sum of the previous two, starting with zero: 0, 1, 1, 2, 3, 5, 8, 13, 21, 34... As the numbers in the sequence get larger, the ratio between them gets ever closer to the Golden Ratio of 1.6180399... Named after Leonardo Fibonacci (c. 1170-1250), one of the greatest mathematicians in history.

Fibonacci Trinity: Leonardo Fibonacci (c. 1170-1250) introduced the following history-shaping trinity to the West in the 13th century (*coined by the authors*):

    1. the Hindu/Arabic numbers (1, 2, 3, 4, 5, 6, 7, 8, 9)
    2. the concept of zero **0**
    3. the use of the decimal point

First 15% Principle: Quality pioneer Dr. W. Edwards Deming's principle that 85% of the results in any given endeavor lie in the First 15% (the front end) of the process or journey. Used in conjunction with the 21-Day Successful New Habit Cycle.

FIT (Fibonacci Interval Training): A Golden Ratio enhancement of the HIT (High Intensity Training) workout system. By utilizing alternating numbers from the Fibonacci Sequence to demarcate workout/resting periods over days and weeks and also within single total high intensity workouts, we can greatly augment the impact and results of exercise efforts. *Coined by the authors.*

Fractal: Any part that reflects the shape or pattern of a whole, e.g., a stalk of broccoli is similar to the larger bunch of broccoli from which it was taken. Fractal geometry, like the Golden Ratio, is present everywhere, at all scales in man, Nature and the Universe. Fractals convey essentially the same principle as the hologram. The Golden

Ratio is a master fractal, operating at all scales throughout the Universe.

Fractal Cognition™: The theory of Accelerated Quantum Learning (AQL), which posits that the brain has the ability to rapidly recreate a whole concept or body of knowledge on a larger scale from any similar yet smaller pattern or piece of information. Fractal Cognition is similar to the fact that any piece of a hologram always reflects the whole from which it came. *Coined by co-author Matthew Cross.*

Generation PHI™: A new generation of centenarians and supercentenarians that reach their longevity potential through the application of the Golden Ratio Lifestyle Diet. *Coined by co-author Robert Friedman, M.D.*

Gluten: A sticky, glue-like component of the protein found in grains such as wheat, rye and barley and thus in many common foods (grains such as quinoa, buckwheat, amaranth and millet are gluten-free). In gluten sensitive people, it can contribute to inflammation, poor digestion, fatigue, weight gain and many health ailments.

God's Code: Another way of describing the Divine Code. The Code is omnipresent at micro and macro levels throughout all creation.

Golden Ratio Lifestyle Diet (GRLD): Comprehensive approach to living that leverages 5 unique cornerstones to support optimum health, happiness and longevity: 1. The holistic, true concept of diet: *everything* we do in a day, not just eating (see Diet). 2. The Hoshin Success Compass™ master prioritization sequencing system for best alignment of the core drivers of health and longevity. 3. The Golden Ratio and accompanying Nature's Secret Nutrient (NSN). 4. The First 15% principle, in that 85% of the results we get in any endeavor originate predominantly in the "First 15%"—the front end—of the journey. 5. The Be Your Own Doctor principle, in that we must take primary responsibility and command of our health and longevity.

Golden Ratio/Golden Mean/Golden Cut/Sacred Cut/Phi: The ratio of a small part to a large part or vice-versa which equals 0.618:1 or 1.618:1 respectively. The ratio appears between adjacent numbers in the Fibonacci Sequence, which ever more closely approximates 1.618:1 or 0.618:1 as one moves up or down the Sequence.

Golden Olympic Training (GOT) Ratio: A balanced approach to working out followed by many Olympians and elite athletes which splits workouts into Golden Ratio training percentages, e.g., 40% endurance, 30% strength, 30% flexibility. The larger training segment (40%) is tuned to one's chosen sport.

Golden Rectangle: Any rectangle whose length-to-width ratio equals 1.618:1, the Golden Ratio. Commonly seen in the shape of playing cards, index cards, debit/credit cards, Apple's classic iPod®, etc.

Goldene Schnitt: Der Goldene "Schnitt" is German for the Golden Cut or Golden Ratio. It also just happens to rhyme with the English word *Sh-t*. The phrase is used to denote ideal, healthy bowel movements of about 1.6 times per day.

Golden Spiral: A logarithmic spiral, as seen in a spiral sea shell or galaxy spiral, where each consecutive full turn of the spiral is in 1.618:1 ratio to the previous.

Golden Star: Any equiangular five-pointed star or pentagram, which reflects the Golden Ratio in its design, in that each line bisects the other at its Golden Ratio points.

High Intensity Training (HIT): Maximal bursts of exertion with minimal repetition, followed by longer than usual recuperation periods. Pioneered by Nautilus exercise equipment designer Arthur Jones. When the exertion/rest segments are tuned to the Fibonacci Sequence, we get the FIT system (Fibonacci Interval Training).

Homo Fatruvius: see *Fatruvian Man*.

Homo Vitruvius: The Golden Ratio's evolutionarily ideal evolved human being, inspired and symbolized by Leonardo Da Vinci's famous drawing: the *Vitruvian Man*. *Coined by co-author Robert Friedman, M.D.*

Hoshin Success Compass™: The master Japanese strategic planning>prioritization> action system guiding the world's greatest companies. Used to reveal the relative Foundation>Action>Result (FAR) priorities of the health and longevity Success Drivers in this book. *From the book of the same title by co-author Matthew Cross.*

Inflammation: A non-specific immune response to injury or irritation with the hallmarks of pain, swelling, redness and heat. Inflammation can also be chronic, low-grade and silent and is suspected of being at the root of many diseases.

IronApe Green Smoothie: A raw green power drink, inspired from Victoria Boutenko's research into the chimpanzee's Golden Ratio based diet. This high ORAC blend augments energy and normalizes bowel function.

Kaizen: Japanese for Continuous Improvement, especially the practice of consistent, small and manageable steps of improvement. Inspired by the teachings of American quality genius Dr. W. Edwards Deming and his legendary contributions to Japanese world quality leadership. Kaizen is a close relative of and integrates both the First 15% principle and the Hoshin process. When applied to habit change, Kaizen's small, easy steps approach supports sustainable progress towards successful new habit adoption.

Macro-Macro-Nutrients: Nutrients needed in much larger amounts than the smaller requirements of the classical macro and micronutrients such as proteins, fats, carbohydrates, vitamins, minerals, enzymes, etc. Macro-Macro-Nutrients are things like air, water, sleep, good posture, exercise, happiness and inner peace.

Markov Chain: A mathematical system that describes transitions from one state to another (from a finite or countable number of possible states) in a chainlike manner. It is a random process characterized as memoryless (i.e. exhibiting the Markov property): *the next state depends only on the current state and not on the entire past.* Markov Chains have many applications as statistical models of real-world processes. *Named for Russian mathematician Andrey Markov.*

Maslow's Hierarchy of Human Needs: A pyramidal ladder representation of human needs, ranging from physiological at the bottom to self-actualization at the capstone. The Golden Ratio Lifestyle Diet has a similarly shaped pyramidal hierarchy, with Air at the bottom and optimal Longevity at the top. Named for humanistic psychologist Abraham Maslow (1908-1970).

Millionaire's MAP™: An interactive game for exercising your imagination and preparing your heart and mind to allow greater wealth and abundance. The game involves journaling the daily spending of increasing amounts of money on paper, according to the Fibonacci Sequence. *From the book by co-author Matthew Cross.*

Nature's Secret Nutrient™ (NSN): An infinitely self-replenishing, Fibonacci/Golden Ratio-based nutritional supplement/turbo-charger, obtained only by learning and applying the Golden Ratio Lifestyle Diet principles. Nature's Secret Nutrient has no mass, no calories, is tasteless, has no expiration date, never spoils and is free for life! *Coined by co-author Robert Friedman, M.D.*

ORAC: An anagram for Oxygen Radical Absorbance Capacity: a measure of the antioxidant potential of foods. High ORAC foods include spices, fruits and vegetables.

Order From Chaos: A 6-step system for personal and professional organization, created by author Liz Davenport; from her bestselling book. The system's key sequenced steps are: 1. The Cockpit Office; 2. Air Traffic Control System; 3. Pending File; 4. Decide NOW; 5. Prioritize Ongoingly; 6. OPEN your day, CLOSE your day, CLEAN OFF YOUR DESK at the end of your day. The system greatly increases order and productivity, simultaneously reducing waste, frustration and stress.

Pandiculation: A natural yawn and stretch reflex that automatically resets your oxygen and CO_2 levels, equalizes ear pressure, lengthens muscles, relieves stiffness and increases blood and lymphatic circulation. This Golden Ratio reset is the most primal form of yoga stretching (asana) and breathing (pranayama).

Paradigm: A model used to describe a particular set of assumptions about reality; our mindset, mental map or theory that shapes how we see and interpret our world.

Pattern Recognition: The ability to see and create meaningful new understandings and insights from seemingly unrelated pieces of data or information. A key skill for higher intelligence; also a component of the *Fractal Cognition System.*

PHI Φ: The 21st letter of the Greek alphabet and another popular term for the Golden Ratio 1.618 : 1.0. Coined by American mathematician Mark Barr, after the first Greek letter in the name of Phidias, the Greek sculptor who lived around 450 BC.

Phyllotaxis: Phyllotaxis or phyllotaxy refers to the arrangement of leaves, stems and seeds on plants. The basic patterns are alternate, opposite, whorled or spiral. They invariably mirror the Golden Spiral and/or the Fibonacci Sequence/Ratio. Phylotaxis with one "L" is the name of the living Golden Ratio-based artwork by Jonathan Harris.

Resveratrol: A supernutrient found in grapes, red wine, berries and Japanese knotweed that can slow the aging process by the same genetic mechanism as caloric reduction, via activation of the SIRT-1 "skinny" gene.

Rₓ: A symbol originally used by Leonardo Fibonacci to designate square roots; later used world-wide as the universal medical/healing symbol for prescriptions.

SENS: Strategies for Engineered Negligible Senescence. A tissue repair strategy for human rejuvenation, prevention of age-related decline and extended lifespan. *Coined by maverick English longevity researcher Aubrey de Grey.*

Socionomics: The Golden Ratio-based Elliott Wave Principle as applied to the human moods that underlie all social, cultural and political phenomena. *Concept developed by Elliott Wave International founder Robert Prechter, Jr.*

Synergy: Describes the desirable state where two or more single elements come together to form a "greater whole" which exceeds the sum of the parts. Example: the 5 individual elements of the Golden Ratio Lifestyle Diet come together to form a breakthrough system for optimum health and longevity. *Coined by Divine Code/ Golden Ratio genius R. Buckminster Fuller.*

Unity Principle: A function of Reality that brings together apparent diversity into a harmonious whole. A prime function of the Golden Ratio/Divine Code.

Vesica Piscis: Latin for "Vessel of the Fish," it is the most basic and important construction in sacred geometry, with multiple profound spiritual connections. It is formed when the circumference of two identical circles each pass through the center of the other and is variously linked with Christ, astrological symbolism and the scared canon of ancient wisdom.

Vital Capacity (VC): The total amount of air that can be breathed out, after a maximal inbreath. This one lung function is the #1 predictor of longevity; that is, the higher your Vital Capacity, the greater your projected longevity.

Vitruvian Man: Leonardo Da Vinci's masterpiece drawing synthesizing art and science by depicting an idealized human in two simultaneous poses, both inscribed in a circle and square. The drawing is replete with Golden Ratio elements and as such serves as an icon for the Golden Ratio Lifestyle Diet.

Vitruvian Woman: The commissioned-by-the-author's counterpart of *The Vitruvian Man,* by contemporary artist Chloe Hedden. When the *Divine Code Vitruvian Woman* is overlaid side-by-side with the *Vitruvian Man,* the dynamic balance necessary for the creation of the sacred Vesica Piscis is created.

W.A.M.: An anagram for Water–Ante–Meridiem. In the Diet, this is the nostrum to drink at least one tall glass of water in the morning (A.M.), upon arising.

Zen Alarm Clock: The beautiful alarm clocks designed by Stephen McIntosh of Now & Zen (www.Now-Zen.com). They gently awaken you with a series of soft tones that follow a decreasing Fibonacci Sequence, a pleasing stimulation in sync with your innate Golden Ratio nature.

Authors' Favorite Nutritional Supplements (short list)

Targeted nutritional supplements can play an important role in supporting greater Golden Ratio balance, robust health and longevity. The following are among the author's favorites. Note: None of the statements accompanying any of the products listed here have been evaluated by the Food and Drug Administration. These products are not intended to diagnose, treat or cure any disease. Please consult with your health provider before using any of these products.

Life Extension Foundation Products: 800-544-4440, Discount Code LA. www.LEF.org/LA
Branched Chain Amino Acids
Complete B-Complex
COQ10 Ubiquinol (electron transport energy optimizer)
DHEA (main anti-aging adrenal hormone)
Endothelial Defense with Full-Spectrum Pomegranate (blood vessel protection)
Gamma E Tocopherol
Life Extension Mix (Super Multi)
Low-Dose Aspirin
Mega Green Tea Extract
Melatonin
Natural Female Support (recommended for women)
Optimized Carnitine (amino acid which optimizes fatty acid metabolism)
PQQ Caps (mitochondrial regenerator)
Pregnenolone (mother of adrenal hormones)
Super Absorbable Tocotrienols (vitamin E compounds)
Super Curcumin (super anti-inflammatory)
Super Digestive Enzymes
Super MiraForte (male support)
Super Omega-3 (EPA & DHA)
Ultra Natural Prostate
Velvet Deer Antler (growth factors)
Vitamin C with Quercetin
Vitamin D-3 with Sea Iodine

To sign up for a free trial Life Extension membership (which includes *Life Extension* magazine) and receive discounts on blood tests and a wide range of scientifically supported supplements (including all those listed above), call: 1-800-544-4440, mention Discount Code LA or visit www.LEF.org/LA

Dr. Richard Schulze Products: www.herbdoc.com
Formulas #1, #2, #3 (herbal laxative formulas; can all be used in conjunction);
SuperFood Plus (great vitamin and mineral herbal concentrate powder; can be used as a general condiment and smoothie boost)

continued on next page

Miscellaneous Products (available online or at health food stores)

Kyolic (brand) Aged Garlic Extract

Magna-Calm (Magnesium Citrate)

Aloe Vera Gel (organic; Lily of the Desert brand)

Bee Pollen (raw; ApiTherapy brand)

Concentrace Trace Mineral Drops (Trace Minerals Research brand)

Garlic: AlliUltra AC-23 Allicin Powder Caps (therapeutic potency; AlliMax brand)

Lecithin Granules (fat emulsifier/choline and inositol source; Lewis Labs brand)

Liqui-Dulse Drops (iodine supplement; Bernard Jensen brand)

Mushroom: Host Defense Stamets 7 (immune system booster; Fungi Perfecti brand)

Olive Leaf Extract (immune system booster; Gaia Herbs brand; extract or caps)

Oregano Extract (anti-viral factor; Gaia Herbs brand; extract or caps)

Echinacea Supreme (immune system booster; Gaia Herbs brand; extract or caps)

Probiotics: healthy digestive system bacteria balance/immunse system support
  (New Chapter brand; Jarrow Formulas brand)

Vitamin B-15/Pangamic Acid (energy/endurance booster; Good 'N Natural brand)

Longevity Plus: www.longevityplus.com

Bio-En'R-G'y C (high quality vitamin-C product)

Zeo Gold (best oral chelation formula)

Beyond B-12 with advanced folate complex

Other Highly Recommended Supplement Companies

Life-Enhancement (Durk Pearson/Sandy Shaw/Jonathan Wright, M.D. products):
  www.life-enhancement.com

Allergy Research Group (innovative, cutting edge supplements):
  www.allergyresearchgroup.com

Mercola (high quality supplements and lifestyle products): www.Mercola.com

Gaia Herbs (premium quality organic and wildcrafted herbal extracts and formulas)

Omega-3/Essential Fatty Acid Oils

Nordic Naturals (brand) Cod Liver Oil/Orange Flavor

Carlson's (brand) Cod Liver Oil/Lemon Flavor

Dr. Sears' OmegaRx (brand); pharmaceutical-grade fish oil: www.zonediet.com

Swanson's Viobin (brand) Wheat Germ Oil: natural Vitamin E source/endurance booster

---

Golden Ratio Lifestyle Diet Products

Authors Robert and Matthew have formulated a unique selection of Golden Ratio Lifestyle Diet products for enhanced Energy, Sleep, Detox and Golden Ratio Nutrition. All are custom formulated according to the Golden Ratio and the core principles in this book. Coming soon to GoldenRatioLifestyle.com

---

RECOMMENDED WEBSITES

Anastasia Soare's Golden Ratio eyebrow products: www.Anastasia.net

Ann Louise Gittleman, the First Lady of Nutrition and Fat Flush pioneer: www.AnnLouise.com

ANDI Food Scale: www.EatRightAmerica.com

Bee Therapy - HoshinDo Healing Arts Institute, Santa Fe, NM: www.hoshindohealingartsinstitute.org

Blood Test for Omega Score™ from Life Extension Foundation: http://tinyurl.com/7p9d6gg

Blood Test for Vitamin D from Life Extension Foundation: http://tinyurl.com/6naey42

Blood Tests for health & longevity from Life Extension Foundation: 1-800-544-4440; Discount Code LA.

Body Bridge: www.BodyBridge.com

BrainSync.com: Acclaimed audio programs for meditation, relaxation and life enhancement.

Bruce Mandelbaum, Master Acupuncturist/Massage Therapist (NYC/CT): 203.733.5812

Chris Johnson, Performance Coach: www.OnTargetLiving.com

Cosmetic Toxicity check site: www.CosmeticsDataBase.com

Dave Scott (6-time Hawaiian Ironman Champion) Coaching: www.DaveScottInc.com

David Ison: Sound therapy pioneer. Beautiful, effective programs. www.TheIsonMethod.com

DEX-II Spinal Decompression System: www.EnergyCenter.com

Divine Code site for companion Golden Ratio book: www.TheDivineCode.com

Dr. Joseph Mercola's World's #1 Natural Health website: www.mercola.com

Dr. Phil Nuernberger, Mindfulness & Inner Strength Coach: www.MindMaster.com

Dr. Richard Schulze, N.D.'s books/products (SuperFood, Detox, etc.): www.HerbDoc.com

Elaine Petrone's Miracle Medicine Ball Method™: www.ElainePetrone.com

Fashion Code, Sara and Ruth Levy: www.TheFashionCode.com

Food Pesticide List: www.FoodNews.com

FreeWillAstrology: Rob Breszny's poetic, inspiring, funny and enlightening weekly forecasts.

Gary Null, health and natural healing champion: www.GaryNull.com

Golden Ratio Calipers. hand-made in brass or stainless steel: http://holyholo.com/caliper.htm

Golden Ratio video/Nature By Numbers: www.etereaestudios.com

Gurumarka, Master Yogi, Breathing, Lifestyle Coach: www.BreathIsLife.com

iPhone/iPad/iPod Upright System: www.apple.com/iphone/appstore/

Jackie Summers blog on love and life wisdom: www.jackfrombkln.com

Juiceman Jay Kordich: www.Juiceman.com

Kevin Trudeau, natural cures advocate: www.KevinTrudeau.com

LifeExtension: Resource for wellness, health supplements and anti-aging: www.LEF.org/LA

Ma Back Roller: www.TheMaRoller.com

Mark Allen (6-time Hawaiian Ironman Champion) Coaching: www.MarkAllenOnline.com

Medicine Balls: www.SPRI.com

MedX Core Spinal Fitness System: www.CoreSpinalFitness.com

Mike Adams, the Health Ranger: www.NaturalNews.com

ORAC foods list: http://tinyurl.com/yrmfse

Radiation alerts: www.nuc.berkeley.edu/UCBAirSampling
         www.radiationnetwork.com   www.blackcatsystems.com/RadMap/map.html

Robert Kaehler, Flexibilty/Performance Coach: www.CoachKaehler.com

Sifu Rob Moses, PhysioStix Fitness Sticks: www.GoldenSpiralWellness.com

TED.org: fantastic resource of health, longevity and general wisdom; free video format.

William Kaye, Master Rolfer (NYC/CT): www.WilliamKayeRolfing.com

Xylitol toothcare/sweetener products: www.EpicDental.com

Zen Alarm Clocks: www.Now-Zen.com

RECOMMENDED READING

GOLDEN RATIO

The Divine Code of Da Vinci, Fibonacci, Einstein & YOU, by Matthew Cross and Robert Friedman, M.D.

The Divine Code Genius Activation Quote Book, by Matthew Cross and Robert Friedman, M.D.

The DaVinci Code, by Dan Brown; especially chapter 20 (on PHI)

The Wave Principle of Human Social Behavior and the New Science of Socionomics, by Robert R. Prechter, Jr.

The Elliott Wave Principle, by A.J. Frost and Robert R. Prechter, Jr.

The New View Over Atlantis, by John Michell

AIR & BREATH

Breathe, You Are Alive: The Sutra on the Full Awareness of Breathing, by Thich Nhat Hanh

Science of Breath, by Rama, Rudolph Ballentine and Alan Hymes

Breathing: The Master Key to Self Healing, by Andrew Weil (Audio CD)

Flood Your Body With Oxygen, by Ed McCabe

WATER & HYDRATION

Water for Health, for Healing, for Life: You're Not Sick, You're Thirsty, by Fereydoon Batmanghelidj, M.D.

Like Water for Chocolate, by Laura Esquivel, Thomas and Carol Christensen

NUTRITION

Mastering the Zone, by Barry Sears, Ph.D.

YOU: On A Diet Revised Edition: The Owner's Manual for Waist Management, by Michael Roizen, M.D., and Mehmet Oz, M.D.

Eat Right For Your Type, by Dr. Peter J. D'Adamo

The Fat Flush Plan, by Ann Louise Gittleman

Dr. Schulze's 20 Steps to a Healthier Life, by Dr. Richard Schulze

The Omega Rx Zone, by Dr. Barry Sears

The Kind Diet, by Alicia Silverstone

Green For Life, by Victoria Boutenko

The Alternate Day Diet, by James Johnson, M.D.

The Joy of Juicing: Creative Cooking With Your Juicer, Gary Null, Ph.D.

Diet For A New America, by John Robbins

On Target Living Nutrition, by Chris Johnson

Sugar Blues, by William Dufty

The Juiceman's Power of Juicing by Jay Kordich

Forks Over Knives: The Plant-Based Way To Health, by Gene Stone

User's Guide to Propolis, Royal Jelly, Honey, & Bee Pollen, by C. Leigh Broadhurst, Ph.D

POSTURE & EXERCISE

Spiral~Chi (DVD), by Robert Friedman, M.D.

ABCore Workout, (DVD) by Matthew Cross

Living Yoga, by Christy Turlington

Spiral Fitness (DVD), by Rob Moses

Let's Get Moving (DVD), by Chris Johnson

A.M./P.M. Yoga (DVD), by Rodney Yee

Consistent Winning, by Dr. Ron Sandler

Active Isolated Stretching: The Mattes Method, by Aaron L. Mattes

High Intensity Training The Mike Mentzer Way, by Mike Mentzer

Holographic Golf, by Larry Miller

DETOXIFICATION

There Are No Incurable Diseases: Dr. Schulze's 30-Day Cleansing & Detoxification Program, by Dr. Richard Schulze, N.D.

*Create Powerful Health Naturally
with Dr. Schulze's 5-Day Liver Detox,*
by Dr. Richard Schulze, N.D.

The Cure for All Diseases, by Dr. Hulda Clark

The Miracle of Fasting, by Paul C. Bragg

Guess What Came to Dinner and *Zapped,*
by Ann Louise Gittleman, Ph.D., C.N.S.

HAPPINESS & INNER PEACE

Happy For No Reason, by Marci Shimnoff

The How of Happiness, by Sonja Lyubomirsky

*US: Transforming Ourselves and the
Relationships that Matter Most,* by Lisa Oz

Live The Life You Love, by Barbara Sher

The 4-Hour Workweek, by Tim Ferriss

The Millionaire's MAP, by Matthew Cross

The Four Agreements, by Don Miguel Ruiz

The Warrior Sage, by Dr. Phil Nuernberger

Lessons of a Lakota, by Billy Mills
1964 Olympic 10k Running Champion

The Prophet, by Kahlil Gibran

The Astonishing Power of Emotions,
by Esther & Jerry Hicks

*Switch: How To Change Things When
Change Is Hard,* by Chip and Dan Heath

*The Spontaneous Healing of Belief: Shattering
the Paradigm of False Limits,* by Greg Braden

Anatomy of An Illness, by Norman Cousins

The Stress of Life, by Hans Selye

The Politics of Happiness, by Derek Bok

Your Brain at Work, by David Rock

*One Small Step Can Change Your Life:
The Kaizen Way,* by Robert Maurer, Ph.D

The 80/20 Principle, by Richard Koch

Order From Chaos, by Liz Davenport

*What Color Is Your Parachute? A Practical
Manual for Job-Hunters and Career-Changers*
by Richard N. Boles

The Sacred Earth, by Courtney Milne

Sacred Earth: Places of Peace and Power,
by Martin Gray

*Wholeliness: Embracing the Sacred Unity That
Heals Our World,* by Carmen Harra, Ph.D.

*Journeys on the Edge: Living a Life that
Matters,* by Walt Hampton

*Catching The Big Fish: Meditation,
Consciousness & Creativity,* by David Lynch

*Transcendence: Healing and Transformation
Through Transcendental Meditation,*
by Norman Rosenthal, M.D.

*Ecstasy Is A New Frequency: Teachings of the
Light Institute,* by Chris Griscom

Chicken Soup for the Soul, by Jack Canfield
and Mark Victor Hansen

The Alchemist, by Paulo Coelho

*The Vortex: Where the Law of Attraction
Assembles All Cooperative Relationships,* by
Esther and Jerry Hicks

*No Matter What!: 9 Steps to Living the Life You
Love,* by Lisa Nichols

NATURAL BEAUTY & ATTRACTION

YOU: Being Beautiful, by Michael Roizen, M.D.,
and Mehmet Oz, M.D.

*How To Make People Like You in 90 Seconds
Or Less,* by Nicholas Boothman

*Lindsay Wagner's New Beauty:
The Acupressure Facelift,* by Lindsay Wagner

The Function of The Orgasm,
by Dr. Wilhelm Reich

*Skeletal Types: Key to unraveling the mystery
of facial beauty and its biologic significance,*
by Dr. Yosh Jefferson

LONGEVITY

*Counterclockwise: Mindful Health and the
Power of Possibility,* by Dr. Ellen Langer

*Ending Aging: The Rejuvenation Breakthroughs
That Could Reverse Human Aging in Our
Lifetime,* by Aubrey de Grey and Michael Rae

*The Blue Zone: Lessons for Living Longer
from the People Who've Lived the Longest,*
by Dan Buettner

- continued next page -

RECOMMENDED READING, CONT.

LONGEVITY, continued

RealAge: Are You As Young As You Can Be?
by Dr. Michael Roizen

*Relaxation Revolution: Enhancing Your
Personal Health Through the Science and
Genetics of Mind Body Healing,*
Herbert Benson, M.D.

The Divine Code of Life, Kazuo Murakami

Forever Young: Introducing the Metabolic Diet,
Nicholas Perricone, M.D.

*Healthy at 100: The Scientifically Proven
Secrets of the World's Healthiest and
Longest-Lived Peoples,* by John Robbins

*Younger Next Year: Live Strong, Fit, and Sexy -
Until You're 80 and Beyond,* by Chris Crowley
and Henry S. Lodge

The Ageless Body, by Chris Griscom

*Fantastic Voyage: Live Long Enough
To Live Forever,* by Ray Kurzweil

The Cure For All Diseases,
by Hulda Clark, Ph.D. N.D.

Molecules of Emotion, by Candice Pert, Ph.D.

The Biology of Belief, by Bruce Lipton, Ph.D.

Become Younger, by Dr. Norman W. Walker

Whole Body Dentistry, by Dr. Mark Briener

Age Less, Live More, by Bernardo LaPallo

Secrets of the Superyoung, by Dr. David Weeks

MISCELLANEOUS

The Hoshin Success Compass,
by Matthew Cross

How To Think Like Leonardo Da Vinci
(especially the Da Vinci Diet section),
by Michael J. Gelb

Fingerprints of the Gods, by Graham Hancock

*The New Economics of Business, Industry and
Government,* by Dr. W. Edwards Deming

Whole Body Dentistry, by Dr. Mark Briener

Revitalizing Your Mouth, by Dr. David Frey

*Awaken the Giant Within: How to
Take Immediate Control of Your Mental,
Emotional, Physical and Financial Destiny!*
by Anthony Robbins

*The Path of Energy: Awaken Your Personal
Power and Expand Your Consciousness,*
by Dr. Synthia Andrews, N.D.

*Harmony: A New Way of Looking at Our
World,* by HRH Charles, The Prince of Wales,
with Tony Juniper and Ian Skelly

Innovate Like Edison, by Michael Gelb

Summerhill: A New View of Childhood,
by A.S. Neill

*Dumbing Us Down: The Hidden Curriculum of
Compulsory Schooling,* by John Taylor Gatto

*Sounding the Inner Landscape:
Music As Medicine,* by Kay Gardner

*Conscious Circles: A Presentation by Colin
Andrews (DVD),* by Colin Andrews

Quality or Else!, by Clare Carwford-Mason
and Lloyd Dobyns

The Late, Great Pennsylvania Station,
by Lorraine B. Diehl

Rich Dad Poor Dad, by Robert T. Kiyosaki

*The Art of Leading: 3 Principles for
Predictable Performance Improvement,*
by Wally Hauck, Ph.D.

The Power of Alpha Thinking, by Jess Stearn

Ancient Aliens (History Channel; DVD set)

If You Love This Planet, by Dr. Helen Caldicott

Man 1, Bank 0, by Patrick Combs

Out of the Transylvania Night,
by Aura Imbarus

Beekeeping For Dummies, by Howland
Blackiston and Kim Flottum

*The Joy Of Ritual: Spiritual Recipes to
Celebrate Milestones, Ease Transitions, and
Make Every Day Sacred,* by Barbara Biziou

Bibliography & Picture Credits

Every effort has been made to assure complete and correct attribution.
Any omissions or errors will be corrected upon notification.

Authors' Notes, Introduction, Preface & Chapter 1

1618 Combination Lock, American flag, starfish/sand dollar, Einstein: wikipedia.org

Adolph Weinman's Day and Night twin maidens adorning clock from NYC's original Penn Station: wikipedia.com; customized by M. Cross and T. Reczek

Brocolli, Divine Code Pulse Graph, Parthenon: *The Golden Mean Book* (Stephen McIntosh), http://www.now-zen.com

Romanesco, Great Pyramid, Parthenon, wine glass, nautilus, ram, wave, galaxy, rocket, butterfly, tennis court, smoke spirals: iStockphoto.com

Skeleton, by T. Reczek after:
http://upload.wikimedia.org/wikipedia/commons/2/21/Skelett-Mensch-drawing.jpg

Mandelbrot by T. Reczek after W. Beyer:
http://en.wikipedia.org/wiki/File:Mandel_zoom_00_mandelbrot_set.jpg

Golden Ratio rectangular grid, pentagram with angles: T. Reczek

Golden Ratio/Divine Code overview page: concept/design by M. Cross; input from R. Friedman, M.D.; rendered by T. Reczek; thumbnail pictures from/created by wikipedia.org, T. Reczek, author's collection, Steven McIntosh

5 Key Aspects of the Golden Ratio Lifestyle Diet Venn diagram: concept by M. Cross and R. Friedman, M.D.; designed by T. Reczek and M. Cross

Hoshin Kanri Japanese characters: T. Reczek

Deming Prize: Courtesy of JUSE/Japan

Hoshin Success Compass™ logo: Designed by M. Cross; rendered by T. Reczek

FAR Pyramid and FAR Flow Diagram: Designed by M. Cross; rendered by T. Reczek

Fibonacci statue: photo by Robert Prechter, Sr., courtesy Robert Prechter, Jr., *The Elliott Wave Principle*

Excerpt from article on Lisa Oz in *Life Extension* magazine, August 2011

The Birth of Venus, lungs, bronchi, oxygen, phytoplankton, Houdini, Edison: www.wikipedia.org

http://en.wikipedia.org/wiki/File:Lungs_open.jpg

Lung volume graph: T. Reczek, after Vihsadas, http://en.wikipedia.org/wiki/File:LungVolume.jpg

Vital Capacity vs. age graph: from the Framingham Study, 1948-1968, adapted by T. Reczek, (after Walford: Beyond the 120-Year Diet, originally from Kannel and Hubert, 1982.)

Biosphere 2: User: Gleam 8/9/99, http://en.wikipedia.org/wiki/File:Biosphere2_1.jpg

Dog stretching: Robert Friedman, M.D.

Birkel DA, Edgren L., *Hatha yoga: improved vital capacity of college students*, Altern Ther Health Med. (2000) Nov.

Prechter, Robert R., Jr., *Pioneering Studies in Socionomics*, New Classics Library, pp. 278-293, (2003)

Walford, Roy, M.D., *Beyond the 120-Year Diet : How to Double Your Vital Years*, Da Capo Press, (2000)

http://thelongestlistofthelongeststuffatthelongestdomainnameatlong last.com/long56.html

Lung graphic: Mariana Ruiz Villarreal "LadyofHats", e-mail: mrv_taur@gmx.net

Lightbulb: iStockPhoto.org; da Vinci filament concept by Robert Friedman, M.D. and Matthew Cross; rendered by Tom Reczek, 618Design.com

David Blaine: http://en.wikipedia.org/wiki/David_Blaine

Harry Houdini: http://en.wikipedia.org/wiki/File:HarryHoudini1899.jpg

The Pattern by John Michell; courtesy of the artist

CHAPTER 2

Stilles Mineralwasser, photographer: Walter J. Pilsak, Waldsassen, Germany. http://en.wikipedia.org/wiki/File:Stilles_Mineralwasser.jpg

Fat Vitruvian man: Commisioned by the authors: ChloeHedden.com

Vitruvain man: www.lucnix.be, http://en.wikipedia.org/wiki/File:Da_Vinci_Vitruve_Luc_Viatour.jpg

Vitruvian Man body water compartments: by Matthew Cross; rendered by T. Reczek

Water drops: Emmanuel Torres. wwwFacebook.com/staticsolo

www.wikipedia.org/wiki/Alkahest

F. Batmanghelidj, *Your Body's Many Cries for Water*, Global Health Solutions, Inc.; Third Edition edition, November 1, 2008

David Fleming, MD, Richard Jackson, MD, MPH, Jim Pirkle, MD, PhD, Second National Report on Human Exposure to Environmental Chemicals, CDC National Center for Environmental Health, January 2003

Giovanni Iazzetti, Enrico Rigutti, Atlas of Anatomy, Giunti Editorial Group, Taj Books, 1/05

Kordich, Jay, *The Juiceman's Power of Juicing: Delicious Juice Recipes for Energy, Health, Weight Loss, and Relief from Scores of Common Ailments*, William Morrow Cookbooks, (2007)

AP Probe Finds Drugs in Drinking Water, Associated Press, 3/9/08

Perricone, M.D., Nicholas, *The Perricone Weight-Loss Diet*, Ballantine Books (April 10, 2007)

Null, Ph.D., Gary, *The Joy of Juicing: Creative Cooking With Your Juicer*, Avery Trade; Rev Upd edition (May 31, 2001).

CHAPTER 3

http://commons.wikimedia.org/wiki/File:The_Sleeping_Innocence.jpg

http://apod.nasa.gov/apod/ap001127.html

Moon phases: iStockphoto.com

Brainwaves: M. Cross

Clock, pinecone: R. Friedman, M.D.

Zen alarm clock: courtesy www.now-zen.com

Chepesiuk, Ron: *Missing the Dark: Health Effects of Light Pollution*, 2/2/2009 www.medscape.com

Demas, TJ.,Statland BE, *Serum caffeine half-lives*, Am J Clin Pathol. 1980 Mar;73(3):390-3

PN Prinz, et.al., *Higher plasma IGF-1 levels are associated with increased delta sleep in healthy older men*, Department of Psychiatry and Behavioral Sciences, University of Washington, Seattle, USA, Journals of Gerontology Series A: Biological Sciences and Medical Sciences, Vol 50, Issue 4 M222-M226

Stevens, Richard G. et.al., *The Role of Environmental Lighting and Circadian Disruption in Cancer and Other Diseases*, Environmental Health Perspectives, Volume 115, Number 9, September 2007

Trichopoulos, Dimitrios, MD, et.al., *Siesta in Healthy Adults and Coronary Mortality in the General Population*, Arch Intern Med. 2007;167(3):296-301

http://www.smh.com.au/news/National/Sleep-deprivation-is-torture Amnesty/2006/10/03/1159641317450.html

http://en.wikipedia.org/wiki/Sleep_deprivation

www.boston.com/business/globe/articles/2007/11/30/night_shift_a_probable_carcinogen/

http://www.sleepgrounded.com/

http://en.wikipedia.org/wiki/File:Die_H%C3%A4ngematte.jpg

"A light on at night can put you in a dark mood." Daily Mail. 11/18/10.http://www.dailymail. co.uk/health/article-1330721/A-light-night-dark-mood.html

Usain Bolt picture: Wikipedia.org, by Erik van Leeuwen

REM sleep data: www.webmd.com/sleep-disorders/excessive-sleepiness-10/sleep-101, www.sleepdex.org/

Mark Allen: Rich Cruse, courtesy of Mark Allen, MarkAllenOnline.com

CHAPTER 4

http://en.wikipedia.org/wiki/File:C-reactive_protein.png

http://commons.wikimedia.org/wiki/File:Darwin_fish_ROF.svg

Healthy/unhealthy cell pic courtesy Chris Johnson; OnTargetLiving.com

Image of the Buddha 2-3th century CE: British Museum. Personal photograph 2005. {GDFL} PHGCOM. http://commons.wikimedia.org/wiki/File:EmaciatedBuddha.JPG

http://commons.wikimedia.org/wiki/File:Grape_in_napa.jpg

Boyer, Jeanelle and Liu, Rui Hai, Apple Phytochemicals and their Health Benefits, Nutrition Journal, 2004, 3:5 doi:10.1186/1475-2891-3-5

apples, http://whfoods.org/genpage.php?tname=foodspice&dbid=15

Farzaneh-Far R; JAMA. 303(3):250-257;2010

Stomach 62% full by R. Friedman, M.D. after: http://commons.wikimedia.org/wiki/File:Gray1050-stomach.png.

Hands Cupped with Cherries: iStockPhoto.com

Golden Ratio Diet Decoder graph: concept/design by M. Cross; input from R. Friedman, M.D.; rendered by T. Reczek

http://en.wikipedia.org/wiki/File:Cholesterol.svg; BorisTM

Sun in Celestia by: Runar Thorvaldsen, http://upload.wikimedia.org/wikipedia/commons/b/b3/Celestia_sun.jpg

DNA courtesy Stephen McIntosh, *The Golden Mean Book*

DNA UV mutation.gif: www.wikepedia.org

Tropics of Cancer/Capricorn:
www.worldatlas.com/ UV map of the world: www.earthobservatory.gov

Plates/golden ratio, carrot: R. Friedman, M.D.

http://upload.wikimedia.org/wikipedia/commons/a/a2/Creation-of-adam.PNG

www.wellcorps.com/Explaining-The-Hidden-Meaning-Of-Michelangelos-Creation-of-Adam.html

http://en.wikipedia.org/wiki/File:Iceberg_with_hole_near_sanderson_hope_2007-07-28_2.jpg

Bougnoux, Philippe and Chajès, Veronique, *Omega–6/Omega–3 Polyunsaturated Fatty Acid Ratio and Cancer*, World review of nutrition and dietetics , 2003, vol. 92, pp. 133-151, Karger, Basel, SUISSE

Broadhurst, CL, Cunnane SC, Crawford MA., *Rift Valley lake fish and shellfish provided brain-specific nutrition for early Homo*, Br J Nutr. 1998 Jan;79(1):3-21

Hamazaki T, Okuyama H. *The Japan Society for Lipid Nutrition recommends to reduce the intake of linoleic acid. A review and critique of the scientific evidence.* World Rev Nutr Diet. 2003;92:109-132

Pasinetti GM, et.al., *Calorie restriction attenuates Alzheimer's disease type brain amyloidosis in Squirrel monkeys (Saimiri sciureus)*, J Alzheimers Dis. 2006 Dec;10(4):417-22

Pella, Daniel, et al., *Effects of an Indo-Mediterranean Diet on the Omega–6/Omega–3 Ratio in Patients at High Risk of Coronary Artery Disease: The Indian Paradox*, World review of nutrition and dietetics, 2003, vol. 92

Scholl, Johannes G., http://www.bmj.com/cgi/eletters/332/7544/752#130637

Simopoulos, AP, *The importance of the ratio of omega-6/omega-3 essential fatty acids*, Biomed Pharmacother. 2002 Oct;56(8):365-79

Linus Pauling Inst., Membrane Structure and Function,
http://lpi.oregonstate.edu/infocenter/othernuts/omega3fa/

http://www.smh.com.au/news/national/more-fat-people-in-world-than-there-are-starving-study-finds/2006/08/14/1155407741532.html

http://www.zonediet.com/EATING/HowtoMakeaZoneMeal/tabid/82/Default.aspx

http://www.chimphaven.org/chimps-facts.cfm

http://www.naturalnews.com/022792_food_raw_food_smoothies.html

http://www.sciencedaily.com/releases/2006/10/061013104633.htm

http://tinyurl.com/5d3auf

USDA/Oxygen Radical Absorbance Capacity (ORAC) of Selected Foods – 2007;
http://tinyurl.com/yrmfse

http://commons.wikimedia.org/wiki/File:Four_temperament.PNG

Oxygen Radical Absorbance Capacity (ORAC) of Selected Foods; 2007; http://tinyurl.com/yrmfse

Jack Lalanne: http://en.wikipedia.org/wiki/File:Edjackfn.jpg

CHAPTER 5

Spine with Golden Ratios by T. Reczek after:
http://en.wikipedia.org/wiki/File:Spinal_column_curvature.png

Skeleton, by T. Reczek after:
http://upload.wikimedia.org/wikipedia/commons/2/21/Skelett-Mensch-drawing.jpg

Pelvic, temporal, sphenoid bones with spirals by T. Reczek: after Mees, L.F.C.;
Secrets of the Skeleton: Form in Metamorphosis, Anthroposophic Press; September 1984

Forearm, hand Golden Ratios: R. Friedman

David statue grids: T. Reczek after, http://en.wikipedia.org/wiki/File:Michelangelos_David.jpg

http://upload.wikimedia.org/wikipedia/commons/7/75/Posture_types_(vertebral_column).jpg,
V-Ugnivenko, author

Hartmann, O.J., *Dynamische Morphologie*; courtesy Scott Olsen, author of *The Golden Section:
Nature's Greatest Secret*, (navel pic)

http://en.wikipedia.org/wiki/File:Computer_Workstation_Variables.jpg, Integrated Safety
Management, Berkeley Lab

Poor posture/computer, osteoporosis, backbend: iStockphoto.com

Source: Briñol, Pablo, Petty, Richard E., Wagner, Benjamin; *Body posture effects on self-
evaluation: A self-validation approach. European Journal of Social Psychology: Volume 39, Issue 6*,
October 2009, Pages: 1053-1064.

No Sitting Zone graphic: by Matthew Cross; rendered by T. Reczek

coccyx, seated chakras, caduceus: www.wikipedia.org

618 caduceus: T. Reczek

Carpenter's level: http://commons.wikimedia.org/wiki/File:DetalleNivelDeBurbuja.jpg

CHAPTER 6

Heart spiral muscle: J. Bell Pettigrew / The Bakken, Minneapolis, MN

Electrocardiogram Golden Ratios: T. Reczek after Agateller (Anthony Atkielski), http://
en.wikipedia.org/wiki/File:SinusRhythmLabels.svg

Golden Ratio WorkoutWave™ graph concept/design by M. Cross; input from R. Friedman,
M.D., rendered by T. Reczek; inspired by Sandler, Dr. Ronald D.; Dennis D. Lobstein; *Consistent
Winning: A Remarkable New Training System that Lets You Peak on Demand*, Rodale Press;
October 1992

Elliott Wave graph by: Prechter, Robert R., Jr. and Frost, A.J.; *Elliott Wave Principle:
Key to Market Behavior*, John Wiley & Sons, Ltd.; 1979

Bjorn Borg/spiral forehand: Author's collection

Rob Moses, David Carradine, Shaolin Monk, PhysioStix: Courtesy of Rob Moses,
www.GoldenSpiralWellness.com

http://commons.wikimedia.org/wiki/File:Grade_1_hypertension.jpg; Author: Steven Fruitsmaak

Speedometer: M. Cross, R. Friedman, M.D. and T. Reczek

Fahey, Thomas D., Swanson, George D., Medicina Sportiva, 12 (4): 124-128, 2008,
*A Model for Defining the Optimal Amount of Exercise Contributing to Health and Avoiding
Sudden Cardiac Death*

Jackicic, John M.; *Effects of Exercise Duration and Intensity on Weight Loss in Overweight,
Sedentary Women: A Randomized Trial*; JAMA 290 (Sept. 10, 2003): 1,323-30

Sandler, Dr. Ronald D.; Dennis D. Lobstein; *Consistent Winning: A Remarkable New Training*

System that Lets You Peak on Demand, Rodale Press; October 1992

Steinberg, Steve, *Men's Journal Magazine*, March 2004, on Baron Davis

Ulmer, Ph.D., Hanno, et al, George Clooney, the cauliflower, the cardiologist, and phi, the golden ratio., 13 December 2009, BMJ 2009;339:b4745

Heart graphic: Mariana Ruiz Villarreal "LadyofHats", e-mail: mrv_taur@gmx.net

Novak Djokovic picture from Wikipedia.org, by Wikipedia user Stefan1991

Man doing sit-ups on Swiss ball: Cerasela Feraru

Yoga stretch: iStockphoto.com

CHAPTER 7

Pulse-oximeter in Golden Ratio: R. Friedman, M.D.

http://en.wikipedia.org/wiki/File:Triathlon_pictogram.svg; Thadius856 (SVG conversion) & Parutakupiu (original image)

http://en.wikipedia.org/wiki/File:Badstuga,_efter_illustration_i_Acerbis_Travels,_Nordisk_familjebok.png

http://www.feinberg.northwestern.edu/nutrition/factsheets/fiber.html

www.HerbDoc.com: website of Dr. Richard Schulze

Mercola, J., *The No Grain Diet*, Plume, March 30, 2004

Sanjoaquin MA, Appleby PN, Spencer EA, Key TJ., *Nutrition and lifestyle in relation to bowel movement frequency: a cross-sectional study of 20630 men and women in EPIC-Oxford*, Public Health Nutrition: 7(1), 77–83, 2003

Santana-Rios, Ph.D., Gilberto, Fiber Facts, http://lpi.oregonstate.edu/sp-su99/santana.html

Well Being Journal Vol. 7, No. 5 ~ September/October 1998

Data for calculating soluble/insoluble ratios was taken from the following two sources; in the event of conflicting measurements, the ratio closest to the Golden Ratio was the default selection:
   1. Anderson JW. Plant Fiber in Foods. 2nd ed. HCF Nutrition Research Foundation Inc.,1990
   2. http://whfoods.org/

CHAPTER 8

Happiness pie graphs, Golden Ratio peace symbol, Golden Ratio work-reduction graph, 80/20 Principle graph, Order From Chaos Golden Ratio desk graph: T. Reczek

DNA molecule courtesy Stephen McIntosh, *The Golden Mean Book*

New Jeruselem Golden Ratio sculpture: Andrew Rodgers, http://en.wikipedia.org/wiki/File:Golden_Ratio.jpg

The New Jerusalem (Tapestry of the Apocalypse): http://en.wikipedia.org/wiki/File:La_nouvelle_J%C3%A9rusalem.jpg

New Jerusalem painting: Michell, John, *The Dimensions of Paradise: The Proportions and Symbolic Numbers of Ancient Cosmology*; Adventures Unlimited Press (May 2, 2001)

Mona Lisa, Vitruvian Man, Leonardo Da Vinci: www.wikepedia.org

DNA mandala: Computer Graphics Lab/UCSF

Ferriss, Timothy, *The 4-Hour Workweek: Escape 9-5, Live Anywhere, and Join the New Rich*; Crown (April 24, 2007)

www.gobankingrates.com/history-of-the-40-hour-work-week-and-its-effects-on-the-economy/

Lipton, Bruce H., Ph.D., *The Biology of Belief: Unleashing the Power of Consciousness, Matter, & Miracles*; Hay House; illustrated edition (September 15, 2008)

Lyubomirsky, Sonja, *The How of Happiness: A New Approach to Getting the Life You Want;* Penguin; Reprint edition, December 30, 2008

Murakami, Kazuo, *The Divine Code of Life: Awaken Your Genes and Discover Hidden Talents*; Atria Books/Beyond Words (April 28, 2006)

Pert, Candace, Ph.D., *Molecules Of Emotion: The Science Between Mind-Body Medicine, Scribner* (1999)

Shimoff, Marci, *Happy for No Reason: 7 Steps to Being Happy from the Inside Out;* Free Press, (March 3, 2009)

What the Bleep Do We Know!?, 20th Century Fox, (2004), Actors: Marlee Matlin, Barry Newman, Elaine Hendrix, Armin Shimerman, Robert Bailey, Jr., John Ross Bowie. Directors: Betsy Chasse, Mark Vicente, William Arntz, Producers: William Arntz, Betsy Chasse

http://en.wikipedia.org/wiki/Itzamna

en.wikipedia.org/wiki/Hot_chocolate

http://en.wikipedia.org/wiki/File:Cacao-pod-k4636-14.jpg

http://en.wikipedia.org/wiki/File:God_D_Itzamna.jpg

CHAPTER 9

Sean Connery: Alan Light,
http://commons.wikimedia.org/wiki/File:Sean_Connery_1980_Crop.jpg

Marilyn Monroe: http://commons.wikimedia.org/wiki/File:Marilyn_Monroe,_The_Prince_and_the_Showgirl,_1.jpg

Brad Pitt and Angelina Jolie: http://commons.wikimedia.org/wiki/File:Fcad3.jpg

Monica Dean: Courtesy of and Copyright ©Monica Dean; photo credit: Giuliano Bekor

Christy Turlington: Courtesy of PETA; photo by Steven Klein

Golden Ratio Calipers: R. Friedman, M.D.; Calipers available from Javier Holodovsky at:
www.holyholo.com/caliper.htm

Anastasia Soare, Brow with Caliper Lines: Courtesy of Anastasia,
www.anastasia.net/help.php?section=goldenratio

Anastasia Golden Ratio browser: T. Reczek, after: http://anastasia.net/index.php

Michelangelo's David: modified by T. Reczek after
http://en.wikipedia.org/wiki/File:Michelangelos_David.jpg

Teeth with calipers: courtesy Dr. Eddie Levin / www.goldenmeangauge.co.uk

Venus de Milo: http://en.wikipedia.org/wiki/File:Venus_de_Milo_Louvre_Ma399_n4.jpg

Adonis: http://en.wikipedia.org/wiki/File:Adonis3.jpg

Julia Roberts: http://en.wikipedia.org/wiki/File:Julia_Roberts_in_May_2002.jpg

George Clooney: http://commons.wikimedia.org/wiki/File:George.Clooneywiki1.jpg

Mona Lisa: http://en.wikipedia.org/wiki/File:Mona_Lisa.jpg

Khalil Gibran: http://en.wikipedia.org/wiki/File:Khalil_Gibran.jpg

Orgasm graph, Chocolate pie graph: T. Reczek

Inspiral® Condom: Inspral.com

Chocolate bars: iStockPhoto.com

Lindsay Wagner: http://en.wikipedia.org/wiki/File:Lindsay_Wagner_July08.jpg

Roses, front and back: M. Cross

Buddha footprint: http://en.wikipedia.org/wiki/File:Buddha-Footprint.jpeg

Ackerman, Diane, *A Natural History of the Senses*, Vintage (September 10, 1991)

http://commons.wikimedia.org/wiki/File:Adonis_Mazarin_Louvre_MR239.jpg

Boothman, Nicholas, *How To Make People Like You in 90 Seconds or Less*, Workman Publishing Company; Reprint edition (July 2, 2008)

Breiter, Hans, Etcoff, Nancy et.al, *Beautiful Faces Have Variable Reward Value*, Neuron, Volume 32, Issue 3, 537-551, 8 November 2001

Brown, Patricia Leigh, *The 'Leonardo' of Condoms*, The New York Times, 4.11.99

Cleese, John and Bates, Brian, *The Human Face*, DK ADULT; 1 edition (July 1, 2001)

Davis, Jeanie, *Men Who Dance Well May Be More Desirable As Mates*, WebMD.com, 12.21.05

Jefferson,Y., *Skeletal Types: Key to unraveling the mystery of facial beauty and its biologic significance*. J Gen Orthod. 1996 Jun;7(2):7-25

Mehrabian, Albert, *Nonverbal Communication*, Aldine Transaction (February 28, 2007)

http://en.wikipedia.org/wiki/Speculation_about_Mona_Lisa

www.oprah.com/article/oprahshow/20090304-tows-female-sex-study/6

http://en.wikipedia.org/wiki/File:Venus_de_Milo_Louvre_Ma399_n4.jpg

Reich, Wilhelm, Carfagno, Vincent R. *The Function of the Orgasm: Discovery of the Orgone (Discovery of the Orgone, Vol 1)*, Farrar, Straus and Giroux (May 1, 1986)

CHAPTER 10

Fountain of Youth: Lucas Cranach, http://en.wikipedia.org/wiki/File:Lucas_Cranach_d._%C3%84._007.jpg

Aquaporins: http://en.wikipedia.org/wiki/File:Aquaporin-Sideview.png

Jeanne Calment: http://en.wikipedia.org/wiki/File:JeanneCalmentaged40.jpg

Nautilus shell: iStockphoto.com

Andersen, Helle R., et.al., *Low activity of superoxide dismutase and high activity of glutathione reductase in erythrocytes from centenarians*, Age and Ageing, 1998; 27: 643-648

Census, http://www.census.gov/compendia/statab/cats/births_deaths_marriages_divorces/life_expectancy.html

Flanagan, Patrick, MD. (MA), *Hydrogen.... Longevity's Missing Link*, Nexus December, 1994—January 1995

Gavrilov, Leonid A. & Gavrilova, Natalia S. *The Biology of Life Span: A Quantitative Approach*; New York: Harwood Academic Publisher, (1991)

Human life expectancy, http://entomology.ucdavis.edu/courses/hde19/lecture3.html

Jean Calment, http://www.nytimes.com/2009/01/27/science/27agre.html?pagewanted=1&_r=1

Robbins, John, *Healthy at 100: The Scientifically Proven Secrets of the World's Healthiest and Longest-Lived Peoples*, Ballantine Books (August 28, 2007)

Walford, Roy L. M.D., *Beyond The 120-Year Diet*; Da Capo Press; Revised and Expanded edition (August 7, 2000).

Whitney, Craig R., Jeanne Calment, *World's Elder, Dies at 122*, The New York Times, 8/5/97

Buettner, Dan, *The Blue Zone: Lessons for Living Longer from the People Who've Lived the Longest*, National Geographic; Reprint edition (April 21, 2009).

Dean, Josh, *The Longevity Expedition*, National Geographic Adventure Magazine, June/July, 2009

Buettner, Dan, *Grecian Formula*, National Geographic Adventure Magazine, October, 2009

Casselman, Anne, *Long-Lived Costa Ricans Offer Secrets to Reaching 100*, National Geographic Adventure Magazine, April 2008

http://science.nasa.gov/headlines/y2006/images/telomeres/caps_med.jpg

http://en.wikipedia.org/wiki/File:Telomere_caps.gif

Skloot, Rebecca, *The Immortal Life of Henrietta Lacks*, Crown; 1 edition, (February 2, 2010)

Benson, M.D., Herbert, *Relaxation Revolution: Enhancing Your Personal Health Through the Science and Genetics of Mind Body Healing*, Scribner; 1 edition (June 22, 2010).

http://en.wikipedia.org/wiki/Longevity_traditions#Biblical

http://commons.wikimedia.org/wiki/File:Foster_Bible_Pictures_0021-2.jpg

http://upload.wikimedia.org/wikipedia/commons/b/b8/Aubrey_de_Grey.jpg

http://en.wikipedia.org/wiki/Itzamna

http://en.wikipedia.org/wiki/Hot_chocolate

http://en.wikipedia.org/wiki/File:Cacao-pod-k4636-14.jpg

http://en.wikipedia.org/wiki/File:God_D_Itzamna.jpg

Eternal Clock, by Robbert van der Steeg, http://www.flickr.com/photos/robbie73/3387189144/

Farzneh-Far, Ramin, M.D., etal., *Association of Marine Omega-3 Fatty Acid Levels With Telomeric Aging in Patients With Coronary Heart Disease*. JAMA. 2010;303(3):250-257.

Songs of Spring: http://commons.wikimedia.org/wiki/File:William-Adolphe_Bouguereau_-_Chansons_de_printemps.jpg

CHAPTER 11

Fibbonacci Running Track: M. Cross, rendered by T. Reczek from iStockPhoto.com

21-Day Quick-Start Checklist: Designed by and Copyright ©2011 by Matthew Cross; rendered by T. Reczek

ABOUT THE AUTHORS, HOSHIN MEDIA/PRODUCTS

Robert Friedman, M.D.: Photo by Kim Jew

Matthew Cross: Photo by Diana Doroftei

All Hoshin Media book covers: Designed by M. Cross; rendered by T. Reczek

Spiral-Chi DVD cover: R. Friedman

ACKNOWLEDGEMENTS

We are grateful to the many "Geniuses of the Code" who have elucidated various aspects of the Golden Ratio/Divine Code over time and made our road easier to travel. The two Leonardos—Fibonacci and Da Vinci—were of particular inspiration during the writing of this book. We undoubtedly felt the same excitement that they did when new Golden Ratio insights come rushing in. In this age there are also certain individuals whose work kindled the activation and focus of the Golden Ratio Lifestyle Diet principles in us. In particular we would like to acknowledge: John Michell, Dr. Ronald Sandler, Robert Prechter, Jr., Dr. W. Edwards Deming, Marshall Thurber, Dr. Barry Sears, Anastasia Soare, Dr. Richard Schulze, Dr. Yosh Jefferson, Dr. Mehmet Oz, Dr. Michael Roizen, Dr. Ellen Langer, Aubrey de Gray, Dan Buettner, Michael J. Gelb and Dr. Joseph Juran being among the modern giants on whose shoulders we stand. A very special thanks is also in order to our good friend and Golden Ratio genius Stephen McIntosh, who graciously contributed key illustrations and insights.

We couldn't have completed this book without the support of our two beautiful Vitruvian Women: Arihanto Luders and Diana Doroftei. They were our Nature's Secret Nutrients who sustained us in so many ways during this journey. Our other secret nutrients that gave us the stamina to finish this book were aspects of the Golden Ratio Lifestyle Diet itself, including: IronApe Green Smoothies, deep breathing, raw vegetable juice, DNA Power Fuel,™ organic/Dagoba chocolate bars, green tea, Spiral~Chi, Golden Ratio breathing, hanging upside-down, running 5K races, midnight oil burning, Korean sports massage at Paradise Spa (Stamford, Connecticut), mountain hikes, Starbucks, Beatles music and... well, you get the idea.

Special thanks to: Our master graphic designer Tom Reczek of 618Design.com who once again embodied the essence of the Golden Ratio in his collaboration on this book's beautiful cover design and Golden Ratio layouts and also for his excellent research and suggestions. Thanks also to artist Chloe Hedden, whose inspired rendition of the comissioned *Divine Code Vitruvian Woman* stands shoulder to shoulder (literally) with Da Vinci's *Vitruvian Man*. We would also like to thank and acknowledge iStockPhoto.com and Wikipedia.org as the source for many of the high-quality illustrations in this book. Wikipedia.org was also a crucial provider of copyright-free material, which has greatly enhanced this work. As lead contributing editor, Diana Doroftei added great insights and value to the book; Maxine "eagle eyes" Friedman, Lou Savary, Vicki Melian-Morse and Chris Johnson also contributed their excellent editorial input and suggestions.

In the spirit of saving the best for last, we thank *you*, dear reader. The opportunity to share this life-transforming material with you is a great honor and delight. We look forward to meeting you on our blog at: www.GoldenRatioLifestyle.com

ABOUT THE AUTHORS

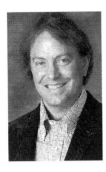

Robert Friedman, M.D.

practiced nutritional and preventive medicine in Santa Fe, New Mexico for twenty five years before turning his attention to the application of the Golden Ratio to health and longevity.

He co-authored with Matthew Cross *The Divine Code of Da Vinci, Fibonacci, Einstein & YOU*, a 660 page tour-de-force on the Golden Ratio, which allows anyone to access the Code and apply it in their chosen field. That book's success inspired two other Golden Ratio-based books: *The Divine Code Genius Activation Quote Book* and *The Golden Ratio Lifestyle Diet*. Dr. Friedman is also the originator of the Spiral-Chi Evolutionary Movement system based on spinal and spiral wave motions. Spiral-Chi has been compared to a synthesis of yoga and tai-chi and emphasizes tuning in to one's spiral nature for regeneration and rejuvenation. Dr. Friedman can be reached at DrBob@GoldenRatioLifestyle.com. Follow him on Twitter: @BobFriedmanMD • *www.about.me/robertfriedmanm.d.*

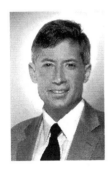

Matthew Cross

is President of Leadership Alliance, an international consulting firm providing breakthrough strategies for growth and transformation. Matthew is a Deming Quality Scholar, Hoshin Kanri strategic alignment specialist, thought leader and speaker who works with Fortune 100 companies around the world.

Matthew began researching the practical applications of the Golden Ratio at age 12. In addition to co-authoring *The Golden Ratio Lifestyle Diet, The Divine Code of Da Vinci, Fibonacci, Einstein & YOU* and *The Divine Code Genius Activation Quote Book* with Robert Friedman, M.D., Matthew is the author of *The Millionaire's MAP, The Hoshin Success Compass* and *Be Your Own President*. He is also an ancient history explorer and competitive athlete (running and tennis), with a deep belief in everyone's unique genius and unlimited potential. Matthew can be reached at: MCross@GoldenRatioLifestyle.com. Follow him on Twitter: @MatthewKCross • *www.about.me/matthewcross*

The authors are available for speaking presentations and interviews.

INDEX

B

Baba, Meher   246
Backbend, Golden Spiral   164
Bangladesh   193
Barban, John   282
Barefoot   169, 170
Barr, Mark   345
Barrymore, Drew   234
Basal Metabolic Rate (BMR)   92
Baseball   309
Bashour, Dr. Mounir   279
Batmanghelidj, Dr. Fereydoon   74-6
Beatles, The   25, 114
Bees   148
Bee Pollen   148
Beets, stamina booster   142
Begin, Menachem   89, 90
Benson, Dr. Herbert   261, 305-06
Berlin, Irving   301
Berry, Halle   267
Beverly Hills, CA   280
Bhajan, Yogi   135
Bieske, Nicole   90
Binoche, Juliette   288
Biodynamics Corporation   79
Bioelectrical Impedence Analysis   78
Biology of Belief   234
Biology of Transcendence   182
Biomarkers of aging   309
Bionic Woman, The   290
Biosphere   59, 60, 122, 126
Birth of Venus, The   50
Blaine, David   57
Blenders (Blendtek, Vitamix)   142
Blood Clotting   149
Blood Pressure   100, 111, 198, 200, 207,
    212, 308-09
Blood Sugar Levels   112, 139, 149, 212
Blood Tests   149, 153
Blue Heron Foundation, The   270
Blue Zones, Longevity   176, 306-07
Blue Zones: Lessons for Living Longer   306
Body Bridge   171
Body Composition   78
Body Composition Analysis (BCA)   77
Body Language   292
Body Mass Index (BMI)   81
Body Symmetry (Golden Ratio)   158
Body Water Percentage   79, 80, 299
Bok, Derek   233
Bolt, Usain   98, 192
Bond, James   266
Bono   4
Boothman, Nicholas   292
Borg, Bjorn   196
Born to Run   169

Botticelli, Sandro   50
Bougnoux, Philppe   117
Bouguereau, William-Adolphe   228, 316
Boutenko, Victoria   120-21, 142, 344
Bowel movement   215-16, 218, 221
Bowflex   206
BPA   84
Brain   123, 136, 138
Brain synchronization   209
Brain Waves   93, 95-6
Breakfast first   139
Breath awareness   253
Breath/breathing (Golden)   63-4, 67, 221, 227
Breiter, Dr. Hans   274
Breuning, Walter   301
Briener, Dr. Mark   281
Broccoli   45
Bronchiole   54
Brooklyn, NY   282
Brown, Dan   5, 173
Brown, Dr. William   282
Buddha   39, 42, 64, 123, 295
Buddha's footprint   295
Burnout   189
Burns, George   301
Business Insider   97
Buttar, Rashid   213-14
Buttener, Dan   306-8
Butterfly Effect   38, 164, 286

C

C-Reactive Protein (CRP)   114, 116, 149, 154
Cacao/cocoa   321-22
Caduceus   165-7
Caffeine   103, 222
Caldicott, Dr. Helen   218
Calipers (Golden Ratio)   341
Calment, Jeanne   86, 300-01, 304-05, 307, 315
Caloric Reduction   122-23, 125, 147, 298,
    307-08, 345
Caloric Restriction Society   122
Calorie Decoder   152
Calories   191
Campbell, Naomi   268
Candle gazing exercise   252, 254
Carbohydrates/Proteins/Fats   110-13, 116,
    140-41, 152-53
Carbon Dioxide/CO2   54, 56-7, 119, 212
Cardiovascular disease   115
Carlisle, Kitty   301
Carlson's Norwegian Cod Liver Oil   120
Carradine, David   197
Case Western Reserve University   91
Catapult effect   185-6
Caucasus Mountains   298, 307
CDC (Center for Disease Control)   214

D

Q

R

X

Y

Z

NOTES

NOTES

NOTES

NOTES

FROM HOSHIN MEDIA

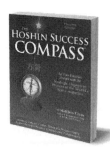

The Hoshin Success Compass™

Map Your Way to Success with the Strategic Alignment
Process of the World's Greatest Companies.

By Matthew Cross

Hoshin Media, 2012; illustrated workbook. • $24.95

www.HoshinSuccessCompass.com

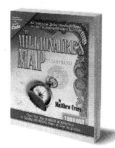

The Millionaire's MAP™

Chart Your Way to Wealth & Abundance by
Tapping the Infinite Power of Your Imagination.

By Matthew Cross

Hoshin Media, 2010; 144 pages, illustrated workbook. $24.95

www.MillionairesMap.com

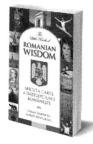

The Little Book of Romanian Wisdom

Discover the Unique Wisdom of Romania.

By Diana Doroftei & Matthew Cross

Hoshin Media, 2011; illustrated. • 12.95

www.RomanianWisdom.com

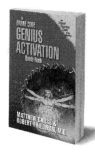

The Divine Code Genius
Activation Quote Book

Activate your Innate Genius with these
Classic Divine Code/Golden Ratio Quotes.

By Matthew Cross & Robert Friedman, M.D.

Hoshin Media, 2011; illustrated. 13.95

www.TheDivineCode.com

Be Your Own President

An Interactive Handbook for Personal
& Professional Leadership and Transformation.

By Matthew Cross

Hoshin Media, 2012; illustrated workbook. $19.95

62 Smashing Success Secrets, Tools & Strategies

Simple, Profound Keys for Activating & Living
Your Full Passion & Potential in Life and Business.

By Matthew Cross

Hoshin Media, 2012; illustrated. $14.95

ABCore Medicine Ball Workout Video

An interactive Medicine Ball exercise program for
strengthening and balancing your abdominal/core.
Easy, fun and great results.

By Matthew Cross

Hoshin Media, 2012; DVD 34 min. $13.95

SPIRAL~CHI DVD FROM ROBERT FRIEDMAN, M.D.

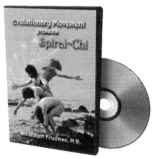

Evolutionary Movement

Learn How to Combine Spinal Waves And Spirals
for the Ultimate in Stretching and Strengthening.
The Next Evolution in Movement Therapy.

With Robert Friedman, M.D.

DVD 43 min. $29.95 order at

www.TheDivineCode.com

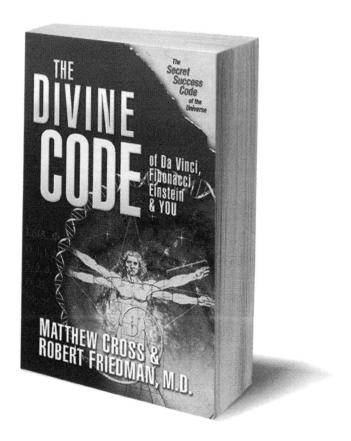

A Tour de Force Adventure into the Secret
Success Code of the Universe: The Golden Ratio

A treasure chest encyclopedia, 10 years in the making, on the history, pioneering geniuses and practical applications of PHI/the Golden Ratio 1.618:1. The Master Design Code of the Universe, the Golden Ratio is a golden key to great wisdom, health, happiness and success at all levels of life.

*In **The Divine Code** Matthew Cross and Dr. Robert Friedman take one of Creation's greatest secrets and make it accessible, engaging and fun.*

**Michael J. Gelb, best-selling author of *Da Vinci Decoded* and
*How To Think Like Leonardo Da Vinci***

Hoshin Media, 2009 - 660 pages, over 600 illustrations • $29.95

Made in the USA
Charleston, SC
13 November 2012